Bladder Cancer

Editor

GURU P. SONPAVDE

HEMATOLOGY/ONCOLOGY CLINICS OF NORTH AMERICA

www.hemonc.theclinics.com

Consulting Editors
GEORGE P. CANELLOS
EDWARD J. BENZ Jr

June 2021 • Volume 35 • Number 3

ELSEVIER

1600 John F. Kennedy Boulevard ● Suite 1800 ● Philadelphia, Pennsylvania, 19103-2899

http://www.theclinics.com

**HEMATOLOGY/ONCOLOGY CLINICS OF NORTH AMERICA Volume 35, Number 3
June 2021 ISSN 0889-8588, ISBN 13: 978-0-323-76451-3**

Editor: Stacy Eastman
Developmental Editor: Ann Gielou M. Posedio

Hematology/Oncology Clinics (ISSN 0889-8588) is published bimonthly by Elsevier Inc., 360 Park Avenue South, New York, NY 10010-1710. Months of issue are February, April, June, August, October, and December. Business and Editorial Offices: 1600 John F. Kennedy Blvd., Ste. 1800, Philadelphia, PA 19103–2899. Customer Service Office: 3251 Riverport Lane, Maryland Heights, MO 63043. Periodicals postage paid at New York, NY and at additional mailing offices. Subscription prices are $456.00 per year (domestic individuals), $1150.00 per year (domestic institutions), $100.00 per year (domestic students/residents), $480.00 per year (Canadian individuals), $100.00 per year (Canadian students/residents), $1213.00 per year (Canadian institutions) $547.00 per year (international individuals), $1213.00 per year (international institutions), and $255.00 per year (international students/residents). International air speed delivery is included in all *Clinics* subscription prices. All prices are subject to change without notice. **POSTMASTER:** Send address changes to *Hematology/Oncology Clinics of North America*, Elsevier Health Sciences Division, Subscription Customer Service, 3251 Riverport Lane, Maryland Heights, MO 63043. Customer Service (orders, claims, online, change of address): Elsevier Health Sciences Division, Subscription **Customer Service, 3251 Riverport Lane, Maryland Heights, MO 63043. Tel: 1-800-654-2452 (U.S. and Canada); 314-447-8871 (outside U.S. and Canada). Fax: 314-447-8029. E-mail: journalscustomerservice-usa@elsevier.com (for print support); journalsonlinesupport-usa@elsevier.com (for online support)**.

Reprints. For copies of 100 or more, of articles in this publication, please contact the Commercial Reprints Department, Elsevier Inc., 360 Park Avenue South, New York, New York 10010-1710; Tel.: 212-633-3874, Fax: 212-633-3820, E-mail: reprints@elsevier.com.

Hematology/Oncology Clinics of North America is covered in *MEDLINE/PubMed (Index Medicus), EMBASE/ Excerpta Medica, and BIOSIS.*

Contributors

CONSULTING EDITORS

GEORGE P. CANELLOS, MD
William Rosenberg Professor of Medicine, Department of Medical Oncology, Dana-Farber Cancer Institute, Boston, Massachusetts, USA

EDWARD J. BENZ Jr, MD
Professor, Pediatrics, Richard and Susan Smith Professor, Medicine, Professor, Genetics, Harvard Medical School, President and CEO Emeritus, Office of the President, Dana-Farber Cancer Institute, Boston, Massachusetts, USA

EDITOR

GURU P. SONPAVDE, MD
Bladder Cancer Director, Lank Center for Genitourinary Oncology, Dana-Farber Cancer Institute, Associate Professor of Medicine, Harvard Medical School, Boston, Massachusetts, USA

AUTHORS

JOSEPH A. CLARA, MD
Cellular and Molecular Therapeutics Branch, National Heart, Lung, and Blood Institutes, National Institutes of Health, Bethesda, Maryland, USA

HAMED AHMADI, MD
Department of Urology, University of Southern California/Norris Comprehensive Cancer Center, Los Angeles, California, USA

RICK BANGS, MBA
Bladder Cancer Patient Advocate, SWOG, Advocate, Bladder Cancer Advocacy Network, Pittsford, New York, USA

JOAQUIM BELLMUNT, MD, PhD
Department of Medical Oncology, Beth Israel Deaconess Medical Center, Harvard Medical School, Boston, Massachusetts, USA

PETER C. BLACK, MD
Vancouver Prostate Centre, University of British Columbia, Vancouver, Canada

KELLY K. BREE, MD
Department of Urology, The University of Texas MD Anderson Cancer Center, Houston, Texas, USA

NATHAN A. BROOKS, MD
Department of Urology, The University of Texas MD Anderson Cancer Center, Houston, Texas, USA

FAN CHENG, MD
Department of Urology, Renmin Hospital of Wuhan University, Wuhan, China

SHIVIRAM CUMARASAMY, MD
Department of Urology, Icahn School of Medicine at Mount Sinai, New York, New York, USA

SIAMAK DANESHMAND, MD
Department of Urology, University of Southern California/Norris Comprehensive Cancer Center; Professor of Urology (Clinical Scholar), USC/Norris Comprehensive Cancer Center, USC Institute of Urology, Los Angeles, California, USA

VINAY DUDDALWAR, MD
Department of Radiology, University of Southern California, Los Angeles, California, USA

JASON A. EFSTATHIOU, MD, DPhil, FASTRO, FACRO
Professor, Harvard Medical School, Department of Radiation Oncology, Massachusetts General Hospital, Boston, Massachusetts, USA

MATTHEW D. GALSKY, MD
Division of Oncology, Department of Medicine, Icahn School of Medicine at Mount Sinai, New York, New York, USA

BRENDAN J. GUERCIO, MD
Department of Medicine, Memorial Sloan Kettering Cancer Center, New York, New York, USA

GOPA IYER, MD
Department of Medicine, Memorial Sloan Kettering Cancer Center, Associate Professor, Weill Cornell Medical College, New York, New York, USA

ASHISH M. KAMAT, MD
Professor of Urologic Oncology, Wayne B. Duddlesten Professor of Cancer Research, Department of Urology, The University of Texas MD Anderson Cancer Center, Houston, Texas, USA

DAVID J. KONIECZKOWSKI, MD, PhD
Assistant Professor, The Ohio State University, Department of Radiation Oncology, James Cancer Hospital, Columbus, Ohio, USA

YOHANN LORIOT, MD, PhD
Département de médecine oncologique, ISNERM U981, Université Paris-Saclay, Gustave Roussy Institute, Villejuif, France

AI-HONG MA, MD, PhD
Department of Biochemistry and Molecular Medicine, University of California, Davis, Sacramento, USA

JOSHUA MA
Vancouver Prostate Centre, University of British Columbia, Vancouver, Canada

DAVID J. McCONKEY, PhD
Director, Johns Hopkins Greenberg Bladder Cancer Institute, Professor, Brady Urological Institute, Baltimore, Maryland, USA

MATTHEW MOSSANEN, MD, MPH
Division of Urology, Brigham and Women's Hospital, Dana Farber Cancer Institute, Assistant Professor, Harvard Medical School, Boston, Massachusetts, USA

KENT W. MOUW, MD, PhD
Assistant Professor, Harvard Medical School, Department of Radiation Oncology, Dana-Farber Cancer Institute, Brigham and Women's Hospital, Boston, Massachusetts, USA

ROSA NADAL, MD
Cellular and Molecular Therapeutics Branch, National Heart, Lung, and Blood Institutes, National Institutes of Health, Bethesda, Maryland, USA

CHONG-XIAN PAN, MD, PhD, MS
Department of Medicine, Brigham and Women's Hospital, Harvard Medical School, Boston, Massachusetts, USA; VA Boston Healthcare System, West Roxbury, Massachusetts, USA

DIPEN JAYSUKHLAL PAREKH, MD, MCh
Professor and Chair, Department of Urology, Director of Robotic Surgery, The Victor A. Politano Endowed Chair in Urology, Member Sylvester Cancer Center, University of Miami Miller School of Medicine, Chief Operating Officer, University of Miami Health System, Miami, Florida, USA

JOHN L. PFAIL, BS
Department of Urology, Icahn School of Medicine at Mount Sinai, New York, New York, USA

DIANE ZIPURSKY QUALE, JD
Co-founder/Director, Bladder Cancer Advocacy Network, Bethesda, Maryland, USA

JONATHAN E. ROSENBERG, MD
Professor, Weill Cornell Medical College, Department of Medicine, Memorial Sloan Kettering Cancer Center, MSK Sidney Kimmel Center for Prostate and Urologic Cancers, New York, New York, USA

ALEXANDER C. SMALL, MD
Department of Urology, Icahn School of Medicine at Mount Sinai, New York, New York, USA

GURU P. SONPAVDE, MD
Bladder Cancer Director, Lank Center for Genitourinary Oncology, Dana-Farber Cancer Institute, Associate Professor of Medicine, Harvard Medical School, Boston, Massachusetts, USA

CONSTANCE THIBAULT, MD
Medical Oncology Department, European Georges Pompidou Hospital, APHP.5, Paris, France

BEGOÑA P. VALDERRAMA, MD
Hospital Universitario Virgen del Rocio, Sevilla, Spain

VIVEK VENKATRAMANI, MS, MCh
Consultant Uro-oncologist and Robotic Urologist, Nanavati Super-Specialty Hospital, Mumbai, India; Visiting Assistant Professor, Department of Urology, University of Miami Miller School of Medicine, Miami, Florida, USA

SHAOMING ZHU, MD
Department of Urology, Renmin Hospital of Wuhan University, Wuhan, China; Division of Hematology and Oncology, Department of Internal Medicine, School of Medicine, University of California, Davis, Sacramento, USA

ZHENG ZHU, PhD
Department of Medicine, Brigham and Women's Hospital, Harvard Medical School, Boston, Massachusetts, USA

Contents

been tested with the intent of improving locoregional disease control, there currently is no role for this modality in routine care. Perioperative systemic therapy is used with the intent of reducing the risk of systemic recurrence. Robust trial evidence supports the use of neoadjuvant cisplatin-based chemotherapy, with adjuvant chemotherapy offered as an alternative if neoadjuvant therapy is not administered. Perioperative immunotherapy represents the next frontier in perioperative therapy. Further biomarker development is required to guide treatment in individual patients.

Transurethral resection of bladder tumor remains the cornerstone of non–muscle invasive bladder cancer management, proper risk stratification, and appropriate selection of adjuvant therapy. A single, postoperative dose of intravesical chemotherapy is used for low-risk patients; patients with high-grade, high-risk disease should receive intravesical bacillus Calmette-Guérin (BCG) induction and maintenance therapy. For patients who develop BCG-unresponsive disease, cystectomy remains the standard of care. Pembrolizumab and valrubicin are approved in the BCG failure setting and as alternative treatments to cystectomy. Nadofaragene firadenovec, vicinium, hyperthermic chemotherapy, and various combination therapies are under investigation as treatment options for patients in the salvage setting.

Cystoscopic examination remains the gold standard technique for initial diagnosis of bladder cancer (BCa). Despite significant progress in enhanced cystoscopic techniques, blue light cystoscopy and narrow band imaging are the only ones well supported by high-level evidence and, if available, should be used during initial staging of BCa. Multiparametric MRI could be an important imaging tool in local staging of BCa. With ever-expanding targeted therapy and immunotherapy options in both muscle-invasive and non–muscle-invasive BCa, molecular subtyping could become an essential part of initial histologic staging in the near future.

The cornerstone for diagnosis and treatment of bladder and upper tract urothelial carcinoma involves surgery. Transurethral resection of bladder tumors forms the basis of further management. Radical cystectomy for invasive bladder carcinoma provides good oncologic outcomes. However, it can be a morbid procedure, and advances such as minimally invasive surgery and early recovery after surgery need to be incorporated into routine practice. Diagnostic ureteroscopy for upper tract carcinoma is needed in cases of doubt after cytology and imaging studies. Low-risk cancers can be managed with conservative endoscopic surgery without compromising oncological outcomes; however, high-risk disease necessitates radical nephroureterectomy.

Bladder-preserving trimodality therapy (TMT), consisting of trans-urethral bladder tumor resection followed by concurrent chemoradiotherapy, is an established standard of care for patients with muscle-invasive bladder cancer. For appropriately selected patients, TMT offers oncologic outcomes comparable to radical cystectomy while preserving the patient's native bladder. Optimal TMT outcomes require careful patient selection, which is currently based on clinical and pathologic factors. The role of immune checkpoint blockade (ICB) in TMT is currently being investigated in several on-going clinical trials. In the future, molecular features associated with response to TMT or ICB may further improve patient selection and guide post-treatment surveillance.

For the last decade, biology of urothelial tumorigenesis has been widely explored, helping to better understand the molecular pathways in urothelial carcinoma (UC). Until recently, no targeted therapies have been approved in UC. However, several new molecules have shown promising results in metastatic UC: fibroblast growth factor receptor inhibitors, conjugated antibodies, PARP inhibitors, and antiangiogenics. In this article, the authors review the targeted therapies that are being evaluated in bladder UC.

Bladder cancer remains a common and insidious disease in the United States. There have been several advances in the understanding of the biology of bladder cancer, novel diagnostic tools, improvements in multidisciplinary care pathways, and new therapeutics for advanced disease over the past few decades. Clinical trials have demonstrated efficacy for new treatments in each disease state, but additional work is needed to advance the effectiveness of bladder cancer care. Real world data provide critical information regarding patterns of care, adverse events, and outcomes helping to bridge the efficacy versus effectiveness gap.

At diagnosis, more than 70% of bladder cancers (BCs) are at the non–muscle-invasive bladder cancer (NMIBC) stages, which are usually treated with transurethral resection followed by intravesical instillation. For the

HEMATOLOGY/ONCOLOGY CLINICS OF NORTH AMERICA

SERIES OF RELATED INTEREST

Surgical Oncology Clinics of North America
https://www.surgonc.theclinics.com/

THE CLINICS ARE AVAILABLE ONLINE!
Access your subscription at:
www.theclinics.com

Preface

Management of Bladder Cancer: The First Inning of a New Era of Rapid Advances

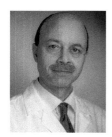

Guru P. Sonpavde, MD
Editor

The management of bladder cancer has witnessed several multidisciplinary advances in the past few years (**Fig. 1**). This issue of the *Hematology/Oncology Clinics of North America* takes the reader on an exciting journey highlighting the recent advances. Metastatic urothelial carcinoma (mUC) is generally incurable. Cisplatin-based combination chemotherapy yields a median survival of 14 to 15 months and 5-year overall survival (OS) of 5% to 15%, suggesting some potential cures.[1] The therapeutic landscape for mUC has been transformed with the advent of PD-1/L1 inhibitors for progressive disease in postplatinum patients. Pembrolizumab yielded an impressive 2-year OS rates of 26.9% (vs 14.3% with taxane or vinflunine chemotherapy) in the intent-to-treat (ITT) population regardless of PD-L1 expression.[2] While the objective response rate (ORR) was higher with pembrolizumab (21.1% vs 11.0%), the most impressive aspect of outcomes may be the prolonged median duration of response greater than 2 years (vs 4.4 months with chemotherapy). Pembrolizumab and atezolizumab are also approved as first-line therapy for cisplatin-ineligible patients with high tumor PD-L1 expression and platinum-ineligible patients, although phase 3 trials have not demonstrated improved survival with this approach.[3,4] Indeed, the DANUBE phase 3 trial could not demonstrate improved OS for durvalumab in patients with PD-L1 high tumors, and with durvalumab combined with tremelimumab versus gemcitabine-platinum in unselected patients.[5] Furthermore, the combination of PD-1/L1 inhibitors with platinum-based chemotherapy for metastatic disease has not been successful in improving survival.[6,7] The combination of atezolizumab with gemcitabine-platinum (IMvigor130) modestly improved progression-free survival (PFS) to 8.2 versus 6.3 months (hazard ratio [HR], 0.82; 95% confidence interval [CI], 0.70–0.96; 1-sided $P = .007$). However, an improvement in OS has not

Hematol Oncol Clin N Am 35 (2021) xiii–xx
https://doi.org/10.1016/j.hoc.2021.03.001
0889-8588/21/© 2021 Published by Elsevier Inc.

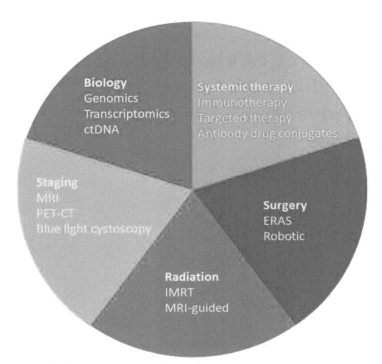

Fig. 1. Advances in the management of bladder cancer.

been demonstrated for combining either atezolizumab or pembrolizumab with gemcitabine-platinum (KEYNOTE361). The landmark Javelin Bladder-100 phase 3 trial demonstrated that first-line switch-maintenance avelumab following responding or stable disease on 4 to 6 cycles of platinum-based chemotherapy improved survival compared with best supportive care (BSC) significantly in the overall ITT population regardless of tumor PD-L1 expression (median OS 21.4 vs 14.3 months; HR, 0.69; 1-sided P = .0005).[8] In addition, prolonged OS was even more impressive in patients with PD-L1–positive tumors (HR, 0.56; P = .0003). PFS was also extended with avelumab plus BSC versus BSC (HR, 0.62; 95% CI, 0.52, 0.75) in the ITT population as well as the PD-L1 high population (HR, 0.56; 95% CI, 0.43, 0.73). These data have already had a practice-changing impact.

Advances have occurred for the therapy of postplatinum and PD-1/L1 inhibitor–treated patients with the accelerated regulatory Food and Drug Administration approval of an antibody drug conjugate (ADC). Enfortumab vedotin (EV), a Nectin-4 targeting ADC, yielded an ORR of 44% (95% CI, 35.1% to 53.2%), including 12% complete responses in 125 patients following platinum-based chemotherapy and PD-1/L1 inhibitors in a phase 2 trial.[9] The median PFS and OS were 5.8 and 11.7 months, respectively. Encouraging responses were seen even in patients with liver metastases and those with no response to prior PD-1/L1 inhibitor therapy. Subsequently, the EV301 phase 3 trial demonstrated improved OS (median 12.88 vs 8.97 months; HR, 0.70; P = .001), PFS (median 5.55 vs 3.71 months; HR, 0.62; P<.001), and ORR (40.6% vs 17.9%).[10] Moreover, EV exhibited similar activity in a phase 2 trial, including a cohort of platinum-naïve mUC patients who were cisplatin-ineligible following a PD-1/L1 inhibitor with ORR of 52% and a median duration of response of 10.9 months, suggesting EV may represent an alternative to carboplatin-based chemotherapy in this population.[11] Another ADC, sacituzumab govitecan, which targets Trop2, has shown preliminary promise in the same setting.[12,13] In the TROPHY U-01 trial, sacituzumab govitecan demonstrated promising activity in 113 patients following platinum and an immune checkpoint inhibitor with an ORR of 27% and median duration of response of 5.9 months.

Erdafitinib, an oral FGFR inhibitor, is the first targeted agent approved for metastatic disease and is applicable to ~15% of postplatinum patients with activating genomic alterations in FGFR2 or FGFR3. In a phase 2 trial enrolling 99 patients, ORR with erdafitinib was observed in 40%, accompanied by a median PFS of 5.5 months, and median OS of 13.8 months.[14] An ongoing phase 3 trial is attempting to validate the activity of erdafitinib. Targeted agents for HER2-driven tumors have shown preliminary promise, which has led to early trials evaluating potent HER2 inhibitors, such as trastuzumab deruxtecan, a novel ADC.[15] PARP inhibitors and epigenetic modifiers have been preliminarily disappointing in unselected or selected patients.[16,17]

Moreover, combinations of active agents are undergoing evaluation. The combination of EV and pembrolizumab exhibited promising activity as first-line therapy for cisplatin-ineligible mUC.[18] An ongoing phase 3 trial is developing this novel combination of EV and pembrolizumab in the first-line setting (EV-302 trial). The combination of VEGF/FGFR inhibitors and PD-1/L1 inhibitors has also shown preliminary promise. One phase 3 trial (LEAP) is evaluating the combination of lenvatinib and pembrolizumab as first-line therapy for metastatic cisplatin-ineligible urothelial carcinoma. The optimal sequencing of active agents needs investigation, although these efforts may need to rely on retrospective analyses and real-world datasets.

Neoadjuvant cisplatin-based combination chemotherapy is established for muscle-invasive bladder cancer (MIBC).[19] Genomic profiling for DNA damage repair (DDR) genes and the basal gene expression subtype has been reported to be associated with pathologic complete remission in retrospective studies.[20-22] The phase 2 RETAIN BLADDER trial suggested the feasibility of using clinical and genomic factors in patients with MIBC to pursue a surveillance approach in those with DDR alterations and clinical complete remission after neoadjuvant chemotherapy.[23] Data supporting neoadjuvant chemotherapy from MIBC have commonly been extrapolated to upper tract urothelial carcinoma (UTUC). For the first time, a definitive phase 3 trial (POUT trial) demonstrated improved outcomes with adjuvant gemcitabine-platinum for pT20 UTUC with improved disease-free survival (DFS) and an HR of 0.45 (P = .0001).[24] The debate continues regarding the role of adjuvant gemcitabine-carboplatin for cisplatin-ineligible patients where the benefit appeared less impressive (with the caveat of an underpowered subanalysis of this cohort). An exciting and potentially practice-changing impact was demonstrated recently using adjuvant nivolumab for muscle-invasive urothelial carcinoma after radical surgery (CHECKMATE274 phase 3 trial) with an improvement in DFS versus placebo, both in the overall population (median 21.0 vs 10.9 months; HR, 0.70; P = .0006) and in those with tumor PD-L1 $\geq$ 1% (median not reached vs 10.8 months; HR, 0.53; P = .0004).[25] The nonurothelial recurrence-free survival and distant metastasis-free survival were also significantly better in the overall and PD-L1 high populations. Toxicities were manageable and consistent with previous reports, and there was no deterioration of health-related quality of life. These data will also lead to an interesting debate regarding the role of adjuvant gemcitabine-carboplatin or nivolumab for cisplatin-ineligible UTUC. Previously, applying atezolizumab to the adjuvant setting following radical cystectomy for high-risk muscle invasive disease did not improve outcomes in the IMvigor010 phase 3 trial.[26] However, an interesting retrospective analysis demonstrated that those with minimal residual disease detected by postoperative tumor-informed circulating tumor–DNA profiling may be able to identify patients likely to benefit from atezolizumab.[27] Similar efforts to evaluate pembrolizumab in the adjuvant setting are ongoing in the AMBASSADOR trial. Neoadjuvant PD-1/L1 inhibitors alone (for cisplatin-ineligible or cisplatin-refusing patients) or combined with cisplatin-based chemotherapy preceding radical cystectomy have exhibited promising activity, and phase 3 trials are attempting to confirm a role for these approaches.[28,29] The incorporation of PD-1/L1 inhibitors in bladder-preserving trimodal chemoradiation approaches is being evaluated in ongoing phase 3 trials.

Therapy for nonmuscle invasive bladder cancer (NMIBC) has also enjoyed advances with the approval of systemic pembrolizumab for rigorously defined Bacillus Calmette-Guérin (BCG)-unresponsive high-risk disease. The complete response rate in 96 patients (KEYNOTE057 trial) with high-risk BCG-unresponsive NMIBC with carcinoma in situ was 41%, and median response duration was 16.2 months.[30] Moreover, other promising intraluminally delivered agents are emerging, including nadofaragene firadenovec (nonreplicating adenovirus vector harboring the human IFN alpha2b gene), vicinium (a recombinant fusion protein of an anti-EpCAM antibody linked to a variant of Pseudomonas exotoxin A), and N-803 (an interleukin-15 superagonist) for high-risk BCG-unresponsive disease.[31-33] Mitomycin gel was approved for low-grade UTUC based on complete response in 41 of 71 patients (58%), who were scheduled to receive 6 weekly treatments, including 46% who had durable complete response at 12 months.[34]

Innovations in surgery, staging, and radiation are also occurring. Blue light cystoscopy has improved the sensitivity of detection of malignancy, although further studies are ongoing to evaluate efficacy and cost-effectiveness to justify universal adoption.[35] Multiparametric MRI and fluorodeoxyglucose–PET imaging may warrant further evaluation to enhance clinical staging of muscle-invasive disease.[36,37] A surgical innovation is enhanced recovery after surgery protocols in the setting of radical cystectomy, which may improve the quality of life of patients.[38] Robotic cystectomy was noninferior to open cystectomy for 2-year PFS and quality of life in the phase 3 RAZOR trial.[39] Finally, the emergence of intensity-modulated radiation therapy and use of MRI to plan radiotherapy may improve the therapeutic index of radiotherapy for MIBC.

Despite these advances in therapy, it is important to not lose sight of the fact that metastatic disease is generally incurable, and clinical trials should be considered a standard of care for all settings of the disease. The critically important first step that begets advances is the understanding of tumor biology. Novel clinical prognostic factors have been presented in the setting of PD-L1 inhibitors following platinum-based chemotherapy.[40] The Cancer Genome Atlas project has shed light on the enormous heterogeneity of tumor biology, high mutation burden, and multiple potential driver alterations in subsets of patients.[41] However, dynamic changes in tumor and microenvironment following therapy need to be better understood for insights into resistance and new therapeutic targets. Noninvasive molecular monitoring employing cell-free DNA profiling studies of plasma and urine may provide avenues to better understand mechanisms of resistance, new therapeutic targets, and minimal residual disease.[42] Precision medicine that leverages molecular information from multiple platforms may be necessary for optimal patient selection. The combination of molecular and clinical factors may also warrant exploration to develop precision medicine.[43,44] These exciting recent advances have set the stage for the next round of progress.

Guru P. Sonpavde, MD
Lank Center for Genitourinary Oncology
Dana-Farber Cancer Institute, D924
Harvard Medical School
450 Brookline Avenue
Boston, MA 02215, USA

E-mail address:
gurup_sonpavde@dfci.harvard.edu

REFERENCES

1. von der Maase H, Sengelov L, Roberts JT, et al. Long-term survival results of a randomized trial comparing gemcitabine plus cisplatin, with methotrexate, vinblastine, doxorubicin, plus cisplatin in patients with bladder cancer. J Clin Oncol 2005;23:4602–8.
2. Fradet Y, Bellmunt J, Vaughn DJ, et al. Randomized phase III KEYNOTE-045 trial of pembrolizumab versus paclitaxel, docetaxel, or vinflunine in recurrent advanced urothelial cancer: results of > 2 years of follow-up. Ann Oncol 2019; 30(6):970–6.
3. Balar AV, Galsky MD, Rosenberg JE, et al. Atezolizumab as first-line treatment in cisplatin-ineligible patients with locally advanced and metastatic urothelial carcinoma: a single-arm, multicentre, phase 2 trial. Lancet 2017;389:67–76.
4. Vuky J, Balar AV, Castellano D, et al. Long-term outcomes in KEYNOTE-052: phase II study investigating first-line pembrolizumab in cisplatin-ineligible patients with locally advanced or metastatic urothelial cancer. J Clin Oncol 2020; 38:2658–66.
5. Powles T, van der Heijden MS, Castellano D, et al. Durvalumab alone and durvalumab plus tremelimumab versus chemotherapy in previously untreated patients with unresectable, locally advanced or metastatic urothelial carcinoma (DANUBE): a randomised, open-label, multicentre, phase 3 trial. Lancet Oncol 2020; 21:1574–88.
6. Galsky MD, Arija JAA, Bamias A, et al. Atezolizumab with or without chemotherapy in metastatic urothelial cancer (IMvigor130): a multicentre, randomised, placebo-controlled phase 3 trial. Lancet 2020;395:1547–57.
7. Alva A, Csoszi T, Ozguroglu M, et al. Pembrolizumab (P) combined with chemotherapy (C) vs C alone as first-line (1L) therapy for advanced urothelial carcinoma (UC): KEYNOTE-361. Ann Oncol 2020;31(suppl 4).
8. Powles T, Park SH, Voog E, et al. Maintenance avelumab + best supportive care (BSC) versus BSC alone after platinum-based first-line (1L) chemotherapy in advanced urothelial carcinoma (UC): JAVELIN Bladder 100 phase III interim analysis. J Clin Oncol 2020;38:LBA1.
9. Rosenberg JE, O'Donnell PH, Balar AV, et al. Pivotal trial of enfortumab vedotin in urothelial carcinoma after platinum and anti-programmed death 1/programmed death ligand 1 therapy. J Clin Oncol 2019;37:2592–600.
10. Powles T, Rosenberg JE, Sonpavde GP, et al. Enfortumab vedotin in previously treated advanced urothelial carcinoma. N Engl J Med 2021.
11. Balar AVMB, Rosenberg JE, et al. EV-201 cohort 2: enfortumab vedotin in cisplatin-ineligible patients with locally advanced or metastatic urothelial cancer

who received prior PD-1/PD-L1 inhibitors. J Clin Oncol 2021;39(suppl 6). Abstract 394.

12. Tagawa ST, Balar A, Petrylak DP, et al. Initial results from TROPHY-U-01: a phase 2 open-label study of sacituzumab govitecan in patients (pts) with metastatic urothelial cancer (MUC) after failure of platinum-based regimens (PLT) or immunotherapy. Ann Oncol 2019;30(suppl 5):v851–934.

13. Loriot Y, Balar A, Petrylak DP, et al. TROPHY-U-01 cohort 1 final results: a phase II study of sacituzumab govitecan (SG) in metastatic urothelial cancer (mUC) that has progressed after platinum (PLT) and checkpoint inhibitors (CPI). Ann Oncol 2020;31(suppl 4):S1142–215.

14. Loriot Y, Necchi A, Park SH, et al. Erdafitinib in locally advanced or metastatic urothelial carcinoma. N Engl J Med 2019;381:338–48.

15. Choudhury NJ, Campanile A, Antic T, et al. Afatinib activity in platinum-refractory metastatic urothelial carcinoma in patients with ERBB alterations. J Clin Oncol 2016;34:2165–71.

16. Grivas P, Loriot Y, Feyerabend S, et al. Rucaparib for recurrent, locally advanced, or metastatic urothelial carcinoma (mUC): results from ATLAS, a phase II open-label trial. J Clin Oncol 2020;38(suppl 6). Abstract 440.

17. Grivas P, Mortazavi A, Picus J, et al. Mocetinostat for patients with previously treated, locally advanced/metastatic urothelial carcinoma and inactivating alterations of acetyltransferase genes. Cancer 2019;125:533–40.

18. Rosenberg JE, Flaig TW, Friedlander TW, et al. Study EV-103: preliminary durability results of enfortumab vedotin plus pembrolizumab for locally advanced or metastatic urothelial carcinoma. J Clin Oncol 2020;38(suppl 6). Abstract 441.

19. Grossman HB, Natale RB, Tangen CM, et al. Neoadjuvant chemotherapy plus cystectomy compared with cystectomy alone for locally advanced bladder cancer. New Engl J Med 2003;349:859–66.

20. Liu D, Plimack ER, Hoffman-Censits J, et al. Clinical validation of chemotherapy response biomarker ERCC2 in muscle-invasive urothelial bladder carcinoma. JAMA Oncol 2016;2:1094–6.

21. Plimack ER, Dunbrack RL, Brennan TA, et al. Defects in DNA repair genes predict response to neoadjuvant cisplatin-based chemotherapy in muscle-invasive bladder cancer. Eur Urol 2015;68:959–67.

22. Seiler R, Ashab HAD, Erho N, et al. Impact of molecular subtypes in muscle-invasive bladder cancer on predicting response and survival after neoadjuvant chemotherapy. Eur Urol 2017;72:544–54.

23. Geynisman DM, Abbosh P, Ross EA, et al. A phase II trial of risk enabled therapy after initiating neoadjuvant chemotherapy for bladder cancer (RETAIN BLADDER): interim analysis. J Clin Oncol 2021;39(suppl 6). Abstract 397.

24. Birtle A, Johnson M, Chester J, et al. Adjuvant chemotherapy in upper tract urothelial carcinoma (the POUT trial): a phase 3, open-label, randomised controlled trial. Lancet 2020;395:1268–77.

25. Bajorin DF, Witjes JA, Gschwend J, et al. First results from the phase 3 CheckMate 274 trial of adjuvant nivolumab vs placebo in patients who underwent radical surgery for high-risk muscle-invasive urothelial carcinoma (MIUC). J Clin Oncol 2021;39(2021suppl 6). Abstract 391.

26. Hussain SA, Lester JF, Jackson R, et al. Phase II randomized placebo-controlled neoadjuvant trial of nintedanib or placebo with gemcitabine and cisplatin in locally advanced muscle invasive bladder cancer (NEO-BLADE). J Clin Oncol 2020;38(suppl 6):2020. Abstract 438.

27. Powles T, Assaf ZJ, Davarpanah N, et al. Clinical outcomes in post-operative ctDNA-positive muscle-invasive urothelial carcinoma (MIUC) patients after atezolizumab adjuvant therapy. ESMO Immuno-Oncology Virtual Congress 2020 (9-12 December).

28. Powles T, Kockx M, Rodriguez-Vida A, et al. Clinical efficacy and biomarker analysis of neoadjuvant atezolizumab in operable urothelial carcinoma in the ABACUS trial. Nat Med 2019;25:1706–14.

29. Necchi A, Raggi D, Gallina A, et al. Updated results of PURE-01 with preliminary activity of neoadjuvant pembrolizumab in patients with muscle-invasive bladder carcinoma with variant histologies. Eur Urol 2020;77:439–46.

30. Balar AV, Kulkarni GS, Uchio EM, et al. Keynote 057: phase II trial of Pembrolizumab (pembro) for patients (pts) with high-risk (HR) nonmuscle invasive bladder cancer (NMIBC) unresponsive to Bacillus Calmette-Guérin (BCG). J Clin Oncol 2019;37:350.

31. Boorjian SA, Dinney C, SUO Clinical Trials Consortium. Safety and efficacy of intravesical nadofaragene firadenovec for patients with high-grade, BCG unresponsive nonmuscle invasive bladder cancer (NMIBC): results from a phase III trial. J Clin Oncol 2020;38(suppl 6). Abstract 442.

32. Shore NO, O'Donnell M, Keane T, et al. PD03-02 phase 3 results of vicinium in BCG-unresponsive non-muscle invasive bladder cancer. J Urol 2020;203(suppl 4):e72.

33. Chamie K, Chang S, Gonzalgo ML, et al. Phase II/III clinical results of IL-15RαFc superagonist N-803 with BCG in BCG-unresponsive non-muscle invasive bladder cancer (NMIBC) carcinoma in situ (CIS) patients. J Clin Oncol 2021;39(suppl 6). Abstract 510.

34. Kleinmann N, Matin SF, Pierorazio PM, et al. Primary chemoablation of low-grade upper tract urothelial carcinoma using UGN-101, a mitomycin-containing reverse thermal gel (OLYMPUS): an open-label, single-arm, phase 3 trial. Lancet Oncol 2020;21:776–85.

35. Lotan Y, Chaplin I, Ahmadi H, et al. Prospective evaluation of blue-light flexible cystoscopy with hexaminolevulinate in non-muscle-invasive bladder cancer. BJU Int 2021;127:108–13.

36. Necchi A, Bandini M, Calareso G, et al. Multiparametric magnetic resonance imaging as a noninvasive assessment of tumor response to neoadjuvant pembrolizumab in muscle-invasive bladder cancer: preliminary findings from the PURE-01 Study. Eur Urol 2020;77:636–43.

37. Einerhand SMH, van Gennep EJ, Mertens LS, et al. 18F-fluoro-2-deoxy-D-glucose positron emission tomography/computed tomography in muscle-invasive bladder cancer. Curr Opin Urol 2020;30:654–64.

38. Vlad O, Catalin B, Mihai H, et al. Enhanced recovery after surgery (ERAS) protocols in patients undergoing radical cystectomy with ileal urinary diversions: a randomized controlled trial. Medicine (Baltimore) 2020;99:e20902.

39. Parekh DJ, Reis IM, Castle EP, et al. Robot-assisted radical cystectomy versus open radical cystectomy in patients with bladder cancer (RAZOR): an open-label, randomised, phase 3, non-inferiority trial. Lancet 2018;391:2525–36.

40. Sonpavde G, Manitz J, Gao C, et al. Five-factor prognostic model for survival of post-platinum patients with metastatic urothelial carcinoma receiving PD-L1 inhibitors. J Urol 2020;204:1173–9.

41. Robertson AG, Kim J, Al-Ahmadie H, et al. Comprehensive molecular characterization of muscle-invasive bladder cancer. Cell 2017;171:540–56.e25.

42. Agarwal N, Pal SK, Hahn AW, et al. Characterization of metastatic urothelial carcinoma via comprehensive genomic profiling of circulating tumor DNA. Cancer 2018;124:2115–24.
43. Nassar AH, Mouw KW, Jegede O, et al. A model combining clinical and genomic factors to predict response to PD-1/PD-L1 blockade in advanced urothelial carcinoma. Br J Cancer 2020;122:555–63.
44. Galsky MD, Saci A, Szabo PM, et al. Nivolumab in patients with advanced platinum-resistant urothelial carcinoma: efficacy, safety, and biomarker analyses with extended follow-up from CheckMate 275. Clin Cancer Res 2020;26:5120–8.

The Epidemiology of Bladder Cancer

Matthew Mossanen, MD, MPH

KEYWORDS

- Epidemiology • Risk factors • Bladder cancer

KEY POINTS

- Bladder cancer is a complex disease with numerous potential risk factors. Risk factors can be external (environmental exposures) or endogenous (inherent to the patient).
- Smoking is the most common risk factor, and many patients with bladder cancer may be active smokers. For active smokers with bladder cancer, discussion of smoking cessation may be an impactful way to improve overall health and oncologic outcomes during bladder cancer treatment.
- Environmental risk factors for bladder cancer include occupational exposure (rubber, diesel, painting dyes, coal, rubber) and contaminated drinking water that has arsenic.
- Endogenous risk factors for bladder cancer are older patients (late 70s), men, and Caucasian race.
- Many risk factors exist and careful history-taking discussing prior treatments and exposures is critical.

BACKGROUND

In the United States (US) in 2019 there were more than 80,000 new cases of bladder cancer diagnosed and more than 17,000 deaths.[1,2] Bladder cancer is the fourth most common cancer in men and accounts for approximately 5% of all new cancer diagnoses in the US.[3] At initial presentation, 70% to 75% will have stage I to II disease, 20% to 30% will have stage II to III disease, and 5% to 10% will have stage IV disease, which can be locally invasive or metastatic (5%).[2–4] Of this 70% to 75%, approximately 10% will be carcinoma in situ (CIS)[5] (**Fig. 1**). The majority, approximately 90%, of bladder cancer cases are urothelial cell carcinoma, and the remaining are composed of other nonurothelial histology.[6] The most common risk factor for bladder cancer is smoking, which accounts for more than 50% of all cases.[7,8] In addition to smoking, there are other risk factors that can increase the risk of bladder cancer. Many of these risk factors can affect general patient health and their oncologic

Division of Urology, Brigham and Women's Hospital and Dana Farber Cancer Institute, Harvard Medical School, 45 Francis Street, Boston, MA 02115, USA
E-mail address: MMossanen@BWH.harvard.edu
Twitter: @MattMossanen (M.M.)

Hematol Oncol Clin N Am 35 (2021) 445–455
https://doi.org/10.1016/j.hoc.2021.02.001
0889-8588/21/© 2021 Elsevier Inc. All rights reserved.
hemonc.theclinics.com

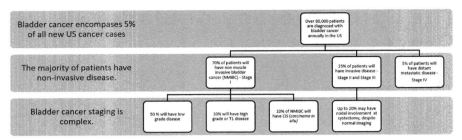

Fig. 1. Bladder cancer staging summary.

outcomes. This article summarizes the epidemiology of bladder cancer and reviews specific risk factors for bladder cancer.

SURVIVAL

The rates of recurrence and progression for nonmuscle invasive tumors can vary depending on 6 clinicopathologic factors, which include number of tumors, size, recurrence rate, T stage, presence of carcinoma in site, and histologic grade. Because of heterogeneity in the complex characterization of noninvasive tumors, 5-year recurrence ranges from 31% to 78% and progression ranges from 1% to 45%.[9] A patient with low-grade Ta typically have rates of recurrence between 25% and 55% although progression is rare.[5] CIS is associated with an average risk of progression of approximately 50% within 5 years of diagnosis.[10] Between 40% and 80% of patients with CIS may develop muscle invasive disease when left untreated.[11] For patients with high-grade T1 bladder cancer, 5-year recurrence, progression, and cancer-specific survival are 42%, 21%, and 87%.[12] After cystectomy, 5-year overall survival varies by pathologic stage, with less than or equal to pT2N0 (organ confined) disease being 62% and 49% for greater than pT2N0 (nonorgan confined).[13] Distant metastatic disease occurs in 25% of patients with organ-confined disease, 37% with nonorgan confined, and 51% with lymph node involvement.[13] At cystectomy, approximately 25% of patients will have lymph node involvement, which corresponds to 5-year recurrence rates of 35%.[14] Patients with lymph node involvement have a 26% 5-year overall survival.[13] Among all patients undergoing cystectomy, 30% may have recurrence, which occurs at a median of 12 months.[14] For patients with distant metastatic disease 5-year survival is dismal at approximately 5%.[2,15]

RISK FACTORS

There are many risk factors for bladder cancer (**Box 1**). During an initial assessment of a patient with bladder cancer a careful discussion and history assessment is important. Particular focus should include social history with details regarding occupational background and discussion of any environmental exposure history.

Smoking

Smoking is the most common risk factor for bladder cancer, and the proportion of the incidence of bladder cancer attributable to smoking, referred to as the population attributable risk, is approximately 50% to 60% for both men and women.[7,8] Smokers have a 3- to 5-fold higher risk of bladder cancer, with increasing risk suggested in those with increasing duration and pack years of smoking.[8,16–20] Bladder cancer is

> **Box 1**
> **Overview of risk factors for bladder cancer**
>
> **Smoking**
> Active smokers, former smokers, second-hand smoke exposure
>
> **Occupational**
> Dyes, paints, rubber, fuels, textiles, asphalt, glass
>
> **Environmental**
> Arsenic in well water, pesticides in agriculture, Agent Orange
>
> **Iatrogenic**
> Pelvic radiation history or cyclophosphamide chemotherapy
>
> **Inflammatory or infectious**
> Chronic urinary tract infections, long-term urinary catheter use, schistosomiasis
>
> **Dietary**
> Increased red and processed meat, decreased fruit and vegetables, low hydration

one of the most common cancers due to smoking and is the second most common tobacco-associated malignancy, second to lung cancer.[21–23]

The relationship between smoking history and bladder cancer risk is complex. A meta-analysis of 83 papers reported the relative risk (RR) for bladder cancer is increased among all smokers (RR = 2.58, 95% confidence interval [CI] 2.37–2.80) with a higher rate for current smokers (RR = 3.47, 3.07–3.91) than for former smokers (2.04, 1.85–2.25).[16] Moreover, all smokers (including current and former) had a higher risk of bladder cancer mortality when compared with nonsmokers.[16] Lastly, second smoking was also associated with an increased risk of bladder cancer (RR 1.40, 1.04–1.88).[16] Smokers who quit have a lower risk of bladder cancer when compared with current smokers (hazard ratio = 0.61, 0.40–0.94), and the risk of bladder cancer may decline by 25% within the first 10 years of cessation and continue to decline, although this value may never reach the level of nonsmokers.[18] Patients who quit for more than 10 years have lower rates of bladder cancer than those who quit for 1 to 4 years or 5 to 9 years; however, even for those who quit for more than 10 years the risk remains elevated in comparison to never smokers.[7] An examination of previously published studies from several prospective US cohorts found that for current smokers relative to never smokers there is an approximately 3-fold increased risk of bladder cancer (95% CI, 2.45–3.54).[7]

Tobacco products contain nicotine and carcinogens, and although nicotine is toxic and addictive, it is the carcinogens in tobacco smoke that can result in DNA mutations, resulting in tumors that are ultimately tobacco-induced cancers.[17] In vitro exposure of bladder cancer cells to tobacco smoke carcinogens has shown increases in levels of DNA damage due to hypermethylation, and also smokers with high-grade bladder cancer have higher levels of DNA hypermethylation than nonsmokers with low-grade bladder cancer.[24] In fact, smokers with bladder cancer have a unique urinary metabolomic signature, suggesting smoking is a key factor in the pathogenesis of tumor growth.[24,25] Evaluation of smoking intensity and duration has suggested higher grade and stage disease in those with more extensive histories and in particular those who smoke more than 60 cigarettes per day.[26]

Smoking is associated with poorer outcomes after radical cystectomy cumulative smoking exposure has been linked to numerous negative clinical outcomes, including more advanced stage of disease, lymph node involvement, disease recurrence, cancer-specific mortality, and overall mortality.[27] Smoking status may also predict worse outcomes after neoadjuvant chemotherapy. In one study, former smokers were twice as likely and current smokers 4 times as likely to show no response (ypT2-4 ypN+) after cisplatin-based neoadjuvant chemotherapy.[28] Also, smokers undergoing radical cystectomy have more surgical complications after surgery including increased rates of reoperation in the immediate postoperative period.[29] A meta-analysis of 17 studies examined more than 13,000 patients after radical cystectomy and reported that active smokers had worse clinical outcomes including increased overall and cancer-specific mortality and increased cancer recurrence after cystectomy.[30] Moreover, nonsmokers were found to have higher rates of complete response to neoadjuvant chemotherapy than active smokers.[30]

For patients who are active smokers, the time of a bladder cancer diagnosis may be a valuable opportunity to engage in smoking cessation. Of note, smokers with a new bladder cancer diagnosis are 5 times more likely to quit than the average smoker (48% vs 10%, $P<.001$), and urologist advice is one of the most commonly cited reasons for cessation[31]; this highlights the potential role of the oncologist treating patients with bladder cancer should include a discussion of smoking cessation and counseling regarding treatment options.[32]

Age, Gender, and Ethnicity

Age and gender are 2 nonmodifiable risk factors for bladder cancer. Bladder cancer is approximately 3 to 4 times more likely in men than in women.[8,19,33] In part, some of this discrepancy has been attributed to differences in smoking habits and occupational or environmental exposures. Bladder cancer is a disease of the elderly, and more than 80% of cases are diagnosed in patients older than 65 years, and the median age of diagnosis in the US is 73.[1] Approximately 20% of patients are 85 years or older.[3] Data have also suggested that increasing number of new bladder cancer diagnosis are occurring among octogenarians[34] due to an increasing number of elderly in the population. As the population continues to age, an increasing proportion of patients with bladder cancer are elderly in the future. There are also data suggesting bladder cancer is more common in Caucasian patients than in African Americans[35] and that African American patients may have poorer survival due to being diagnosed with later stages at the time of presentation.[36–38]

Occupational

Multiple professions have been associated with an increase in bladder cancer, and incidence due to occupational exposure has been estimated to be between 5% and 18% with exposure to elements including rubber, aluminum, paints, dyes, diesel fuel, metal, textiles, and printing.[8,19] Aromatic amines (beta-naphthylamine) were used during the manufacturing of products including dyes, rubber, and fuels and has been described as a risk factor for bladder cancer.[39] Aromatic amines contaminate the ambient air through tobacco smoke or occupational exposures.[39] In fact, polycyclic aromatic hydrocarbons are present in coal, crude oil, and gasoline and are also produced when coal, wood, gas, tobacco, or garbage are burned, and once contaminated air is breathed in or absorbed by skin exposure the body metabolizes the compound and metabolites, which are then processed and passed into the urine.[40] Occupations with a potentially increased risk of bladder cancer include firefighters, truck drivers, machinists, hair dressers, and farmers.[4] Firefighters may have an increased risk of bladder cancer due to exposure to products of combustion, including polycyclic aromatic hydrocarbons, which has been detected on personal protective equipment (such as helmets and clothing) as well as on bodily surfaces (skin and throat).[41]

Environmental

Drinking well water contaminated with arsenic may be associated with an increased risk of bladder cancer.[42,43] An association between exposure to Agent Orange, a chemical defoliant with concentrations of the carcinogen dioxin, and bladder cancer risk in Veterans from the Vietnam War has also been described.[44] There is also evidence suggesting that pesticide exposure is associated with an increased risk of bladder cancer.[35]

Iatrogenic

The use of cyclophosphamide-induced bladder cancer has been described, and incidence may be as high as 16% at 15 years after time of exposure.[45] Radiation-induced bladder cancers are also described after pelvic radiation used to treat prostate or cervical cancer. These secondary bladder cancers can present after a latency period lasting years 5 to 15 years and can demonstrate more aggressive behavior or advanced stage at the time of diagnosis.[46,47] Several medications have also been linked to bladder cancer, including the diabetes medication pioglitazone[48] and an analgesic known as phenacetin.[49,50]

Genetics

Certain patients may have an increased susceptibility to bladder cancer due to genetic factors.[51] The dynamic interplay between genetic susceptibility and environmental risk factors may account for the variations in bladder cancer epidemiology. Moreover, multiple low-penetrance predisposition genes can account for varying degrees of susceptibility.[51] A study of twin cohorts from Sweden, Denmark, and Finland showed that inherited genetic factors are a minor contributing component to the development of bladder cancer and that environmental factors are a driving factor.[52] Future work may help identify candidate genes that can be incorporated into comprehensive prediction tools to predict clinical outcomes.

Dietary Intake

A meta-analysis determined that although overall meat intake was not related to the risk of bladder cancer, those with high levels of red and processed meat consumption did have an increased risk of bladder cancer when compared with those with the lowest consumption rates.[53] A positive association has been observed between processed meat consumption and bladder cancer, and an increased consumption of red and processed meat may increase the risk of bladder cancer by 25% and 33%, respectively.[54] Alcohol intake has not been shown to increase the risk of bladder cancer.[55] Fruit and vegetable intake may have a protective effect against bladder cancer.[56] Low hydration has also been associated with an increased risk of bladder cancer.[8]

Obesity and Sedentary Lifestyle

A meta-analysis of 11 cohort studies found obesity was associated with a 10% increased risk of bladder cancer.[57] Further work reported that increasing body mass index was associated with a rising risk of bladder cancer in a linear fashion, with the risk increasing by 4% for every 5 kg/m^2 increase.[58] A meta-analysis of 15 studies reported that physical activity was associated with a decreased risk of bladder cancer and that high versus low levels of physical activity may decrease bladder cancer risk by 15%.[59]

Table 1
Risk factors for bladder cancer and possible strategies for modifying or reducing exposure

Risk Factors Category	Consideration for Modifiability
Smoking	Smoking cessation may reduce the risk of bladder cancer For those diagnosed, smoking can be associated with an increased risk with worse oncologic and overall health outcomes
Occupational exposure	Reducing exposure to toxic chemicals in the workplace (paints, dyes, solvents) through appropriate protective equipment may reduce the risk of bladder cancer
Environmental factors	Avoiding consumption of contaminated drinking water may decrease the risk of bladder cancer
Lifestyle	Increased fruit and vegetable consumption and reduced consumption of processed and red meat intake may be associated with a reduced risk of bladder cancer

Infectious or Inflammatory

Patients with schistosomiasis parasitic infections may also have an increased risk of bladder cancer and in particular squamous cell carcinoma of the bladder.[60] Schistosomiasis is endemic to many areas throughout Africa and the Middle-East and often associated with squamous cell carcinoma of the bladder due to chronic infection.[61] Treatment with praziquantel is effective in treating the infection and may help prevent bladder cancer.[61] Indwelling suprapubic tube catheters or chronic urinary tract infections may also lead to long-term inflammation and can be associated with the occurrence of bladder cancer.[62]

Modifiability of Risk Factors for Bladder Cancer

A meta-analysis of risk factors for bladder cancer determined that approximately 82% of total bladder cancer cases could be linked to a specific cause.[63] A proportion of risk

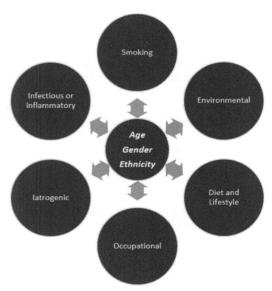

Fig. 2. Multiple factors that have an impact on the risk of developing bladder cancer.

factors for bladder may be modifiable in the sense that exposure can be reduced or even avoided, whereas others are immutable and inherent to the patient.

Certain risk factors for bladder cancer such as smoking or exposure to toxic chemicals may be detrimental to overall health and oncologic outcomes. Determining a patient's exposure history may allow health care providers to provide tailored counsel

Table 2
Epidemiologic overview: a clinical summary of risk factors for bladder cancer

Risk Factor	Clinical Summary	Clinical Tip
Smoking	**Most common risk factor → 50%–60% A subset of patients may have had second-hand exposure, which also increases the risk of bladder cancer.** *Linked to worse oncologic and overall health outcomes including worse responses to neoadjuvant chemotherapy, cancer survival, and recurrence as well as increased surgical complications.*	If patients are active smokers assess willingness to quit and discuss cessation.
Age	**Median age of diagnosis is 73 y and up to 20% of patients may be 85 y or older** *As the US population continues to age, the incidence of bladder cancer may also continue to increase over time.*	Bladder cancer is common in older patients.
Gender	**Men are 3–4 times more likely to develop bladder cancer than women.** *Older men are the most commonly seen patients.*	Bladder cancer occurs more often in men.
Occupational and environmental	**Chemicals or toxic by-products can increase the risk of bladder cancer.** *Exposure to fuels, paints, dyes, oils, or cleaning solvents and contaminated drinking water and discuss professional background (factory worker or firefighter).*	Assess social history and occupational background.
Iatrogenic	**Exposure to certain chemotherapy regimens or radiation.** *Bladder cancer occurrence can have a latency period of many years after these exposures.*	Be cognizant of any prior oncologic treatment history.
Infectious	**Recurrent infectious or indwelling suprapubic tubes.** *Chronic urinary tract irritation or inflammation can increase the risk of bladder cancer.*	Patients with long-term indwelling catheters are at risk.
Lifestyle	**Increased fruit and vegetable consumption and good hydration may be protective.** *Limiting red and processed meat intake may be protective.*	Lifestyle and nutrition counselling are vital.

the individual patient. Providers may be able to make recommendations to decrease the harmful impact of that risk factor through several modifications relating to lifestyle or exposure. **Table 1** describes different risk factors for bladder cancer and possible strategies for modifying or reducing exposure.

The most causative agent associated with bladder cancer is smoking, and thus, smoking cessation represents an opportunity to improve outcomes. However, in practice, most patients may possess multiple risk factors, and there is a dynamic interplay between risk factors for an individual (**Fig. 2**). *Ultimately, multiple factors, including endogenous and environmental, combine in a dynamic interplay to affect the risk of developing bladder cancer.*

SUMMARY AND CLINICS CARE POINTS

- Bladder cancer is a complex disease with numerous potential risk factors. Risk factors can be external (environmental exposures) or endogenous (inherent to the patient) (**Table 2**).
- Smoking is the most common risk factor and many patients with bladder cancer may be active smokers. For active smokers with bladder cancer, discussion of smoking cessation may be an impactful way to improve overall health and oncologic outcomes during bladder cancer treatment.
- Environmental risk factors for bladder cancer include occupational exposure (rubber, diesel, painting dyes, coal, rubber) and contaminated drinking water that has arsenic.
- Endogenous risk factors for bladder cancer are older patients (late 70s), men, and Caucasian race.
- Many risk factors exist, and careful history-taking discussing prior treatments and exposures is critical.

DISCLOSURE

The authors have nothing to disclose.

REFERENCES

1. Howlader N, Noone AM, Krapcho M, et al, editors. SEER Cancer Statistics Review, 1975-2017. Bethesda: National Cancer Institute. https://seer.cancer.gov/csr/1975_2017/, based on November 2019 SEER data submission, posted to the SEER web site, April 2020.
2. Siegel RL, Miller KD, Jemal A. Cancer statistics, 2019. CA Cancer J Clin 2019; 69(1):7–34.
3. Miller KD, Nogueira L, Mariotto AB, et al. Cancer treatment and survivorship statistics, 2019. CA Cancer J Clin 2019;69(5):363–85.
4. Sharma S, Ksheersagar P, Sharma P. Diagnosis and treatment of bladder cancer. Am Fam Physician 2009;80(7):717–23.
5. Nerli RB, Ghagane SC, Shankar K, et al. Low-Grade, Multiple, Ta Non-muscle-Invasive Bladder Tumors: Tumor Recurrence and Worsening Progression. Indian J Surg Oncol 2018;9(2):157–61.
6. Chalasani V, Chin JL, Izawa JI. Histologic variants of urothelial bladder cancer and nonurothelial histology in bladder cancer. Can Urol Assoc J 2009;3(6 Suppl 4):S193–8.
7. Freedman ND, Silverman DT, Hollenbeck AR, et al. Association between smoking and risk of bladder cancer among men and women. JAMA 2011;306(7):737–45.

8. Cumberbatch MGK, Jubber I, Black PC, et al. Epidemiology of Bladder Cancer: A Systematic Review and Contemporary Update of Risk Factors in 2018. Eur Urol 2018;74(6):784–95.
9. Sylvester RJ, van der Meijden AP, Oosterlinck W, et al. Predicting recurrence and progression in individual patients with stage Ta T1 bladder cancer using EORTC risk tables: a combined analysis of 2596 patients from seven EORTC trials. Eur Urol 2006;49(3):466–75 [discussion: 475–7].
10. Tang DH, Chang SS. Management of carcinoma in situ of the bladder: best practice and recent developments. Ther Adv Urol 2015;7(6):351–64.
11. Althausen AF, Prout GR Jr, Daly JJ. Non-invasive papillary carcinoma of the bladder associated with carcinoma in situ. J Urol 1976;116(5):575–80.
12. Martin-Doyle W, Leow JJ, Orsola A, et al. Improving selection criteria for early cystectomy in high-grade t1 bladder cancer: a meta-analysis of 15,215 patients. J Clin Oncol 2015;33(6):643–50.
13. Madersbacher S, Hochreiter W, Burkhard F, et al. Radical cystectomy for bladder cancer today–a homogeneous series without neoadjuvant therapy. J Clin Oncol 2003;21(4):690–6.
14. Stein JP, Lieskovsky G, Cote R, et al. Radical cystectomy in the treatment of invasive bladder cancer: long-term results in 1,054 patients. J Clin Oncol 2001;19(3):666–75.
15. Mar N, Dayyani F. Management of Urothelial Bladder Cancer in Clinical Practice: Real-World Answers to Difficult Questions. J Oncol Pract 2019;15(8):421–8.
16. Cumberbatch MG, Rota M, Catto JW, et al. The role of tobacco smoke in bladder and kidney carcinogenesis: a comparison of exposures and meta-analysis of incidence and mortality risks. Eur Urol 2016;70(3):458–66.
17. Hecht SS. Tobacco carcinogens, their biomarkers and tobacco-induced cancer. Nat Rev Cancer 2003;3(10):733–44.
18. Li Y, Tindle HA, Hendryx MS, et al. Smoking Cessation and the Risk of Bladder Cancer among Postmenopausal Women. Cancer Prev Res (Phila) 2019;12(5):305–14.
19. Saginala K, Barsouk A, Aluru JS, et al. Epidemiology of bladder cancer. Med Sci (Basel) 2020;8(1):177–89.
20. Baris D, Karagas MR, Verrill C, et al. A case-control study of smoking and bladder cancer risk: emergent patterns over time. J Natl Cancer Inst 2009;101(22):1553–61.
21. Boffetta P. Tobacco smoking and risk of bladder cancer. Scand J Urol Nephrol Suppl 2008;(218):45–54.
22. Gandini S, Botteri E, Iodice S, et al. Tobacco smoking and cancer: a meta-analysis. Int J Cancer 2008;122(1):155–64.
23. Theis RP, Dolwick Grieb SM, Burr D, et al. Smoking, environmental tobacco smoke, and risk of renal cell cancer: a population-based case-control study. BMC Cancer 2008;8:387.
24. Jin F, Thaiparambil J, Donepudi SR, et al. Tobacco-Specific Carcinogens Induce Hypermethylation, DNA Adducts, and DNA Damage in Bladder Cancer. Cancer Prev Res (Phila) 2017;10(10):588–97.
25. Putluri N, Shojaie A, Vasu VT, et al. Metabolomic profiling reveals potential markers and bioprocesses altered in bladder cancer progression. Cancer Res 2011;71(24):7376–86.
26. Chamssuddin AK, Saadat SH, Deiri K, et al. Evaluation of grade and stage in patients with bladder cancer among smokers and non-smokers. Arab J Urol 2013;11(2):165–8.

27. Rink M, Zabor EC, Furberg H, et al. Impact of smoking and smoking cessation on outcomes in bladder cancer patients treated with radical cystectomy. Eur Urol 2013;64(3):456–64.
28. Boeri L, Soligo M, Frank I, et al. Cigarette smoking is associated with adverse pathological response and increased disease recurrence amongst patients with muscle-invasive bladder cancer treated with cisplatin-based neoadjuvant chemotherapy and radical cystectomy: a single-centre experience. BJU Int 2019;123(6):1011–9.
29. Reese SW, Ji E, Paciotti M, et al. Risk factors and reasons for reoperation after radical cystectomy. Urol Oncol 2020;38(4):269–77.
30. Cacciamani GE, Ghodoussipour S, Mari A, et al. Association between Smoking Exposure, Neoadjuvant Chemotherapy Response and Survival Outcomes following Radical Cystectomy: Systematic Review and Meta-Analysis. J Urol 2020;204(4):649–60.
31. Bassett JC, Gore JL, Chi AC, et al. Impact of a bladder cancer diagnosis on smoking behavior. J Clin Oncol 2012;30(15):1871–8.
32. Mossanen M, Caldwell J, Sonpavde G, et al. Treating Patients With Bladder Cancer: Is There an Ethical Obligation to Include Smoking Cessation Counseling? J Clin Oncol 2018;36(32):3189–91.
33. Shariat SF, Sfakianos JP, Droller MJ, et al. The effect of age and gender on bladder cancer: a critical review of the literature. BJU Int 2010;105(3):300–8.
34. Schultzel M, Saltzstein SL, Downs TM, et al. Late age (85 years or older) peak incidence of bladder cancer. J Urol 2008;179(4):1302–5 [discussion: 1305–6].
35. Lane G, et al. Persistent muscle-invasive bladder cancer after neoadjuvant chemotherapy: an analysis of Surveillance, Epidemiology and End Results-Medicare data. BJU Int 2019;123(5):818–25.
36. Yee DS, Ishill NM, Lowrance WT, et al. Ethnic differences in bladder cancer survival. Urology 2011;78(3):544–9.
37. Prout GR Jr, Wesley MN, Greenberg RS, et al. Bladder cancer: race differences in extent of disease at diagnosis. Cancer 2000;89(6):1349–58.
38. Prout GR Jr, Wesley MN, McCarron PG, et al. Survival experience of black patients and white patients with bladder carcinoma. Cancer 2004;100(3):621–30.
39. Vineis P, Pirastu R. Aromatic amines and cancer. Cancer Causes Control 1997; 8(3):346–55.
40. Boffetta P, Jourenkova N, Gustavsson P. Cancer risk from occupational and environmental exposure to polycyclic aromatic hydrocarbons. Cancer Causes Control 1997;8(3):444–72.
41. Stec AA, Dickens KE, Salden M, et al. Occupational Exposure to Polycyclic Aromatic Hydrocarbons and Elevated Cancer Incidence in Firefighters. Sci Rep 2018;8(1):2476.
42. Marshall G, Ferreccio C, Yuan Y, et al. Fifty-year study of lung and bladder cancer mortality in Chile related to arsenic in drinking water. J Natl Cancer Inst 2007; 99(12):920–8.
43. Kurttio P, Pukkala E, Kahelin H, et al. Arsenic concentrations in well water and risk of bladder and kidney cancer in Finland. Environ Health Perspect 1999;107(9): 705–10.
44. Mossanen M, Kibel AS, Goldman RH. Exploring exposure to Agent Orange and increased mortality due to bladder cancer. Urol Oncol 2017;35(11):627–32.
45. Talar-Williams C, Hijazi YM, Walther MM, et al. Cyclophosphamide-induced cystitis and bladder cancer in patients with Wegener granulomatosis. Ann Intern Med 1996;124(5):477–84.

46. Sountoulides P, Koletsas N, Kikidakis D, et al. Secondary malignancies following radiotherapy for prostate cancer. Ther Adv Urol 2010;2(3):119–25.
47. Shirodkar SP, Kishore TA, Soloway MS. The risk and prophylactic management of bladder cancer after various forms of radiotherapy. Curr Opin Urol 2009;19(5): 500–3.
48. Kermode-Scott B. Meta-analysis confirms raised risk of bladder cancer from pioglitazone. BMJ 2012;345:e4541.
49. Piper JM, Tonascia J, Matanoski GM. Heavy phenacetin use and bladder cancer in women aged 20 to 49 years. N Engl J Med 1985;313(5):292–5.
50. McCredie M, Stewart JH, Ford JM, et al. Phenacetin-containing analgesics and cancer of the bladder or renal pelvis in women. Br J Urol 1983;55(2):220–4.
51. Gu J, Wu X. Genetic susceptibility to bladder cancer risk and outcome. Per Med 2011;8(3):365–74.
52. Lichtenstein P, Holm NV, Verkasalo PK, et al. Environmental and heritable factors in the causation of cancer–analyses of cohorts of twins from Sweden, Denmark, and Finland. N Engl J Med 2000;343(2):78–85.
53. Wang C, Jiang H. Meat intake and risk of bladder cancer: a meta-analysis. Med Oncol 2012;29(2):848–55.
54. Li F, An S, Hou L, et al. Red and processed meat intake and risk of bladder cancer: a meta-analysis. Int J Clin Exp Med 2014;7(8):2100–10.
55. Pelucchi C, Galeone C, Tramacere I, et al. Alcohol drinking and bladder cancer risk: a meta-analysis. Ann Oncol 2012;23(6):1586–93.
56. Yao B, Yan Y, Ye X, et al. Intake of fruit and vegetables and risk of bladder cancer: a dose-response meta-analysis of observational studies. Cancer Causes Control 2014;25(12):1645–58.
57. Qin Q, Xu X, Wang X, et al. Obesity and risk of bladder cancer: a meta-analysis of cohort studies. Asian Pac J Cancer Prev 2013;14(5):3117–21.
58. Sun JW, Zhao LG, Yang Y, et al. Obesity and risk of bladder cancer: a dose-response meta-analysis of 15 cohort studies. PLoS One 2015;10(3):e0119313.
59. Keimling M, Behrens G, Schmid D, et al. The association between physical activity and bladder cancer: systematic review and meta-analysis. Br J Cancer 2014; 110(7):1862–70.
60. Mostafa MH, Sheweita SA, O'Connor PJ. Relationship between schistosomiasis and bladder cancer. Clin Microbiol Rev 1999;12(1):97–111.
61. Botelho MC, Alves H, Richter J. Halting Schistosoma haematobium - associated bladder cancer. Int J Cancer Manag 2017;10(9):e9430.
62. Sui X, Lei L, Chen L, et al. Inflammatory microenvironment in the initiation and progression of bladder cancer. Oncotarget 2017;8(54):93279–94.
63. Al-Zalabani AH, Stewart KF, Wesselius A, et al. Modifiable risk factors for the prevention of bladder cancer: a systematic review of meta-analyses. Eur J Epidemiol 2016;31(9):811–51.

Molecular Biology of Bladder Cancer
Potential Implications for Therapy

David J. McConkey, PhD

KEYWORDS

- Molecular subtypes • Neoadjuvant • Cisplatin • Immune checkpoint blockade
- FGFR3 • Variant histology

KEY POINTS

- Molecular subtypes are associated with prognosis and may predict clinical outcomes in patients treated with neoadjuvant therapies.
- Gene expression signatures associated with tumor-associated host (stromal) cells also seem to be predictive in patients treated with chemotherapy or immunotherapy.
- DNA damage and repair mutations may also be predictive of response.
- The optimization of existing urine and blood liquid biopsy platforms will be important tools for validating predictions made using pretreatment biopsies.

INTRODUCTION AND HISTORY

Urothelial cancers of the bladder have been grouped historically into disease states characterized by differences in growth patterns (papillary, flat) and/or by depth of invasion (noninvasive, non–muscle invasive [<T2], or muscle invasive [>T2]).[1,2] Beyond these distinctions, early studies demonstrated that most low-grade papillary tumors contain activating *FGFR3* mutations,[2,3] whereas high-grade and flat lesions often contain inactivating mutations in *TP53* and/or *CDKN2A*,[2] and these observations served as the basis for the hypothesis that the 2 bladder cancers tracks are characterized by either Ras pathway activation (papillary) or loss of cell cycle–regulating tumor suppressors (nonpapillary).[1] Studies using microarrays to characterize large-scale gene expression patterns demonstrated that non–muscle invasive bladder cancers (NMIBCs) and muscle-invasive bladder cancers can be distinguished easily from one another by unbiased ("unsupervised") bioinformatics methods,[4–7] providing a molecular and mechanistic basis for the observed association between stage and grade and prognosis. Other work demonstrated that inactivating mutations in chromatin-modifying genes (*KDM6A*, *KMT2D*, etc)[8] and the cohesion complex gene *STAG2*,[8–11]

Johns Hopkins Greenberg Bladder Cancer Institute, 600 North Wolfe Street, Park 219, Baltimore, MD 21287, USA
E-mail address: djmcconkey@jhmi.edu

Hematol Oncol Clin N Am 35 (2021) 457–468
https://doi.org/10.1016/j.hoc.2021.02.009
0889-8588/21/© 2021 Elsevier Inc. All rights reserved.
hemonc.theclinics.com

and activating mutations in the *TERT* promoter[12] are enriched in certain subsets but are common at all stages of disease.[2]

After decades of relative neglect, bladder cancer has become a "hot" topic for basic and translational research investigation. High-throughput sequencing approaches have used to generate robust data collections from fresh and archival formalin-fixed, paraffin-embedded tumor specimens, providing high-resolution portraits of disease heterogeneity and candidate biomarkers for the prediction of sensitivity and/or resistance to systemic therapies.[13-15] Overall, the messenger RNA (mRNA) expression work revealed that bladder cancers can be grouped into mRNA-based molecular subtypes that should probably be treated as distinct disease entities[13,16,17] and that tumor-infiltrating host cells have critically important effects on tumor biology.[16,18,19] In addition, DNA sequencing studies have begun to reveal the nature of the mutagenic "field effects" that are linked to age,[20-23] the action of the APOBEC family of innate immune effector enzymes,[14] and exposure to cigarette smoke carcinogens and other environmental contaminants.[21,22] Inactivating mutations in the genes that encode DNA damage and repair (DDR) enzymes,[24,25] and in particular mutations in *ERCC2*,[26] have been linked to clinical response to neoadjuvant cisplatin-based combination chemotherapy, and tumor mutational burden (TMB) seems to be linked to clinical benefit from immune checkpoint blockade.[27,28] Finally, techniques for measuring circulating tumor cells[29] and cancer-associated DNA alterations in blood[30] seem to have strong prognostic value, and similar methods are being developed for urine.[31,32] These emerging methods for measuring the clinically relevant biological characteristics of bladder cancers are described in greater detail elsewhere in this article.

MOLECULAR HETEROGENEITY OF BLADDER CANCER: MOLECULAR SUBTYPES

Studies performed more than 20 years ago that used array-based mRNA (transcriptome) profiling and unsupervised clustering analyses revealed that human breast cancers can be grouped into intrinsic subtypes, which reflect the gene expression patterns present in normal mammary epithelial cells at different stages of differentiation.[33] Basal-like breast cancers express high-molecular weight cytokeratins (KRT5, 6, and 14) and biomarkers that are associated with cancer stem cells, including TP63, CD44, and the transcription factors that activate epithelial-to-mesenchymal transition (ie, TWIST, SNAI1/2, and ZEB1/2). Luminal breast cancers are characterized by expression of the estrogen receptor and biomarkers associated with terminal differentiation, including FOXA1, GATA3, and CD24. The basal-like and luminal intrinsic subtypes of breast cancer are similar to the estrogen receptor positive/progesterone receptor positive and triple-negative subtypes identified by immunohistochemistry, and, like them, they have prognostic value. Basal-like cancers are associated with advanced stage and metastatic disease at presentation and shorter disease-specific survival. In addition, the intrinsic subtypes are prognostic with respect to systemic therapies—patients with basal-like cancers derive a greater survival benefit from perioperative combination chemotherapy, whereas patients with luminal cancers derive more benefit from adjuvant therapy with estrogen receptor antagonists. A gene expression-based platform (the PAM-50) was developed to assign breast cancers to the intrinsic subtypes and has been integrated into clinical practice.

The identification of mRNA-based molecular subtypes in breast cancer prompted investigators to look for intrinsic subtypes in urothelial bladder cancer. Early studies demonstrated that unsupervised analyses of mRNA expression segregated bladder cancers into subsets that correlated closely with clinical or pathologic stage and grade.[4–6] Subsequently, a group of investigators based at Lund University performed a series of studies that revealed the presence of additional molecular subtypes that they termed urothelial, genomically unstable, infiltrated, and squamous cell carcinoma like, that were not as closely linked to clinical criteria but nevertheless had significant implications for prognosis.[34] Subsequently, several groups in North America undertook independent efforts to identify discrete molecular subtypes of bladder cancer.[13,16,17] They also used unsupervised methods to demonstrate that muscle-invasive bladder cancers can be divided into clusters, and they recognized that the clusters were characterized by expression of some of the same genes that characterize basal-like and luminal breast cancers. Formal bioinformatics cross-comparisons confirmed that the subtypes identified by the Lund group and the others were very similar, and an international working group was established to establish a consensus molecular subtyping approach.[35] In the end, the group settled on a set of 6 consensus subtypes that capture the key biological features of the molecular subtypes identified by the other classifiers (**Fig. 1**). An R package is now publicly available that can be used with any whole transcriptome mRNA expression profile to assign single tumors to 1 of these 6 consensus subtypes.

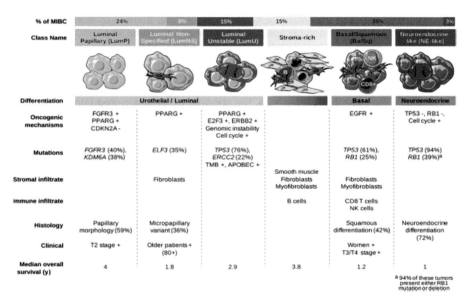

Fig. 1. Summary of the characteristics of the consensus molecular subtypes of bladder cancer. From top to bottom, the following characteristics are presented: proportion of consensus classes in the 1750 tumor samples; consensus class names; schematic graphical representation of tumor cells and their microenvironments (immune cells, fibroblasts, and smooth muscle cells); differentiation-based color scale showing features associated with consensus classes, including a luminal-to-basal gradient and neuroendocrine differentiation; and a table displaying the dominant characteristics such as oncogenic mechanisms, mutations, stromal infiltrate, immune infiltrate, histology, clinical characteristics, and median overall survival. Ba/Sq, basal/squamous; LumNS, luminal nonspecified; LumP, luminal papillary; LumU, luminal unstable; MIBC, muscle-invasive bladder cancer; NE, neuroendocrine; NK, natural killer. (*From* Kamoun, A. *et al.* A Consensus Molecular Classification of Muscle-invasive Bladder Cancer. *Eur Urol* 77, 420-433, https://doi.org/10.1016/j.eururo.2019.09.006 (2020); with permission.)

Tumor molecular subtype membership has implications for prognosis, and it may also be associated with clinical benefit from therapy. Patients with basal tumors are more likely to present with muscle-invasive and metastatic disease,[16] but they also seem to greater more benefit from chemotherapy[36] and immunotherapy.[37] Basal tumors are enriched in women,[16,38] which may contribute to their poorer survival outcomes relative to men. Conversely, patients with luminal papillary tumors tend to have much better prognoses,[14,35] and their tumors are often downstaged by neoadjuvant chemotherapy,[16,36] but they do not seem to gain as much benefit from neoadjuvant chemotherapy as patients with basal tumors do,[36] perhaps because they have less subclinical metastatic disease. The neuroendocrine subtype is relatively rare but particularly interesting.[14,35] It is enriched with neuroendocrine and small cell histopathologic features and expresses histopathologic protein biomarkers that are shared with small-cell lung cancers and neuroendocrine prostate cancers. It is intrinsically clinically aggressive,[14] but may be exceptionally responsive to immunotherapy,[39] although this conclusion remains controversial.[40] Retrospective studies are exploring the effects of chemotherapy in these patients, and prospective clinical trials are being designed to conclusively examine the potential clinical activity of immunotherapy.

To date, most of the work linking molecular subtypes to clinical outcomes has been performed in muscle-invasive and more advanced cancers, but ongoing studies are exploring their potential significance in NMIBCs. Overall, there is consensus that the vast majority of NMIBCs can be assigned to luminal subtypes. The UROMOL project reported the results of an unsupervised analysis of the mRNA expression profiles of a large set (n = 460) of NMIBCs.[15] The results revealed the presence of 3 major clusters, one of which seemed to be early basal like, but true basal/squamous cancers are relatively rare among NMIBCs and seem to be restricted to a small subset of high-grade T1 tumors.[41] Consistent with this idea, the shortest progression-free survival was not associated with the early basal NMIBC subtype (cluster 3), but rather with UROMOL cluster 2, which corresponded fairly closely with the Lund group's genomically unstable luminal molecular subtype and was associated with nearly uniform expression of a CIS-associated gene expression signature.[15] Other studies identified molecular subtypes in cohorts of noninvasive Ta tumors[42] and high-grade T1 tumors[43] that also seemed to have prognostic value. However, there is no evidence yet that the NMIBC molecular subtypes are associated with differential clinical benefit from BCG or other adjuvant therapies, including immune checkpoint blockade, which is now approved by the US Food and Drug Administration for BCG-unresponsive non–muscle-invasive disease. Identifying such predictive biomarkers is a very high priority for ongoing research.

Importantly, emerging studies indicate that molecular subtype membership is not always a stable tumor phenotype. Mapping studies demonstrated that multifocal tumors[44] and distinct regions within solitary tumors[45] express contrasting basal versus luminal gene expression signatures. Furthermore, single-cell RNA sequencing studies demonstrated that molecular subtype membership is highly heterogeneous at the single cell level,[46] with cells corresponding with basal, luminal, and mesenchymal phenotypes coexisting in tumors regardless of bulk tumor molecular subtype. The use of patient-derived tumor organoids provides us with a potentially powerful tool to understand the molecular mechanisms underlying this basal–luminal lineage plasticity. Studies have shown that luminal primary tumors often give rise to basal organoids in ex vivo tissue culture and that they reassume luminal subtype membership after orthotopic reimplantation in immunodeficient mice.[47] Therefore, luminal subtype membership can be controlled by specific tumor–host interactions that should be discoverable through experimentation with organoids.

MOLECULAR HETEROGENEITY OF BLADDER CANCER: STROMAL CELLS

The work on the molecular subtypes of bladder cancer and the clinical success with immune checkpoint blockade in patients spawned interest in defining the possible roles of tumor stromal cells in therapeutic sensitivity and resistance. One of the original molecular subtypes, termed p53-like by the MD Anderson group,[16] luminal infiltrated by TCGA,[14] and infiltrated by the Lund group,[34] is characterized by expression of genes associated with cancer-associated fibroblasts (CAFs) and extracellular matrix proteins. P53-like/infiltrated tumors seem to be relatively quiescent in terms of expression of early and late cell cycle genes, and they were associated with lower rates of response to neoadjuvant chemotherapy (as measured by pathologic downstaging to pT0 or <pT2) in an early study.[16] CAFs can cause quiescence and chemoresistance in preclinical models, so the implication of CAFs in chemoresistance is consistent with our current understanding of cancer biology. However, subsequent studies failed to validate this observation,[36] possibly because different gene expression platforms were used to profile tumors, so the link between CAF infiltration and chemoresistance in bladder cancer has not been independently validated. Plans are underway to perform RNAseq on the tumors that were prospectively collected within the context of SWOG's S1314 (CoXEN) clinical trial of neoadjuvant gemcitabine/cisplatin or dose-dense MVAC[48]; subsequent analyses of the relationship between molecular subtypes and downstaging should resolve the issue.

In contrast, independent efforts to identify RNA-based predictive biomarkers for immune checkpoint blockade implicated CAFs, and in particular, CAF-derived transforming growth factor-β, in resistance,[18] and observation that has been confirmed independently by another group.[19] Analyses of tumors from patients treated with anti- programmed cell death ligand 1 antibodies demonstrated that gene expression signatures associated with effector T cells and IFN-γ were associated with response.[27] Importantly, these associations were not directly linked to the TMB, even though a high TMB (and subsequent high levels of tumor neoantigens) has also been linked to response. Ongoing efforts to characterize tumor immune and stromal landscapes using longitudinal samples and platforms with single-cell spatial resolution should help to determine whether these markers can be used to predict response accurately.

DNA MUTATIONS IN CARCINOGENESIS AND RESPONSE TO THERAPY

Bladder cancer is caused by smoking,[1,2] and mice exposed to the cigarette smoke-like carcinogen N-butyl-N-(4-hydroxybutyl)-N-nitrosamine through their drinking water develop CIS and invasive bladder cancers that share biological properties with human cancers.[49] Like lung cancer, bladder cancer is thought to arise through field cancerization, where environmental exposures cause preneoplastic DNA mutations that predispose cells to subsequent carcinogenesis. Recent whole organ mapping studies using next-generation DNA sequencing revealed some of the key features of this process.[21,22] It seems that, in bladders that do not contain cancer from autopsies, as well as in normal-appearing areas of the urothelium distal from cancer, microscopic clonal expansions can often be detected that contain a subset of the same mutations that are observed in bladder cancers.[21,22] They are enriched with inactivating mutations in chromatin-modifying enzymes, but they rarely (if ever) contain mutations in canonical urothelial cancer oncogenes (ie, FGFR3, HRAS, and ERBB2), major tumor suppressors (TP53, RB1, and CDKN2A), or the TERT promoter. Interestingly, these small clonal expansions correspond roughly in size and number to urothelial stem cell densities, they accumulate with age, and they are associated with the COSMIC age-related single base substitution (SBS) signature 1 (SBS1), APOBEC SBS2 and SBS13, and a novel signature associated with cigarette smoking.[21] This work has important implications for early detection and prevention. For example, it may be possible to detect early field defects using urine liquid biopsies, and it is possible that cancer could be prevented using pharmacologic or genetic approaches to block the effects of the inactivating mutations in chromatin-modifying enzymes. In addition, tests for early cancer detection that assay for mutations in chromatin-modifying enzymes will produce false positives in patients with field defects, whereas mutations in oncogenes, major tumor suppressors, and the TERT promoter may be more specific for cancer.

As introduced elsewhere in this article, early work demonstrated that urothelial bladder cancers progress along 2 distinct tracks associated with different clinical characteristics. The vast majority of noninvasive low-grade papillary Ta tumors never progress to become muscle invasive and metastatic.[2] These tumors essentially all belong to the luminal papillary molecular subtype, but they can be subdivided based on differences in DNA copy number profiles.[42] They usually contain activating mutations in FGFR3 that cause constitutive dimerization and ligand-independent activation, resulting in downstream Ras pathway activation and increased G1-S cell cycle transition.[2] A fraction of them can become high-grade through loss of the cell cycle inhibitors, CDKN2A (p16) and/or TP53, and some can even progress to become highly aggressive. The approximately 15% of muscle-invasive and advanced/metastatic tumors that contain activating FGFR3 mutations (and the subset of cancers that respond to FGFR inhibitors like erdafitinib) presumably arise through this mechanism.[14] It also seems likely that FGFR inhibitors would produce higher response rates in patients with earlier stage disease than the 25% to 40% rates observed in patients with advanced disease.[50] Ongoing clinical trials in patients with low- and intermediate-risk NMIBC are examining this possibility.

Cisplatin causes DNA damage that results in tumor cell death, and defects in DNA repair pathways have been linked to cisplatin sensitivity in cancer. Preclinical studies demonstrated that cisplatin is synthetically lethal (as are PARP inhibitors) in cells with defects in homologous recombination-mediated DNA repair,[51] such as those caused by inactivating mutations in BRCA1/2. In bladder cancer, 1 group reported that inactivating mutations in ERCC2 were enriched in cisplatin-sensitive tumors,[25] whereas another concluded that inactivating mutations in any 1 of 3 DDR genes (RB1, ATM, and FANCC) were associated with sensitivity.[24] Two different prospective studies are underway to test whether patients whose tumors contain DDR mutations can be managed with neoadjuvant chemotherapy and aggressive surveillance without radical surgery. However, 2 other recent retrospective studies failed to validate these observations,[52,53] serving as a cautionary note for the ongoing trials. Attempts to prospectively validate the observations are also currently underway using DNA from the tumors from the S1314/CoXEN clinical trial. The development of better surveillance tools for monitoring subclinical local and systemic disease would help to confirm that cisplatin-based chemotherapy eradicated DDR mutation-positive tumors and facilitate the early introduction of alternative therapies in patients whose tumors are resistant (**Fig. 2**).

Mutations in DDR genes and ERCC2-related SBS5 signatures have also been linked to clinical benefit from immune checkpoint blockade,[54] presumably because they cause higher TMBs and tumor neoantigen production. Increased TMB is also associated with the action of the APOBEC cysteine deaminases, and TMB and APOBEC SBS2 and 13 signatures have been associated with good prognoses independently of immunotherapy.[14] Presumably, the bladder cancers that respond to immunotherapy are the ones that are already being recognized by the adaptive immune

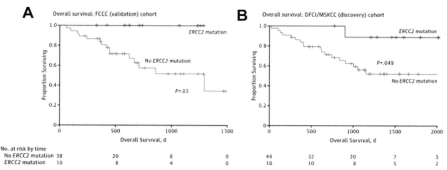

Fig. 2. Overall survival of patients with bladder cancer treated with neoadjuvant cisplatin-based combination chemotherapy whose tumors did or did not contain somatic *ERCC2* mutations. (*A*) Overall survival with and without somatic *ERCC2* mutations in the current (Fox Chase Cancer Center [FCCC]) validation cohort. Kaplan-Meier analysis of overall survival by the presence or absence of a somatic *ERCC2* mutation. There is a statistically significant difference in survival (log-rank test; *P* = .03). (*B*) Overall survival with and without somatic *ERCC2* mutations in a previously reported[25] (Dana Farber Cancer Institute and Memorial Sloan Kettering Cancer Center [DFCI/MSKCC] combined) discovery cohort. Kaplan-Meier analysis of overall survival by the presence or absence of a somatic *ERCC2* mutation. There is a statistically significant difference in survival, log-rank test (*P* = .049). (*From* Liu, D. *et al.* Clinical Validation of Chemotherapy Response Biomarker ERCC2 in Muscle-Invasive Urothelial Bladder Carcinoma. *JAMA Oncol* 2, 1094-1096, https://doi.org/10.1001/jamaoncol.2016.1056 (2016); with permission.)

system; the challenge for ongoing and future efforts is to enhance the effects of immunotherapy in the tumors that are not already infiltrated with and recognized by effector T cells. Strategies to do so include blocking the inhibitory effects of the CAF-associated transforming growth factor-β production described above and potentially by inhibiting FGFR3, expression of which is enriched in luminary papillary tumors that are poorly infiltrated with T cells.[35]

ONGOING STUDIES AND FUTURE DIRECTIONS

Before introducing molecular subtyping into routine clinical practice, the possible relationships between the basal subtype and benefit from chemotherapy and immune checkpoint blockade must be validated prospectively. Preliminary analyses have been performed examining the relationship between molecular subtypes and pathologic downstaging in the S1314 CoXEN trial; consistent with other recent studies, no relationship was observed. There is some concern about how differences in the whole transcriptome mRNA expression platforms might affect subtype assignments, which is being addressed in ongoing studies. In addition, the clinical outcomes data from the trial are still not yet mature enough to examine the association between the basal/squamous subtype and disease-specific survival. As noted elsewhere in this article, the relationship between the presence of DDR alterations and pathologic downstaging is also currently under investigation.

The presence of activating *FGFR3* mutations and fusions is associated with FGFR3 dependency in preclinical models and with clinical benefit from erdafitinib and other clinically available FGFR inhibitors in patients. However, only minorities of patients with advanced disease respond to them, and responses are not very durable. Other preclinical work has provided mechanistic explanations for this acquired resistance, all related to plasticity in tumor cell reliance on particular growth factor receptors, the most notable being EGFR and ERBB2. Biomarkers are needed to prospectively identify the patients with *FGFR3* alterations who will receive benefit and direct the others to alternative therapies. It will also be interesting to see whether FGFR inhibitors are more active in patients with FGFR3 alterations and earlier stage disease.

Signatures associated with immune cell infiltration and IFN pathway activation seem to identify bladder cancers that are more likely to respond to anti-programmed cell death ligand 1 antibodies. However, these signatures and the other available biomarkers (like TMB) are insufficient to stratify patients for therapy. New technologies that enable high-throughput spatial quantitative measurements of specific proteins and mRNAs are currently being applied to bladder cancers collected before therapy, and where possible, at sentinel time points after therapy is initiated. It seems likely that these high-resolution spatial and temporal characterizations of the tumor immune landscape will reveal whether static and bulk tumor measurements have the potential to inform clinical practice (or not).

Finally, better strategies to monitor minimal residual disease would provide powerful support for the use of these and other RNA- and DNA-based pretreatment predictive biomarkers that measure disease biology and heterogeneity. Emerging evidence indicates that levels of circulating tumor DNA[30] and circulating tumor cells[29] are highly prognostic for disease-specific survival, and it seems likely that longitudinal measurements of circulating tumor DNA could be used to measure the systemic effects of neoadjuvant and adjuvant therapies (**Fig. 3**). Likewise, several studies have established that tumor DNA can also be detected in the urine,[31,32] and it is therefore possible that urine tumor DNA could be used not only as a source of biomarkers that could be used to assign and predict clinical benefit from local therapies, but also as a means of measuring residual disease volume directly in the bladder after local surgery. Finally, it may also be possible to use urine as a source of RNA- and cell-based biomarkers for monitoring the response of the local immune system to intravesical and systemic immunotherapies. Continuous improvements in technology will help to accelerate our efforts to understand disease heterogeneity and evolution and improve our ability to deliver precision medicine.

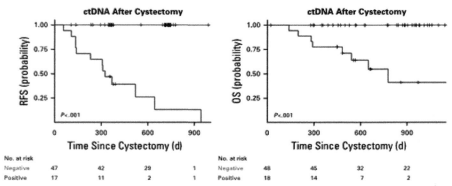

Fig. 3. Prognostic value of circulating tumor DNA (ctDNA) detection. Kaplan-Meier survival analysis shows probability of recurrence-free survival (RFS) and overall survival (OS) stratified by ctDNA status after cystectomy. (*From* Christensen, E. *et al.* Early Detection of Metastatic Relapse and Monitoring of Therapeutic Efficacy by Ultra-Deep Sequencing of Plasma Cell-Free DNA in Patients With Urothelial Bladder Carcinoma. *J Clin Oncol* 37, 1547-1557, https://doi.org/10.1200/JCO.18.02052 (2019); with permission.)

CLINICS CARE POINTS

- There is consensus that bladder cancers can be grouped into RNA-based basal and luminal molecular subtypes.
- The molecular subtypes appear to have prognostic value.
- DNA damage and repair mutations and high tumor mutational burden correlate with clinical benefit from systemic therapies.
- Ongoing prospective studies will determine whether molecular subtypes and DDR mutations can be used to inform clinical management.
- "Plasticity" can cause molecular subtype switching.
- Longitudinal urine and blood "liquid biopsies" hold promise for monitoring MRD and tumor evolution.

DISCLOSURE

Grant support: AstraZeneca, Rainier Pharmaceuticals; advisory boards: Janssen, H3 Biomedicine, Rainier Pharmaceuticals.

REFERENCES

1. Dinney CP, McConkey DJ, Millikan RE, et al. Focus on bladder cancer. Cancer Cell 2004;6(2):111–6.
2. Knowles MA, Hurst CD. Molecular biology of bladder cancer: new insights into pathogenesis and clinical diversity. Nat Rev Cancer 2015;15(1):25–41.
3. Cappellen D, De Oliveira C, Ricol D, et al. Frequent activating mutations of FGFR3 in human bladder and cervix carcinomas. Nat Genet 1999;23(1):18–20.
4. Dyrskjot L, Thykjaer T, Kruhøffer M, et al. Identifying distinct classes of bladder carcinoma using microarrays. Nat Genet 2003;33(1):90–6.
5. Sanchez-Carbayo M, Socci ND, Lozano J, et al. Defining molecular profiles of poor outcome in patients with invasive bladder cancer using oligonucleotide microarrays. J Clin Oncol 2006;24(5):778–89.
6. Blaveri E, Simko JP, Korkola JE, et al. Bladder cancer outcome and subtype classification by gene expression. Clin Cancer Res 2005;11(11):4044–55.
7. Lindgren D, Frigyesi A, Gudjonsson S, et al. Combined gene expression and genomic profiling define two intrinsic molecular subtypes of urothelial carcinoma and gene signatures for molecular grading and outcome. Cancer Res 2010; 70(9):3463–72.
8. Guo G, Sun X, Chen C, et al. Whole-genome and whole-exome sequencing of bladder cancer identifies frequent alterations in genes involved in sister chromatid cohesion and segregation. Nat Genet 2013;45(12):1459–63.
9. Balbas-Martinez C, Sagrera A, Carrillo-de-Santa-Pau E, et al. Recurrent inactivation of STAG2 in bladder cancer is not associated with aneuploidy. Nat Genet 2013;45(12):1464–9.
10. Solomon DA, Kim JS, Bondaruk J, et al. Frequent truncating mutations of STAG2 in bladder cancer. Nat Genet 2013;45(12):1428–30.
11. Taylor CF, Platt FM, Hurst CD, et al. Frequent inactivating mutations of STAG2 in bladder cancer are associated with low tumour grade and stage and inversely related to chromosomal copy number changes. Hum Mol Genet 2014;23(8): 1964–74.

12. Kinde I, Munari E, Faraj SF, et al. TERT promoter mutations occur early in urothelial neoplasia and are biomarkers of early disease and disease recurrence in urine. Cancer Res 2013;73(24):7162–7.
13. Cancer Genome Atlas Research N. Comprehensive molecular characterization of urothelial bladder carcinoma. Nature 2014;507(7492):315–22.
14. Robertson AG, Kim J, Al-Ahmadie H, et al. Comprehensive molecular characterization of muscle-invasive bladder cancer. Cell 2017;171(3):540.e25.
15. Hedegaard J, Lamy P, Nordentoft I, et al. Comprehensive Transcriptional Analysis of Early-Stage Urothelial Carcinoma. Cancer Cell 2016;30(1):27–42.
16. Choi W, Porten S, Kim S, et al. Identification of distinct basal and luminal subtypes of muscle-invasive bladder cancer with different sensitivities to frontline chemotherapy. Cancer Cell 2014;25(2):152–65.
17. Damrauer JS, Hoadley KA, Chism DD, et al. Intrinsic subtypes of high-grade bladder cancer reflect the hallmarks of breast cancer biology. Proc Natl Acad Sci U S A 2014;111(8):3110–5.
18. Mariathasan S, Turley SJ, Nickles D, et al. TGFβ attenuates tumour response to PD-L1 blockade by contributing to exclusion of T cells. Nature 2018;554(7693): 544–8.
19. Wang L, Saci A, Szabo PM, et al. EMT- and stroma-related gene expression and resistance to PD-1 blockade in urothelial cancer. Nat Commun 2018;9(1):3503.
20. Majewski T, Yao H, Bondaruk J, et al. Whole-organ genomic characterization of mucosal field effects initiating bladder carcinogenesis. Cell Rep 2019;26(8): 2241.e4.
21. Lawson ARJ, Abascal F, Coorens THH, et al. Extensive heterogeneity in somatic mutation and selection in the human bladder. Science 2020;370(6512):75–82.
22. Li R, Du Y, Chen Z, et al. Macroscopic somatic clonal expansion in morphologically normal human urothelium. Science 2020;370(6512):82–9.
23. Rozen SG. Mutational selection in normal urothelium. Science 2020; 370(6512):34–5.
24. Plimack ER, Dunbrack RL, Brennan TA, et al. Defects in DNA Repair Genes Predict Response to Neoadjuvant Cisplatin-based Chemotherapy in Muscle-invasive Bladder Cancer. Eur Urol 2015;68(6):959–67.
25. Van Allen EM, Mouw KW, Kim P, et al. Somatic ERCC2 mutations correlate with cisplatin sensitivity in muscle-invasive urothelial carcinoma. Cancer Discov 2014;4(10):1140–53.
26. Li Q, Damish AW, Frazier Z, et al. ERCC2 helicase domain mutations confer nucleotide excision repair deficiency and drive cisplatin sensitivity in muscle-invasive bladder cancer. Clin Cancer Res 2019;25(3):977–88.
27. Rosenberg JE, Hoffman-Censits J, Powles T, et al. Atezolizumab in patients with locally advanced and metastatic urothelial carcinoma who have progressed following treatment with platinum-based chemotherapy: a single-arm, multicentre, phase 2 trial. Lancet 2016;387(10031):1909–20.
28. Necchi A, Raggi D, Gallina A, et al. Updated Results of PURE-01 with preliminary activity of neoadjuvant pembrolizumab in patients with muscle-invasive bladder carcinoma with variant histologies. Eur Urol 2020;77(4):439–46.
29. Chalfin HJ, Glavaris SA, Gorin MA, et al. Circulating Tumor Cell and Circulating Tumor DNA Assays Reveal Complementary Information for Patients with Metastatic Urothelial Cancer. Eur Urol Oncol 2019. https://doi.org/10.1016/j.euo.2019. 08.004.
30. Christensen E, Birkenkamp-Demtröder K, Sethi H, et al. Early detection of metastatic relapse and monitoring of therapeutic efficacy by ultra-deep sequencing of

plasma cell-free DNA in patients with urothelial bladder carcinoma. J Clin Oncol 2019;37(18):1547–57.

31. Christensen E, Birkenkamp-Demtröder K, Nordentoft I, et al. Liquid Biopsy Analysis of FGFR3 and PIK3CA Hotspot Mutations for Disease Surveillance in Bladder Cancer. Eur Urol 2017;71(6):961–9.

32. Springer SU, Chen C-H, Rodriguez Pena MDC, et al. Non-invasive detection of urothelial cancer through the analysis of driver gene mutations and aneuploidy. Elife 2018;7. https://doi.org/10.7554/eLife.32143.

33. Perou CM, Sørlie T, Eisen MB, et al. Molecular portraits of human breast tumours. Nature 2000;406(6797):747–52.

34. Sjodahl G, Lauss M, Lövgren K, et al. A molecular taxonomy for urothelial carcinoma. Clin Cancer Res 2012;18(12):3377–86.

35. Kamoun A, de Reyniès A, Allory Y, et al. A Consensus Molecular Classification of Muscle-invasive Bladder Cancer. Eur Urol 2020;77(4):420–33.

36. Seiler R, Ashab HAD, Erho N, et al. Impact of molecular subtypes in muscle-invasive bladder cancer on predicting response and survival after neoadjuvant chemotherapy. Eur Urol 2017;72(4):544–54.

37. Necchi A, Raggi D, Gallina A, et al. Impact of Molecular Subtyping and Immune Infiltration on Pathological Response and Outcome Following Neoadjuvant Pembrolizumab in Muscle-invasive Bladder Cancer. Eur Urol 2020;77(6):701–10.

38. de Jong JJ, Boormans JL, van Rhijn BWG, et al. Distribution of molecular subtypes in muscle-invasive bladder cancer is driven by sex-specific differences. Eur Urol Oncol 2020;3(4):420–3.

39. Kim J, Kwiatkowski D, McConkey DJ, et al. The cancer genome atlas expression subtypes stratify response to checkpoint inhibition in advanced urothelial cancer and identify a subset of patients with high survival probability. Eur Urol 2019; 75(6):961–4.

40. Batista da Costa J, Gibb EA, Bivalacqua TJ, et al. Molecular Characterization of Neuroendocrine-like Bladder Cancer. Clin Cancer Res 2019;25(13):3908–20.

41. Patschan O, Sjödahl G, Chebil G, et al. A Molecular Pathologic Framework for Risk Stratification of Stage T1 Urothelial Carcinoma. Eur Urol 2015;68(5):824–6 [discussion: 835–6].

42. Hurst CD, Alder O, Platt FM, et al. Genomic subtypes of non-invasive bladder cancer with distinct metabolic profile and female gender bias in KDM6A mutation frequency. Cancer Cell 2017;32(5):701.e7.

43. Robertson AG, Groeneveld CS, Jordan B, et al. Identification of differential tumor subtypes of T1 bladder cancer. Eur Urol 2020;78(4):533–7.

44. Thomsen MBH, Nordentoft I, Lamy P, et al. Comprehensive multiregional analysis of molecular heterogeneity in bladder cancer. Sci Rep 2017;7(1):11702.

45. Warrick JI, Sjödahl G, Kaag M, et al. Intratumoral Heterogeneity of Bladder Cancer by Molecular Subtypes and Histologic Variants. Eur Urol 2019;75(1):18–22.

46. Sfakianos JP, Daza J, Hu Y, et al. Epithelial plasticity can generate multi-lineage phenotypes in human and murine bladder cancers. Nat Commun 2020;11(1):2540.

47. Lee SH, Hu W, Matulay JT, et al. Tumor Evolution and Drug Response in Patient-Derived Organoid Models of Bladder Cancer. Cell 2018;173(2):515.e17.

48. Flaig TW, Tangen CM, Daneshmand S, et al. A randomized phase II study of co-expression extrapolation (COXEN) with neoadjuvant chemotherapy for bladder cancer (SWOG S1314; NCT02177695). Clin Cancer Res 2021. https://doi.org/10.1158/1078-0432.CCR-20-2409.

49. Fantini D, Glaser AP, Rimar KJ, et al. A Carcinogen-induced mouse model reca-pitulates the molecular alterations of human muscle invasive bladder cancer. Oncogene 2018;37(14):1911–25.
50. Loriot Y, Necchi A, Park SH, et al. Erdafitinib in Locally Advanced or Metastatic Urothelial Carcinoma. N Engl J Med 2019;381(4):338–48.
51. Ashworth A, Lord CJ. Synthetic lethal therapies for cancer: what's next after PARP inhibitors? Nat Rev Clin Oncol 2018;15(9):564–76.
52. Taber A, Christensen E, Lamy P, et al. Molecular correlates of cisplatin-based chemotherapy response in muscle invasive bladder cancer by integrated multi-omics analysis. Nat Commun 2020;11(1):4858.
53. Becker REN, Meyer AR, Brant A, et al. Clinical Restaging and Tumor Sequencing are Inaccurate Indicators of Response to Neoadjuvant Chemotherapy for Muscle-invasive Bladder Cancer. Eur Urol 2021;79(3):364–71.
54. Snyder A, Nathanson T, Funt SA, et al. Contribution of systemic and somatic fac-tors to clinical response and resistance to PD-L1 blockade in urothelial cancer: an exploratory multi-omic analysis. Plos Med 2017;14(5):e1002309.

Current Therapy for Metastatic Urothelial Carcinoma

Rosa Nadal, MD[a], Joseph A. Clara, MD[a],
Begoña P. Valderrama, MD[b], Joaquim Bellmunt, MD, PhD[c],*

KEYWORDS

- Urothelial carcinoma • Systemic therapy • Immune checkpoint inhibitors
- Targeted therapy • FGFR inhibitor • Antibody-drug conjugate

KEY POINTS

- Cytotoxic, platinum-based chemotherapy has been the mainstay of treatment for metastatic urothelial carcinoma (UC) for many years. Although still being the starting option for first-line fit patients, several new treatment options have recently shifted the treatment paradigm in other disease settings.
- Five immune checkpoint inhibitors targeting PD-1 or PD-L1 have been approved for metastatic UC within the past 3 to 4 years.
- Maintenance avelumab plus best supportive care significantly prolonged overall survival among patients with UC who had disease that had not progressed with frontline chemotherapy.
- Biomarker-based treatment targeting alterations of FGFR has recently been approved for treatment of metastatic UC that has failed platinum-based chemotherapy.
- An antibody-drug conjugate, enfortumab vedotin, has been approved for treatment of postimmunotherapy and platinum-treated patients.

SYSTEMIC CHEMOTHERAPY IN ADVANCED UROTHELIAL CANCER
First-Line Chemotherapy

The landmark of systemic chemotherapy in metastatic urothelial carcinoma (mUC) was the development of the combination of methotrexate, vinblastine, doxorubicin, and cisplatin (MVAC) (**Fig. 1**). For patients who are cisplatin eligible, MVAC has been associated with considerable activity (response rate [RR] of >50%) and 3-year-survival of 20% to 25%.[1] Furthermore, MVAC was shown to be superior to

[a] Cellular and Molecular Therapeutics Branch, National Heart, Lung, and Blood Institutes, National Institutes of Health, 10 Center Drive, Room 3E-5330, Bethesda, MD 20892, USA;
[b] Hospital Universitario Virgen del Rocio, Avenida Manuel Siurot, s/n, Sevilla 41001, Spain;
[c] Department of Medical Oncology, Beth Israel Deaconess Medical Center, Harvard Medical School, 330 Brookline Avenue, KS 118, Boston, MA 02215, USA
* Corresponding author.
E-mail address: jbellmun@bidmc.harvard.edu

Hematol Oncol Clin N Am 35 (2021) 469–493
https://doi.org/10.1016/j.hoc.2021.02.010
0889-8588/21/© 2021 Elsevier Inc. All rights reserved.

hemonc.theclinics.com

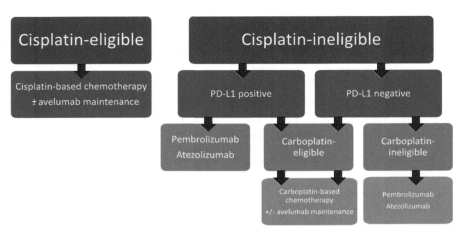

Fig. 1. First-line therapy for mUC.

single-agent cisplatin in a randomized trial establishing the role of combination chemotherapy in advanced urothelial carcinoma (UC). In this US Intergroup trial, 246 patients with advanced disease were randomly assigned to receive cisplatin alone or MVAC. Although the overall response rate (ORR) for MVAC-treated patients was 39%, only 12% of patients receiving cisplatin achieved an objective response. Similarly, the progression-free survival (PFS) and overall survival (OS) favored the classic MVAC arm (10 vs 4.3, and 12.5 vs 8.2 months, respectively).[2] Several regimens similar to MVAC have also been studied,[3–5] with the CISCA regimen (cisplatin, cyclophosphamide, doxorubicin) being the one that was formally compared and found to be inferior to MVAC in a randomized trial.[6]

In an effort to enhance the activity of MVAC, clinical researchers from the European Organization for Research and Treatment of Cancer (EORTC) evaluated the activity of high-dose MVAC made feasible by the use of granulocyte-colony stimulating factor (G-CSF) in comparison with the classical MVAC. This trial reported decreased mucositis and neutropenic fever rates with dose-dense MVAC compared with classic MVAC without an initial influence in survival beyond the initial outcomes observed with MVAC.[7] With longer follow-up (7 years) and acknowledging that in this long period of time other factors might have influenced, the initial results were confirmed with PFS and mortality hazard ratios (HR) of 0.73 and 0.76, respectively, on 2-year and 5-year survival.[8]

Owing to concerns regarding MVAC toxicity, clinical investigators focused on the development of other cisplatin-based combinations mainly with gemcitabine and taxanes. The gemcitabine-cisplatin combination (GC) has been evaluated in different studies that used different administration schedules.[9–11] GC has been compared with MVAC in a randomized phase III randomized trial. This trial showed that GC had somewhat less toxicity with significantly lower rates of neutropenic sepsis and grade 3 or 4 mucositis. RRs for GC compared with MVAC were 49% and 45%, respectively. Median overall survival (mOS) of 14 and 15.2 months and the time to progressive disease were identical in both groups at 7.4 months. Furthermore, there were a statistically significant higher number of patients with a greater than 5% increase in weight in the GC arm and a no-statistically significant reduction in fatigue. Other quality-of-life markers were maintained and were similar in both arms.[12,13] Although this trial was not powered as an equivalency study, GC largely replaced MVAC in practice as the standard of care for patients with metastatic disease.

Regimens of combined paclitaxel or docetaxel and cisplatin have also been developed in the metastatic setting.[14-18] Only the combination docetaxel-cisplatin was compared with G-CSF supported MVAC in a randomized phase III trial. Docetaxel-cisplatin was found to be inferior to MVAC, although the difference in survival did not reach statistical significance because of an imbalance in performance status between the 2 arms.[19]

Triplet combination has also been studied in a phase III study comparing paclitaxel in addition to gemcitabine-cisplatin (PCG) with GC in patients with locally advanced or mUC. PCG led to a higher RR than GC (55.5% vs 43%, respectively), and a 3.1-month survival benefit was observed with a mOS of 15.8 months on PCG versus 12.7 months on GC (HR, 0.85; P = .075).[20] In the same clinical setting, a randomized phase III trial showed that the combination of larotaxel (a semisynthetic taxoid) and cisplatin had inferior outcomes compared with the standard combination of GC.[21]

Platinum-based chemotherapy regimens are associated with a significant toxicity, and ~25% to 50% of patients with mUC are unable to tolerate cisplatin-based therapy owing to renal impairment or poor performance status and various comorbidities[22,23] (**Box 1**). These patients have been traditionally treated with non-cisplatin-based chemotherapy combinations based on data from phase II/III trials. The EORTC led the first trial, which evaluated the optimal first-line metastatic regimen for cisplatin-ineligible patients by comparing gemcitabine and carboplatin (GCb) with the older regimen of methotrexate, carboplatin, and vinblastine. In that study, cisplatin-ineligible criteria were an estimated glomerular filtration rate between 30 and 60 mL/min and/or a performance score of 2. Both the ORR and toxicity profile favored GCb and establishing this regimen as the preferred regimen in cisplatin-ineligible patients.[24] However, GCb is inferior to cisplatin-based chemotherapy owing to lower RRs, shorter durations of response, and decreased OS.[25] In 2 phase II studies of the combination of GCb in mostly untreated patients with mUC, which did not specifically include patients

---

Box 1
Definitions

Fitness for cisplatin-based chemotherapy
  Patients meeting at least one of the following criteria are considered "unfit" for cisplatin treatment[1]:
  • World Health Organization or Eastern Cooperative Oncology Group performance status 2 or Karnofsky performance status of 60% to 70%
  • Creatinine clearance less than 60 mL/min
  • Grade 2 or greater audiometric hearing loss
  • Grade 2 or greater peripheral neuropathy
  • New York Heart Association class III or greater heart failure

Erdafitinib-susceptible FGFR alterations
  Patients are selected for treatment with erdafitinib based on the presence of at least 1 of the following genetic alterations as detected by an FDA-approved companion diagnostic[2,3]:
  • FGFR3 gene mutations (R248C, S249C, G370C, Y373C)
  • FGFR gene fusions (FGFR3-TACC3, FGFR3-BAIAP2L1, FGFR2-BICC1, FGFR2-CASP7)

PD-L1 positivity
  Atezolizumab and pembrolizumab are approved for first-line treatment of cisplatin-ineligible patients whose tumors express PD-L1 as assessed by respective companion diagnostic tests.[4,5]
  • Atezolizumab: SP142 assay, PD-L1–stained tumor-infiltrating immune cells covering ≥5% of the tumor area
  • Pembrolizumab: 22C3 antibody assay, combined positive score ≥10

unfit for cisplatin treatment, RRs of 56% and 59% were reported but with a mOS of 10 months in both studies.[26,27] The combination of paclitaxel and carboplatin has also been studied, and again the mOS was less than 10 months in all studies.[28–32] Non-platinum-based chemotherapy combinations have also been studied. For example, JASINT-1, an international randomized phase II trial, compared vinflunine plus gemcitabine to vinflunine plus carboplatin in cisplatin-intolerant patients. This study reported similar disease control rate, ORR, and OS for both vinflunine-based doublets, whereas hematologic tolerance favored the vinflunine-gemcitabine combination.[33]

Most centers worldwide have considered MVAC or gemcitabine in combination with cisplatin the standard treatments for mUC for cisplatin-eligible patients, and gemcitabine in combination with carboplatin for cisplatin-ineligible patients for almost 2 decades. However, gemcitabine and cisplatin or carboplatin has preferentially been used as a backbone for the addition of other novel agents, including immune checkpoint inhibitors (ICIs), antiangiogenic therapies, or other agents in already reported and active trials underway.

Second-Line Chemotherapy

Although mUC is highly sensitive to chemotherapy, the duration of response is short, and chemotherapy is rarely curative. Until recently, the standard-of-care second-line therapies were docetaxel or paclitaxel in the United States[34] and vinflunine in Europe,[35,36] resulting in only single-digit RR and very modest survival benefit. New treatment options with the potential for more durable remissions have largely replaced the use of chemotherapeutic agents in the second-line setting and beyond (**Fig. 2**).

IMMUNE CHECKPOINT INHIBITORS IN ADVANCED UROTHELIAL CARCINOMA

The immunogenicity of UC has been demonstrated on many fronts. The Cancer Genome Atlas (TCGA) project showed UC to be associated with a high mutational burden, with only lung cancer and melanoma harboring more DNA alterations.[37] In addition, several mutations associated with UC are related to increased immunogenicity,[38] and tumor-infiltrating immune cells have been identified in some UC tumors.[39]

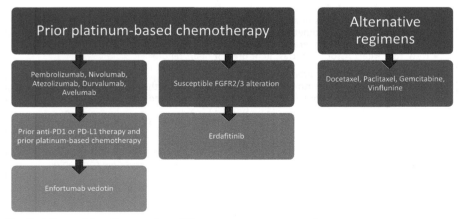

Fig. 2. ≥Second-line therapy for mUC.

Despite the recognized immunogenic nature of a subset of UC tumors, tumor cells are capable of evading the antitumor immune response by exploiting immune checkpoints. Immune checkpoints are cell-surface receptors expressed by immune cells that physiologically aid in protection from autoimmunity, but can also function as a mechanism of tumor-mediated immune suppression.[40,41] The most comprehensively described immune checkpoint axis consists of the programmed cell death-1 (PD-1) receptor and the programmed death ligand-1 (PD-L1). PD-L1 is frequently overexpressed in UC cells, and high PD-1 expression is associated with T-cell exhaustion and correlated with tumor aggressiveness in UC.[42,43] Elucidation of these concepts has formed the basis for the clinical investigation of anti-PD-L1 and anti-PD-1 agents in UC leading to the Food and Drug Administration (FDA) approval of 5 ICIs in the metastatic setting since 2016. The use of specific ICIs is now incorporated into upfront for cisplatin-ineligible patients, subsequent-line therapy after failure to platinum, as well as first-line maintenance irrespective of cisplatin fitness (**Table 1**).

First-Line Immune Checkpoint Inhibition

The accelerated approvals of atezolizumab and pembrolizumab for cisplatin-ineligible patients with advanced UC represented the first approved immunotherapies for this patient population. These approvals were based on single-arm trials demonstrating reasonable objective RRs and favorable durations of response with an acceptable toxicity profile compared with available non-cisplatin-containing chemotherapy regimens. However, based on concerning preliminary reports from 2 phase III trials (IMvigor130 and KEYNOTE-361), the FDA revised the indication for both agents in PD-L1–negative cisplatin-ineligible patients. Both of these agents are now FDA approved for first-line treatment of advanced UC in patients who are unfit for cisplatin-containing chemotherapy and whose tumors express PD-L1 as assessed by companion immunohistochemistry (IHC) assays (see **Box 1**) and in patients who are considered ineligible for any platinum-containing chemotherapy regardless of PD-L1 status.[44]

Atezolizumab is a humanized immunoglobulin G1 (IgG1) monoclonal antibody (mAb) that targets PD-L1.[45] Its approval in the first-line setting was based on the IMvigor210 trial, which demonstrated a durable benefit in a cohort of 119 cisplatin-ineligible, chemotherapy-naïve patients who were treated with atezolizumab as first-line therapy. This cohort of patients saw an ORR of 23% with complete response (CR) rate of 9%, with durable responses in most responders at 17.2 months' median follow-up. mOS was 15.9 months.[46] Pembrolizumab is an IgG4κ mAb that targets PD-1, and similar to atezolizumab, was also granted accelerated approval for use in the first-line setting. The approval was based on the results of the single-arm phase II KEYNOTE-052 study in 370 patients, which demonstrated an ORR of 24% with first-line pembrolizumab.[47] Long-term follow-up has confirmed durable antitumor activity in cisplatin-ineligible patients, with markedly higher and longer-lasting responses and OS seen in patients with PD-L1–positive tumors. ORR for patients with PD-L1–expressing and PD-L1–negative tumors was 47% and 20%, median duration of response was not reached, and mOS was 18.5 months and 9.7 months, respectively, suggesting PD-L1 as a powerful predictive biomarker for response to pembrolizumab in the first-line setting.[48]

Immune Checkpoint Inhibition Following Platinum-Based Chemotherapy

Atezolizumab was the first to demonstrate promising signs of activity in an early phase I study in mUC, which showed safety and an ORR of 26%.[49] Subsequently, the phase II open-label, single-arm IMvigor210 trial demonstrated an ORR of 16%, a favorable toxicity profile, and durable responses in the cohort of patients with advanced UC

Table 1
programmed cell death-1 and programmed death ligand-1 checkpoint inhibitor trials in advanced urothelial cancer

Study Details	Treatment	ORR (%)	RR by PD-L1 (%)	Survival (mo)
Cisplatin-ineligible, first line				
KEYNOTE-052[47] phase II n = 370	Pembrolizumab	24	CPS ≥10%: 39 CPS 1% to <10%: 20 CPS <1%: 11	mPFS: 2 6-mo OS: 67
IMvigor210 (cohort 1)[46] phase II n = 119	Atezolizumab	23	<1% on ICs: 21 1% to <5% on ICs: 21 ≥5%on ICs: 28	mPFS: 2.7 mOS: 15.9
Second line				
KEYNOTE-045[55] phase III n = 542	Pembrolizumab vs physician's choice (vinflunine, paclitaxel, or docetaxel)	21.1 vs 11.4	CPS ≥10%: 21.6 vs 6.7	PFS: 2.1 vs 3.3 OS 10.3 vs 7.4 mOS for CPS ≥10%: 8 vs 5.2
PCD4989 g[49] phase I n = 67	Atezolizumab	26.2	PD-L1 IHC 0–1: 11 PD-L1 IHC 2–3: 43	Not reported
IMvigor210 (cohort 2)[50] phase II n = 310	Atezolizumab	15	<1% on ICs: 8 1% to <5% on ICs: 10 ≥ 5% on ICs: 26	mPFS: 2.1 mOS: 11.4 mDR: 13.7 (not reached)
IMvigor211[53] phase III n = 931	Atezolizumab vs physician's choice (vinflunine, paclitaxel, or docetaxel)	13 vs 13	≥5% on ICs: 23 vs 22	OS for PD-L1 ITT population: 8.6 vs 8.0 OS for PD-L1 ≥5% on ICs: 11.1 vs 10.6
CheckMate 275[58] phase II n = 265	Nivolumab	19.6	≥5% on TCs: 28.4 1%–4% on TCs: 23.8 <1% on TCs: 16.1	mPFS: 2 mOS: 8.7
NCT01693562[63] phase I/II	Durvalumab	17.8	≥25% on TCs and ICs: 27.6 <25% on TCs and ICs: 5.1	mPFS: 1.5 mOS: 8.2
JAVELIN (updated)[66] phase I	Avelumab	16	≥5% on TCs: 24 <5% on TCs: 13	mPFS: 1.6 mOS: 6.5
Maintenance following platinum-based chemotherapy				
JAVELIN Bladder 100[69] phase III n = 700	Avelumab + BSC or BSC alone following first-line platinum-based chemotherapy	N/A	N/A	mOS: 21.4 vs 14.3

Abbreviations: CPS, combined positive score of PD-L1 on immune and tumor cells; IC, inflammatory cell; ITT, intent to treat; mDR, median duration of response; N/A, not applicable; TC, tumor cell.

treated with atezolizumab after progression on platinum-based chemotherapy. mOS was 7.9 months in all patients, and 11.9 months in patients with PD-L1–positive tumors (measured by IHC on tumor-infiltrating immune cells).[50,51] These results led to the accelerated FDA approval in 2016 for patients with locally advanced or mUC whose disease had progressed during or after platinum-containing chemotherapy, or within 12 months of neoadjuvant or adjuvant platinum-containing chemotherapy.[52] Based on these results, a phase III trial (IMvigor211) was conducted, with 931 patients with mUC who had progressed after platinum-based chemotherapy who were randomized to receive atezolizumab or chemotherapy (vinflunine, docetaxel, or paclitaxel according to physician's choice). The primary endpoint of OS was tested hierarchically in prespecified populations: IC2/3 (PD-L1 expression in ≥5% of tumor-infiltrating immune cells), followed by IC1/2/3 (PD-L1 expression in ≥1% of tumor-infiltrating immune cells), followed by the intention-to-treat population. The trial did not meet its primary endpoint of OS in the PD-L1–positive population: in the IC2/3 population, OS did not differ significantly between patients in the atezolizumab group and those in the chemotherapy group (median 11.1 months vs 10.6 months; HR, 0.87; 95% CI: 0.63–1.21; P = .41).[53]

Pembrolizumab received FDA approval in 2017 for patients with locally advanced or mUC in the second-line setting.[54] The results of the open-label phase III KEYNOTE-045 trial, which compared pembrolizumab with chemotherapy in 542 patients with platinum-refractory advanced UC, led to the approval. Chemotherapy consisted of investigator's choice with either paclitaxel, docetaxel, or vinflunine. Pembrolizumab demonstrated superior ORR, OS, and fewer adverse events than chemotherapy in the trial. The OS benefit appeared to be independent of PD-L1 expression. mOS at that time was 10.3 months with pembrolizumab compared with 7.4 months with chemotherapy. As expected, immune-related adverse events (irAEs) were more common with pembrolizumab than with chemotherapy, whereas good quality-of-life endpoint favored the pembrolizumab arm. The study's independent data-monitoring committee recommended the trial be stopped early after it met the coprimary endpoint for OS.[55] Long-term follow-up data showed that survival benefit was maintained at 36 months, with an HR for death of 0.72 (95% CI: 0.59–0.87; P = .00030).[56]

Nivolumab is a fully human IgG4 mAb that targets PD-1.[57] Nivolumab was also granted accelerated FDA approval in 2017 based on the results of the phase II, single-arm CheckMate 275 trial.[58,59] With 33.7 months' minimum follow-up, the trial showed clinically meaningful efficacy and an acceptable safety profile, with an ORR of 20.7% in the entire study population compared with 25.8% in patients with PD-L1 expression of ≥5%.[60] Additional studies corroborated the clinical efficacy and safety of nivolumab in patients with recurrent, advanced UC previously treated with platinum-containing chemotherapy. The phase I/II CheckMate 032 study demonstrated a substantial and durable ORR of 24%, which appeared to be independent of PD-L1 expression on tumor cells.[61]

Durvalumab is an anti–PD-L1 human IgG1 mAb that was granted accelerated approval in 2017 for the treatment of locally advanced or mUC in patients with disease progression during or after treatment with platinum-containing chemotherapy.[62] The approval was based on the updated results from a phase I/II trial with 191 patients with advanced UC who were either cisplatin ineligible or were previously treated with platinum-based chemotherapy that showed antitumor activity and a manageable safety profile, with an ORR of 17.8% in the entire study population and 27.6% in patients with PD-L1–high tumors.[63]

Avelumab is a fully human IgG1λ mAb that targets PD-L1 and is unique among mAbs targeting PD-1 or PD-L1 because it has demonstrated the ability to elicit cell-mediated cytotoxicity in vitro in addition to PD-L1/PD-1 axis blockade.[64] It was granted accelerated FDA approval based on the results of the JAVELIN Solid Tumors study.[65] This phase I trial of avelumab in patients with advanced solid tumors included 44 patients with UC who demonstrated an ORR of 18.2%. A strikingly higher RR (50.0% vs 4.3%) was seen in those with positive PD-L1 expression on tumor cells, defined as 5% or more, compared with patients with PD-L1–negative tumors.[66] An updated pooled cohort with 249 patients also included patients who were platinum chemotherapy naïve. A similar ORR of 17% was noted in the pooled cohort, but the impact of PD-L1 positivity was less marked (24% vs 14%) between those with PD-L1 -positive and -negative tumors.[67]

As a result of these trials, 5 ICIs are now treatment options for advanced UC after chemotherapy failure. With similar mechanisms of action, toxicity profiles, and ORRs among ICIs, pembrolizumab is the only therapy with an OS benefit observed in a randomized phase III trial, to guide treatment decisions.[55] With greater use of ICIs, irAEs present a considerable challenge for patients undergoing therapy. These irAEs can affect a variety of organs and can result in substantial morbidity and even mortality. Overall, any grade irAE occurs in roughly one-quarter of patients treated with ICI, whereas grade 3 to 4 irAEs are noted in approximately 15% of patients.[68]

Immune Checkpoint Inhibitors as First-Line Maintenance Therapy

Very recently, avelumab was also found to prolong survival in patients with locally advanced or mUC when used as first-line maintenance following treatment with platinum-based chemotherapy. The phase III JAVELIN Bladder 100 trial randomized 700 patients who had not progressed following 4 to 6 cycles of first-line platinum-containing chemotherapy to receive avelumab plus best supportive care (BSC) or the latter alone. Maintenance treatment with avelumab resulted in a significantly prolonged OS of 21.4 months in the avelumab group compared with 14.3 months in the BSC alone arm. Among patients with PD-L1–positive tumors, survival was significantly prolonged ($P = .001$) with a mOS that was not reached for avelumab-treated patients compared with 17.1 months for the BSC-alone group. Grade 3 or higher events, most frequently urinary tract infection, anemia, hematuria, fatigue, and back pain, were reported in 47.4% versus 25.5%, respectively.[69] This study formed the basis of the FDA approval for avelumab as first-line switch-maintenance therapy after initial platinum-based chemotherapy, marking a momentous advance with a new first-line standard of care for advanced UC that has not progressed on first-line platinum-based chemotherapy.[70]

Emerging Immunotherapy Combinations

Efforts are being made to identify agents that may have synergistic antitumor activity when combined with ICIs (**Table 2**). Early attempts to combine immune-modulating agents with systemic chemotherapy resulted in a very limited impact on clinical activity. One of the earliest trials using α-interferon with fluorouracil and cisplatin demonstrated an improvement in clinical activity but was more toxic than classic MVAC.[71] With the recent advances in immune checkpoint inhibition, Galsky and colleagues[72] studied the combination of GC with ipilimumab in a phase II trial. The addition of ipilimumab to GC did not appear to have an impact on survival greater than that observed with chemotherapy alone.[72]

Recent data about the combination of immune checkpoint inhibition and chemotherapy have been reported in mUC. The phase III IMvigor130 trial evaluated 1213 untreated patients with locally advanced or metastatic urothelial carcinoma. Patients

Table 2
Selected ongoing phase III trials

Trial	Setting	Arm 1	Arm 2	Arm 3	Primary End Points	NCT
KEYNOTE-361	First-line unresectable/mUC	Pembrolizumab	Pembrolizumab-chemotherapy	—	PFS and OS	NCT02853305
CheckMate-901	First-line unresectable or mUC	Gemcitabine + cisplatin/carboplatin	Nivolumab-ipilimumab	Nivolumab + gemcitabine + cisplatin/carboplatin	OS in cisplatin-ineligible participant and OS in PD-L1(+) participant	NCT03036098
NILE	First-line unresectable or mUC	Gemcitabine + cisplatin/carboplatin	Durvalumab + gemcitabine + cisplatin/carboplatin	Durvalumab + tremelimumab + gemcitabine + cisplatin/carboplatin	PFS and OS	NCT03682068
LEAP-011	First-line unresectable or mUC cisplatin-ineligible with PD-L1 CPS ≥10 or platinum-ineligible	—	Pembrolizumab + placebo	Pembrolizumab + lenvatinib	PFS and OS	NCT03898180
THOR	Platinum-treated with/without ICI-treated mUC with FGFR mutation or fusions/translocations	Erdafitinib	Chemotherapy	Pembrolizumab	OS	NCT03390504
TROPiCs-04	Platinum-treated and ICI-treated mUC	Chemotherapy	Sacituzumab govitecan	—	OS	NCT04527991
EV-302	First-line unresectable/mUC	Chemotherapy	Enfortumab vedotin + pembrolizumab	—	PFS and OS	NCT04223856

Abbreviations: CPS, combined positive score of PD-L1 on immune and tumor cells; NCT, National Clinical Trial.

were randomized into 3 groups: atezolizumab plus platinum-based chemotherapy (group A), atezolizumab alone (group B), and placebo plus platinum-based chemotherapy (group C). The trial met one of its coprimary endpoints of PFS of group A versus C (8.2 vs 6.3 months, respectively, HR, 0.82; 95% CI: 0.70–0.96; P = .007). With a still immature median follow-up of 11.8 months, mOS was 16 months in group A and 13.4 in group C (HR, 0.83; 0.69–1.00; 1-sided P = .027). Because this result did not cross the prespecified interim efficacy boundary for statistical significance (P = .007), no further statistical hypothesis testing was done for group B versus group C. ORR was 47% for group A, 23% for group B, and 44% for group C.[73] A similar phase III trial evaluating the combination of pembrolizumab in association with platinum-based chemotherapy in the first-line setting has recently reported with negative results. KEYNOTE 361 is a phase III trial with a similar design that included 1010 patients with locally advanced or mUC without prior systemic treatment for advanced disease, who were randomized to receive pembrolizumab plus platinum-based chemotherapy, pembrolizumab alone, or platinum-based chemotherapy. The prespecified dual primary endpoints of OS and PFS were not met, with a median progression-free survival (mPFS) in the pembrolizumab and chemotherapy arm of 8.3 versus 7.1 months in the chemotherapy arm (HR, 0.78; 95% CI: 0.65–0.93; P = .003) and a mOS of 17.0 versus 14.3 months, respectively (HR, 0.86; 95% CI: 0.72–1.02; P = .0407).[74] A third randomized phase III study (DANUBE) has explored the role of durvalumab with or without tremelimumab versus platinum-based chemotherapy alone in 1032 patients with untreated unresectable, locally advanced, or mUC. The coprimary endpoints were OS compared between the durvalumab monotherapy versus chemotherapy groups in the population of patients with high PD-L1 expression and between the durvalumab plus tremelimumab versus chemotherapy groups in the intention-to-treat population. With a median follow-up of 41.2 months, the study did not meet either of its coprimary endpoints: in the high PD-L1 population, mOS was 14·4 months in the durvalumab monotherapy group versus 12.1 months in the chemotherapy group (HR, 0·89; 95% CI: 0.71–1.11; P = .30). In the intention-to-treat population, mOS was 15·1 months (13.1–18.0) in the durvalumab plus tremelimumab group versus 12·1 months (10.9–14.0) in the chemotherapy group (HR, 0.85; 95% CI: 0.72–1.02; P = .075).[75] Based on these results, and the role of ICI alone or in combination with chemotherapy in the first-line setting is still not clear. Other phase III trials are ongoing and will help to clarify this uncertainty. The NILE trial (NCT03682068) is evaluating chemotherapy with or without durvalumab alone or in combination with tremelimumab, and the CheckMate901 (NCT03036098) is comparing the combination of nivolumab and ipilimumab versus gemcitabine-platinum in cisplatin-ineligible patients as well as PD-L1 high patients in conjunction with a substudy evaluating standard cisplatin-based chemotherapy with or without nivolumab.

The combination of immunotherapy agents targeting PD-1/PD-L1 along with the immune checkpoint CTLA-4 and/or antiangiogenic agents has also been evaluated. The phase I/II CheckMate 032 study evaluated the efficacy of nivolumab alone or combined with the CTLA-4 inhibitor ipilimumab in platinum-refractory UC patients. ORR was 26% in the nivolumab alone group and highest at 38% in the group that received nivolumab 1 mg/kg and ipilimumab 3 mg/kg (58% in patients with PD-L1 ≥1% by IHC). With a minimum follow-up of 56 months, mPFS and mOS were 4.9 and 15.3 months, respectively.[76] This study demonstrated the potential impact of immunotherapy combinations in advanced UC that are being further investigated in the CheckMate 901 phase III trial (NCT03036098). The combination of durvalumab and tremelimumab has not shown benefit in either ORR or OS compared with standard chemotherapy in first line in DANUBE trial, but mOS was 17.9 months (95% CI: 14.8–24.2) in PD-L1 high population.[75]

Multiple ICIs are currently being investigated in combination with novel immunotherapies to enhance or overcome resistance to PD-1 blockade in patients with advanced solid tumors. For example, preliminary promising data from the ongoing PIVOT-02 trial in mUC patients evaluating NKTR-214, a CD122 agonist, in combination with nivolumab, were recently reported. Best ORR was 48% (13/27) in efficacy-evaluable patients, with a 19% CR rate.[77] Other studies include combinations with GSK3174998, an agonist of OX40, a potent costimulatory tumor necrosis factor receptor expressed on activated $CD4^+$ and $CD8^+$ T cells (NCT02528357); MK-4280, targeting the lymphocyte-activation gene 3 receptor (NCT02720068); TSR-022, an anti–T-cell immunoglobulin and mucin-containing protein-3 antibody (NCT02817633); CDX-1127, targeting CD27, a lymphocyte-specific member of the tumor necrosis factor receptor (NCT02543645), and IPI-549, a potent and selective phosphoinositide-3-kinase-gamma (PI3K-γ) inhibitor (NCT03980041).

The vascular endothelial growth factor receptor-2 (VEGFR-2) antibody ramucirumab combined with pembrolizumab demonstrated modest antitumor activity and good tolerability in previously treated UC patients based on an interim report of an ongoing phase Ia/b trial (NCT02443324).[78] The combination of cabozantinib, a multikinase inhibitor that targets MET, VEGFR, AXL, and RET kinases, with nivolumab or ipilimumab/nivolumab has also demonstrated promising antitumor activity in a phase I trial of genitourinary malignancies, with an impressive ORR of 38.5% with CR in 23.1%, and an mOS of 25.4 months (95% CI: 5.7–41.6 months) for patients with mUC.[79] Similarly, the combination of sitravatinib, a VEGFR inhibitor that also inhibits the TAM group of kinases (Tyro, AXL, MER), or lenvatinib demonstrated promising activity when combined with PD-1 inhibitors (nivolumab or pembrolizumab, respectively) following platinum.[80,81] The ongoing LEAP-011 trial compared first-line pembrolizumab with or without lenvatinib for cisplatin-ineligible patients with PD-L1 high tumors or platinum-ineligible patients. Multiple ongoing trials of additional promising antiangiogenic agents in combination with ICIs, such as cabozantinib combined with atezolizumab or pembrolizumab and apatinib with pembrolizumab, will help elucidate the role of immunotherapy combinations in advanced UC (NCT03170960, NCT03534804, NCT03407976, respectively).

The incorporation of prospective assignment to a specific therapy by tumor genomic alterations has been explored in the BISCAY trial. This trial was an open-label, randomized, multidrug, biomarker-directed, phase Ib study in patients with mUC who have failed at least 1 prior platinum regimen, assessing immunotherapy with durvalumab as monotherapy and in combination with select targeted therapies. Treatment assignment was based on the tumor biomarker profile and included olaparib, a PARP inhibitor; vistusertib, an mTOR inhibitor; AZD4547, an fibroblast growth receptor (FGFR) inhibitor; and AZD1775, a WEE1 inhibitor. Using Foundation One tumor genomic profiling, a total of 391 platinum-refractory patients were screened for prespecified FGFR (targeted with AZD4547), mTOR (targeted with vistusertib), or DNA damage repair (targeted with olaparib) biomarkers. Preliminary results reported an ORR of 20% for AZD4547 alone, 28.6% for AZD4547 plus durvalumab, 35.7% for olaparib plus durvalumab, 24.1% for vistusertib plus durvalumab, and 27.6% for durvalumab monotherapy. Combination therapy regimens displayed higher rates of adverse effects, including higher rates of patients for whom adverse events led to treatment discontinuation (33%–38% for combination regimens, 20% for AZD4547 alone, 10% durvalumab alone).[82]

TARGETING FIBROBLAST GROWTH RECEPTOR IN ADVANCED UROTHELIAL CARCINOMA

Despite the advent of ICIs, only a subset of patients truly benefits, whereas most patients with advanced UC continue to lack effective alternatives to single-agent chemotherapy. One of the most successful molecular targets identified to date is the FGFR family tyrosine kinases, which have been implicated in tumor survival and proliferation.[83] Gene-expression profiling has identified several subtypes of UC with recognizable differences in their propensity to benefit from chemotherapy or immunotherapy.[37,58,84] The luminal I subtype exhibits relatively lower PD-L1 expression and has a lower immune signature than other subtypes. This subtype has been associated with poor response to immunotherapy but is enriched for mutations in the *FGFR* gene, underscoring an attractive therapeutic target in patients who are predicted to have poor responses to ICIs.[50,58] Indeed, as many as 20% of advanced UC patients carry *FGFR* alterations, such as *FGFR2/3* mutations and fusions, which are particularly frequent in the luminal I subtype.[83–85]

Erdafitinib is a potent orally administered inhibitor of FGFR1-4 that demonstrated antitumor activity in preclinical models of various solid tumors.[86] In a first-in-human study, among 23 evaluable patients with *FGFR* alterations, 4 confirmed responses and an unconfirmed partial response were observed. The responses were seen in patients with UC, glioblastoma, and endometrial cancer, all with *FGFR2* or *FGFR3* translocations, and there were no responses noted in patients without *FGFR* alterations. Hyperphosphatemia, a unique pharmacodynamic effect associated with FGFR inhibitors, was observed in all patients receiving at least 4 mg daily, and levels were associated with efficacy. The safety profile was acceptable, with asthenia, dry mouth, nail toxicity, and constipation making up the most common treatment-emergent adverse events after hyperphosphatemia[87]

A subsequent phase II dose-escalation study randomized patients with mUC with prespecific FGFR2 and/or FGFR3 genetic alterations to either continuous or intermittent dosing schedules in the dose-selection phase.[88] At the first interim analysis, the ORR in the continuous dosing arm was superior to that of the intermittent dosing arm (35% vs 24%), establishing continuous dosing of 8 mg/d as the starting dose, with provision for a pharmacodynamically guided dose escalation to 9 mg. A total of 99 heavily pretreated patients with advanced UC were treated in the continuous-regimen group and demonstrated an ORR of 40%. Although only 1 of 22 patients had responded to a prior ICI, a remarkable ORR of 59% was seen with erdafitinib in the group of 22 patients who had previously received immunotherapy. Intriguingly, a retrospective analysis of the IMvigor210 and CHECKMATE-275 trials demonstrated that RRs in FGFR3 were altered and wild-type tumors were similar.[89] Treatment-related adverse events were consistent with prior studies of erdafitinib and were managed primarily by dose adjustments.[90] These results led to FDA approval of erdafitinib in 2019 for the treatment of patients with advanced or mUC with *FGFR2* or *FGFR3* alterations who have progressed following platinum-containing chemotherapy.[91] With a median follow-up of 24 months, updated results of mPFS and mOS were 5.52 and 11.3 months, respectively.[92]

In addition to erdafitinib, other FGFR inhibitors, including rogaratinib, infigratinib, and pemigatinib, have been explored in separate phase I and II trials, with an RR of around 25%, with a toxicity profile consistent with other FGFR inhibitors.[93–95] Results of anti-FGFR3 mAb vofatamab (B-701) monotherapy or in combination with docetaxel have been recently reported, with a confirmed RR of 10% and 33%, respectively.[96]

Additional biomarker studies and combination strategies of targeted therapies combined with ICIs are underway. Vofatamab has been evaluated in a I/II trial in combination with pembrolizumab in 22 patients with previously treated mUC with and without FGFR3 alterations (FIERCE-22 trial). The ORR was 36% in the entire cohort (33% in wild-type tumors and 43% in tumors with FGFR3 alterations).[97] Other combinations under investigation include erdafitinib and certrelimab (an anti–PD-1 mAb) in the NORSE trial (NCT03473743), pemigatinib and pembrolizumab in the FIGTH-205 trial (NCT04003610), and rogaratinib combined with atezolizumab in the FORT-2 trial (NCT03473756), all in phase Ib/II trials. The results of these combination studies have the potential to influence the management of advanced UC.

ANTIBODY-DRUG CONJUGATES IN ADVANCED UROTHELIAL CANCER

A novel class of agents that is very promising includes antibody drug conjugates (ADCs). In advanced UC, enfortumab vedotin (EV), which is composed of an anti–Nectin-4 mAb attached to microtubule-disrupting agent monomethyl auristatin E (MMAE), has been investigated with very promising results.[98] Nectin-4 is a cell-adhesion molecule that is overexpressed in UCs compared with both other cancers and nonmalignant tissues. EV binds to cells that express Nectin-4 with high affinity, triggering the internalization and release of MMAE in target cells. MMAE disrupts microtubule networks, leading to cell-cycle arrest and apoptotic death of Nectin-4–expressing cells. In a phase I trial in previously treated patients with advanced UC, EV was found to have a tolerable safety profile, and an expansion cohort suggested a high degree of antitumor activity in UC. The ORR was 41%; mOS and mPFS were 13.6 and 5.4 months, respectively.[99] In the pivotal single-arm phase II study (EV-201, cohort 1), 125 patients with advanced UC and with prior PD-1/L1 inhibitor and platinum-based therapy received three 1.25 mg/kg doses of EV per 28-day cycle until disease progression or withdrawal from treatment. The primary end point was ORR. Of patients, 90% had visceral disease, 50% had received 3 or more prior systemic therapies, and 80% were anti–PD-1/L1 nonresponders. After a median follow-up duration of 10.2 months, 44% of patients had an objective response (including 12 CR). The estimated mPFS duration at the time of analysis cutoff was 5.8 months, with an estimated mOS duration of 11.7 months. ORRs were generally similar across the various subgroups, including those who had received ≥3 prior lines of therapy. Grade ≥3 treatment-related adverse events were observed in 54% of patients and resulted in treatment discontinuation in 12% of the patients. The most common treatment-related adverse events of any grade included fatigue (50%), any peripheral neuropathy (50%), and alopecia (49%) with no single grade 3 or higher treatment-related adverse events occurring in 10% or more of patients.[100] On December 2019, the FDA granted accelerated approval to EV for patients with advanced or mUC who have previously received anti–PD-1/PD-L1 therapy and a platinum-containing chemotherapy in the neoadjuvant/adjuvant, locally advanced, or metastatic setting.[101]

Very recently, preliminary results of the randomized phase III trial EV-301 comparing EV monotherapy with single-agent chemotherapy in patients with prior platinum and anti–PD-1/L1 therapy have been reported in a press release showing for the first time an OS survival benefit in third-line setting (NCT03474107).

The EV-201 study is also actively enrolling a second cohort (cohort 2) of patients who have received prior anti–PD-1/L1 therapy and are cisplatin ineligible without prior platinum treatment to determine if a similar benefit will be observed. Moreover, EV is being evaluated in a broader population of patients with UC, including the first-line setting, where it is being studied in combination with anti–PD-1 and/or platinum-based therapies. Early data have also shown very promising clinical activity for EV plus pembrolizumab in advanced UC. Interim results of the phase Ib/II EV-103 trial on the combination of EV plus pembrolizumab as first-line therapy led to an ORR of 73%, including a 15.6% CR rate and a 57.8% partial RR in patients previously untreated with locally advanced of mUC who were ineligible for cisplatin-based chemotherapy. Median duration of response had not yet been reached for this population.[102] If future studies continue to hold up these results, the combination could become a platinum-free combination, first-line option for cisplatin-ineligible patients.

Another ADC with a different mechanism of action is sacituzumab govitecan (SG), which consists of the active metabolite of irinotecan, SN-38, linked with a humanized IgG antibody targeted against Trop-2, a cell-surface glycoprotein. SG has also received breakthrough designation for mUC on the basis of 2 different phase II trials in heavily pretreated patients.[103] A phase I/II, open-label, single-arm, multicenter, basket trial investigated the activity of SG in patients with metastatic epithelial malignancies; among 45 patients with mUC, the ORR was 31%, with manageable toxicity profile. Patients with visceral metastasis had an ORR of 27%, whereas patients with prior anti–PD-L1 treatment had an ORR of 23%.[104] TROPHY-U-01 (NCT03547973) is a multicohort, global, open-label, phase 2 study evaluating SG clinical activity in patients with unresectable locally advanced or mUC with measurable disease. The final results of cohort 1 with 113 patients progressing after platinum chemotherapy and immune-checkpoint inhibitors have recently been reported, with an ORR of 27%, and mPFS and mOS were 5.4 and 10.5 months, respectively. Key grade $\geq$3 treatment-related adverse events were neutropenia (35%), anemia (14%), febrile neutropenia (10%), and diarrhea (10%).[105] A randomized phase III trial of SG comparing SG monotherapy with single-agent chemotherapy in patients with prior platinum and anti–PD-1/L1 therapy is now accruing (NCT04527991)

Multiple antibody-drug conjugates are also being developed to target HER2 in UC. HER2 is expressed to varying degrees in urothelial bladder cancer, and an ADC targeting HER2 is a very rational approach. Results of a single-arm, nonrandomized phase II study of RC48-ADC in HER2-positive patients with pretreated mUC were recently reported. This trial enrolled 43 patients and demonstrated an impressive ORR of 51.2%, being greater than 60% in patients with liver metastases and previously treated with anti–PD-1/L1 treatments.[106] Ado-trastuzumab emtansine (T-DM1) is an ADC that is already FDA approved for HER2-positive metastatic breast cancer. Clinical trials testing T-DM1 in mUC have completed enrollment, and results are forthcoming. DS-8201a (trastuzumab deruxtecan) is another ADC with a topoisomerase-1 inhibiting payload targeting HER2 but exhibiting activity against bystander Her2-negative cells owing to a cleavable linker, with early signs of impressive efficacy in breast and gastric cancer, that is being combined with nivolumab in an ongoing trial of patients with breast and bladder cancer expressing HER2 (NCT03523572).

ANTIANGIOGENIC THERAPY IN UROTHELIAL CARCINOMA

Endothelial growth factor levels seem to be prognostic for clinical outcomes in advanced UC, and preclinical evaluation of angiogenesis inhibition demonstrates anticancer activity, which has prompted the development of these therapeutic strategies.[107] Multiple agents targeting the VEGF pathway have been studied as single agents or in combination with traditional chemotherapy.

Single-arm studies have investigated the use of single-agent sorafenib, pazopanib, and sunitinib, demonstrating limited clinical activity.[108–110] After many trials demonstrating limited activity with antiangiogenic therapies for UC, this therapeutic strategy may have found redemption with cabozantinib, which has shown single-agent clinical activity in a phase II study with an encouraging ORR of 19.5% in patients with relapsed or refractory mUC. Extensive correlative analysis in this clinical trial showed that cabozantinib has innate and adaptive immunomodulatory properties providing a rationale for combining cabozantinib with immunotherapeutic strategies.[111] Despite the strong clinical rationale and availability of agents, the efficacy and safety of combinatory regimens with antiangiogenic agents in combination with traditional chemotherapy, such as sunitinib in combination with GC, sorafenib combined with CbG, or vandetanib plus docetaxel, have been met with disappointing results in small phase II trials.[112–114] One of the most encouraging results came from a small phase II trial of paclitaxel plus pazopanib that resulted in a substantial ORR of 54% in patients with advanced pretreated UC, indicating that the antitumor activity with anti-VEGF agents could be achieved in combination with other chemotherapeutic agents.[115]

Two phase III trials have failed to demonstrate survival benefit in advanced UC. The RANGE trial included 530 patients who progressed during or after platinum-based chemotherapy and demonstrated a longer mPFS of 4.1 months with ramucirumab (an IgG1 VEGFR-2 antagonist) plus docetaxel, compared with an mPFS of 2.8 months in the docetaxel-alone arm ($P = .0002$). Unfortunately, ramucirumab plus docetaxel did not demonstrate an OS benefit compared with single-agent docetaxel.[116] The CALGB 90601 phase III trial evaluated the combination of GC with or without bevacizumab (an mAb directed against circulating VEGF) and did not result in improved OS in patients with mUC and no prior treatment of metastatic disease.[117]

TARGETING ENDOTHELIAL GROWTH FACTOR RECEPTOR FAMILY IN ADVANCED UROTHELIAL CARCINOMA

Analysis of TCGA has shown that epidermal growth factor receptor (EGFR) signaling pathways are upregulated in selected advanced UC tumors, with *EGFR* amplification in 11% of UC and *ERBB2* amplification and mutation in 9%.[37] A comprehensive molecular analysis has confirmed that EGFR amplifications (11%), HER2 amplifications (7%), and ERBB3 somatic mutations (11%) are relatively frequent in UC.[118] Lapatinib is a dual tyrosine kinase inhibitor of EGFR and HER2 that showed antitumor activity in a phase II study in a subset of 34 patients with EGFR/HER2-overexpressing tumors.[119] In contrast, in a study of 232 mUC patients who had clinical benefit from frontline chemotherapy and HER1/HER2-positive status confirmed by IHC, no improvement in PFS was found with maintenance lapatinib versus placebo.[120] Afatinib, another dual EGFR and HER2 inhibitor, was suggested to have clinical activity in patients with platinum-refractory advanced UC with *ERBB2* or *ERBB3* genetic alterations detected by quantitative polymerase chain reaction or fluorescent in situ hybridization.[121] However, these results were not confirmed in the phase II LUX-BLADDER-1 study in selected patients with ERBB2/ERRB alterations, which closed prematurely after a futility analysis (NCT02780687).

Combination studies of cytotoxic chemotherapy with ErbB targeted therapies have also been carried out, such as cetuximab combined with CG or paclitaxel, CG plus gefitinib, or ddMVAC in combination with panitumumab. These studies did not demonstrate additional activity with the different combinations but increased toxicity.[122–125] None of these ErbB targeted therapies has translated into clinical practice.

OTHER TARGETED THERAPIES IN ADVANCED UROTHELIAL CARCINOMA

Other pathways frequently dysregulated in bladder cancer are PI3K signaling (altered in 72% of cases), cell-cycle regulation (93%), and chromatin remodeling, including mutations or somatic copy number alterations in histone-modifying genes (89%).[37] However, no significant activity has been obtained with drugs directed against these specific targets, such as everolimus or temsirolimus, palbociclib, or apatorsen.[126–130] PARP inhibitors have acquired special interest in the treatment of advanced UC, because alterations in BRCA1/2 have been described altered in up to 31% of cases.[37] Several clinical trials are currently ongoing with these drugs, both as single agents and in combination.

SUMMARY

Improving systemic treatment for patients with UC has been a challenge in recent years. Currently, advanced UC has multiple treatment options, including traditional cytotoxic chemotherapy, immune-checkpoint inhibitors, and targeted therapies, such as erdafitinib, for patients whose tumors carry *FGFR* alterations, and EV. We have entered an era of excitement and hope for mUC. After decades of paucity in terms of therapeutics available for everyday clinical practice, the increasing under-standing of the biology of UC promises a future of truly effective treatments for our patients.

CONFLICT OF INTEREST STATEMENT

J. Bellmunt has been a consultant for Agensys, Amgen, Astra Zeneca, Bayer, Eisai, Genentech, Janssen, Merck, Novartis, Pfizer, Sanofi, and Seattle Genetics and has received financial support for research from Novartis and Sanofi and royalties for his UpToDate contribution in urothelial tumors. B.P. Valderrama reports personal fees from Astellas Pharma, Novartis, Pfizer, Pierre Fabre, Bayer, Sanofy, Bristol Myers Squibb, and Ipsen. R. Nadal and J. Clara declare no competing interests.

CLINICS CARE POINTS

- Cisplatin-based chemotherapy is still the gold-standard frontline treatment for patients with cisplatin-eligible advanced/metastatic urothelial carcinoma.

- Maintenance avelumab is a new standard of care treatment for patients with advanced/metastatic urothelial carcinoma whose disease did not progress with first-line platinum-based chemotherapy.

- Pembrolizumab has emerged as the standard of care in the treatment of platinum-refractory advanced UC based on level 1 evidence.

- Erdafitinib is a novel targeted therapy approved for FGFR-mutated urothelial cancer.

- Enfortumab vedotin is the first Nectin-4–directed antibody-drug conjugate to receive regulatory approval for the treatment of patients with immune-checkpoint inhibitors, and a platinum-containing chemotherapy experienced urothelial carcinoma.

REFERENCES

1. Sternberg CN, Yagoda A, Scher HI, et al. M-VAC (methotrexate, vinblastine, doxorubicin and cisplatin) for advanced transitional cell carcinoma of the uro-thelium. J Urol 1998;139:461–9.
2. Loerhrer PJ Sr, Einhorn LH, Elson PJ, et al. A randomized comparison of cisplatin alone or in combination with methotrexate, vinblastine, and doxorubicin in patients with metastatic urothelial carcinoma: a cooperative group study. J Clin Oncol 1992;10:1066–73.

3. Mead GM, Russell M, Clark P, et al. A randomized trial comparing methotrexate and vinblastine (MV) with cisplatin, methotrexate and vinblastine (CMV) in advanced transitional cell carcinoma: results and a report on prognostic factors in a Medical Research Council study. Br J Cancer 1998;78:1067–75.
4. Kyriakakis Z, Dimopoulos MA, Kostakopoulos A, et al. Cisplatin, ifosfamide, methotrexate and vinblastine combination chemotherapy for metastatic urothelial cancer. J Urol 1997;158:408–11.
5. Logothetis CJ, Dexeus FH, Chong C, et al. Cisplatin, cyclophosphamide and doxorubicin chemotherapy for unresectable urothelial tumors: the M.D. Anderson Experience. J Urol 1989;141:33–7.
6. Logothetis CJ, Dexeus FH, Finn L, et al. A prospective randomized trial comparing MVAC and CISCA chemotherapy for patients with metastatic urothelial tumors. J Clin Oncol 1990;8:1050–5.
7. Sternberg CN, de Mulder PH, Schornagel JH, et al. Randomized phase III trial of high-dose-intensity methotrexate, vinblastine, doxorubicin, and cisplatin (MVAC) chemotherapy and recombinant human granulocyte colony-stimulating factor versus classic MVAC in advanced urothelial tract tumors: European Organization for Research and Treatment of Cancer Protocol no. 30924. J Clin Oncol 2001;19:2638–46.
8. Sternberg CN, de Mulder P, Schornagel JH, et al. Seven year update of an EORTC phase III trial of high-dose intensity M-VAC chemotherapy and G-CSF versus classic M-VAC in advanced urothelial tract tumours. Eur J Cancer 2006;42:50–4.
9. Von Der Maase H, Andersen L, Crinò L, et al. Weekly gemcitabine and cisplatin combination therapy in patients with transitional cell carcinoma of the urothelium: a phase II clinical trial. Ann Oncol 1999;10:1461–5.
10. Kaufman D, Raghavan D, Carducci M, et al. Phase II trial of gemcitabine plus cisplatin in patients with metastatic urothelial cancer. J Clin Oncol 2000;18:1921–7.
11. Moore MJ, Winquist EW, Murray N, et al. Gemcitabine plus cisplatin, an active regimen in advanced urothelial cancer: a phase II trial of the National Cancer Institute of Canada Clinical Trials Group. J Clin Oncol 1999;17:2876–81.
12. von der Maase H, Hansen SW, Roberts JT, et al. Gemcitabine and cisplatin versus methotrexate, vinblastine, doxorubicin, and cisplatin in advanced or metastatic bladder cancer: results of a large, randomized, multinational, multicenter, phase III study. J Clin Oncol 2000;18:3068–77.
13. Von der Maase H, Sengelov L, Roberts JT, et al. Long-term survival results of a randomized trial comparing gemcitabine plus cisplatin, with methotrexate, vinblastine, doxorubicin, plus cisplatin in patients with bladder cancer. J Clin Oncol 2005;23:4602–8.
14. Dreicer R, Manola J, Roth BJ, et al. Phase II study of cisplatin and paclitaxel in advanced carcinoma of the urothelium: an Eastern Cooperative Oncology Group Study. J Clin Oncol 2000;18:1058–61.
15. Burch PA, Richardson RL, Cha SS, et al. Phase II study of paclitaxel and cisplatin for advanced urothelial cancer. J Urol 2000;164:1538–42.
16. Dimopoulos MA, Bakoyannis C, Georgoulias V, et al. Docetaxel and cisplatin combination chemotherapy in advanced carcinoma of the urothelium: a multicenter phase II study of the Hellenic Cooperative Oncology Group. Ann Oncol 1999;10:1385–8.
17. Sengeløv L, Kamby C, Lund B, et al. Docetaxel and cisplatin in metastatic urothelial cancer: a phase II study. J Clin Oncol 1998;16:3392–7.

18. Garcia del Muro X, Marcuello E, Gumá J, et al. Phase II multicentre study of docetaxel plus cisplatin in patients with advanced urothelial cancer. Br J Cancer 2002;86:326–30.

19. Bamias A, Aravantinos G, Deliveliotis C, et al. Docetaxel and cisplatin with granulocyte colony-stimulating factor (G-CSF) versus MVAC with G-CSF in advanced urothelial carcinoma: a multicenter, randomized, phase III study from the Hellenic Cooperative Oncology Group. J Clin Oncol 2004;22:220–8.

20. Bellmunt J, von der Maase H, Mead GM, et al. Randomized phase III study comparing paclitaxel/cisplatin/gemcitabine and gemcitabine/cisplatin in patients with locally advanced or metastatic urothelial cancer without prior systemic therapy: EORTC Intergroup Study 30987. J Clin Oncol 2012;30:1107–13.

21. Sternberg CN, Skoneczna IA, Castellano D, et al. Larotaxel with cisplatin in the first-line treatment of locally advanced/metastatic urothelial tract or bladder cancer: a randomized, active-controlled, phase III trial (CILAB). Oncology 2013;85:208–15.

22. Galsky MD, Hahn NM, Rosenberg J, et al. A consensus definition of patients with metastatic urothelial carcinoma who are unfit for cisplatin-based chemotherapy. Lancet Oncol 2011;12:211–4.

23. Galsky MD, Hahn NM, Rosenberg J, et al. Treatment of patients with metastatic urothelial cancer "unfit" for cisplatin-based chemotherapy. J Clin Oncol 2011;29:2432–8.

24. De Santis M, Bellmunt J, Mead G, et al. Randomized phase II/III trial assessing gemcitabine/carboplatin and methotrexate/carboplatin/vinblastine in patients with advanced urothelial cancer who are unfit for cisplatin-based chemotherapy: EORTC study 30986. J Clin Oncol 2012;30:191–9.

25. Dogliotti L, Cartenì G, Siena S, et al. Gemcitabine plus cisplatin versus gemcitabine plus carboplatin as first-line chemotherapy in advanced transitional cell carcinoma of the urothelium: results of a randomized phase 2 trial. Eur Urol 2007;52:134–41.

26. Nogué-Aliguer M, Carles J, Arrivi A, et al. Gemcitabine and carboplatin in advanced transitional cell carcinoma of the urinary tract: an alternative therapy. Cancer 2003;97:2180–6.

27. Shannon C, Crombie C, Brooks A, et al. Carboplatin and gemcitabine in metastatic transitional cell carcinoma of the urothelium: effective treatment of patients with poor prognostic features. Ann Oncol 2001;12:947–52.

28. Vaughn DJ, Malkowicz SB, Zoltick B, et al. Paclitaxel plus carboplatin in advanced carcinoma of the urothelium: an active and tolerable outpatient regimen. J Clin Oncol 1998;16:255–60.

29. Redman BG, Smith DC, Flaherty L, et al. Phase II trial of paclitaxel and carboplatin in the treatment of advanced urothelial carcinoma. J Clin Oncol 1998;16:1844–8.

30. Zielinski CC, Schnack B, Grbovic M, et al. Paclitaxel and carboplatin in patients with metastatic urothelial cancer: results of a phase II trial. Br J Cancer 1998;78:370–4.

31. Small EJ, Lew D, Redman BG, et al. Southwest Oncology Group Study of paclitaxel and carboplatin for advanced transitional-cell carcinoma: the importance of survival as a clinical trial end point. J Clin Oncol 2000;18:2537–44.

32. Friedland DM, Dakhil S, Hollen C, et al. A phase II evaluation of weekly paclitaxel plus carboplatin in advanced urothelial cancer. Cancer Invest 2004;22:374–82.

33. De Santis M, Wiechno PJ, Bellmunt J, et al. Vinflunine-gemcitabine versus vinflunine-carboplatin as first-line chemotherapy in cisplatin-unfit patients with

advanced urothelial carcinoma: results of an international randomized phase II trial (JASINT1). Ann Oncol 2016;27:449–54.

34. Sonpavde G, Pond GR, Choueiri TK, et al. Single-agent taxane versus taxane-containing combination chemotherapy as salvage therapy for advanced urothelial carcinoma. Eur Urol 2016;69:634–41.

35. Bellmunt J, Théodore C, Demkov T, et al. Phase III trial of vinflunine plus best supportive care compared with best supportive care alone after a platinum-containing regimen in patients with advanced transitional cell carcinoma of the urothelial tract. J Clin Oncol 2009;27:4454–61.

36. Bellmunt J, Fougeray R, Rosenberg JE, et al. Long-term survival results of a randomized phase III trial of vinflunine plus best supportive care versus best supportive care alone in advanced urothelial carcinoma patients after failure of platinum-based chemotherapy. Ann Oncol 2013;24:1466–72.

37. Weinstein JN, Akbani R, Broom BM, et al. Comprehensive molecular characterization of urothelial bladder carcinoma. Nature 2014;507:315–22.

38. Lawrence MS, Stojanov P, Polak P, et al. Mutational heterogeneity in cancer and the search for new cancer-associated genes. Nature 2013;499:214–8.

39. Sharma P, Shen Y, Wen S, et al. CD8 tumor-infiltrating lymphocytes are predictive of survival in muscle-invasive urothelial carcinoma. Proc Natl Acad Sci U S A 2007;104:3967–72.

40. Fife BT, Bluestone JA. Control of peripheral T-cell tolerance and autoimmunity via the CTLA-4 and PD-1 pathways. Immunol Rev 2008;224:166–82.

41. Bardhan K, Anagnostou T, Boussiotis VA. The PD1:PD-L1/2 pathway from discovery to clinical implementation. Front Immunol 2016;7:550.

42. Barber DL, Wherry EJ, Masopust D, et al. Restoring function in exhausted CD8 T cells during chronic viral infection. Nature 2006;439:682–7.

43. Nakanishi J, Wada Y, Matsumoto K, et al. Overexpression of B7-H (PD-L1) significantly associates with tumor grade and postoperative prognosis in human urothelial cancers. Cancer Immunol Immunother 2007;56:1173–82.

44. Suzman DL, Agrawal S, Ning YM, et al. FDA approval summary: atezolizumab or pembrolizumab for the treatment of patients with advanced urothelial carcinoma ineligible for cisplatin-containing chemotherapy. Oncologist 2019;24:563–9.

45. Lee HT, Lee JY, Lim H, et al. Molecular mechanism of PD-1/PD-L1 blockade via anti-PD-L1 antibodies atezolizumab and durvalumab. Sci Rep 2017;7:5532.

46. Balar AV, Galsky MD, Rosenberg JE, et al. Atezolizumab as first-line treatment in cisplatin-ineligible patients with locally advanced and metastatic urothelial carcinoma: a single-arm, multicentre, phase 2 trial. Lancet 2017;389:67–76.

47. Balar AV, Castellano D, O'Donnell PH, et al. First-line pembrolizumab in cisplatin-ineligible patients with locally advanced and unresectable or metastatic urothelial cancer (KEYNOTE-052): a multicentre, single-arm, phase 2 study. Lancet Oncol 2017;18:1483–92.

48. Vuky J, Balar AV, Castellano D, et al. Long-term outcomes in KEYNOTE-052: phase II study investigating first-line pembrolizumab in cisplatin-ineligible patients with locally advanced or metastatic urothelial cancer. J Clin Oncol 2020; 38(23):2658–66.

49. Powles T, Eder JP, Fine GD, et al. MPDL3280A (anti-PD-L1) treatment leads to clinical activity in metastatic bladder cancer. Nature 2014;515:558–62.

50. Rosenberg JE, Hoffman-Censits J, Powles T, et al. Atezolizumab in patients with locally advanced and metastatic urothelial carcinoma who have progressed following treatment with platinum-based chemotherapy: a single-arm, multi-centre, phase 2 trial. Lancet 2016;387:1909–20.

51. Loriot Y, Rosenberg JE, Powles TB, et al. Atezolizumab (atezo) in platinum (plat)-treated locally advanced/metastatic urothelial carcinoma (mUC): updated OS, safety and biomarkers from the Ph II IMvigor210 study. Ann Oncol 2016;266–95.

52. U.S.FDA: atezolizumab for urothelial carcinoma. Available at: https://www.fda.gov/drugs/resources-information-approved-drugs/atezolizumab-urothelial-carcinoma.

53. Powles T, Durán I, van der Heijden MS, et al. Atezolizumab versus chemotherapy in patients with platinum-treated locally advanced or metastatic urothelial carcinoma (IMvigor211): a multicentre, open-label, phase 3 randomised controlled trial. Lancet 2018;391:748–57.

54. U.S. FDA: pembrolizumab (Keytruda): advanced or metastatic urothelial carcinoma. Available at: https://www.fda.gov/drugs/resources-information-approved-drugs/pembrolizumab-keytruda-advanced-or-metastatic-urothelial-carcinoma.

55. Bellmunt J, de Wit R, Vaughn DJ, et al. Pembrolizumab as second-line therapy for advanced urothelial carcinoma. N Engl J Med 2017;376:1015–26.

56. Necchi A, Fradet Y, Bellmunt J, et al. Three-year follow-up from the phase 3 KEYNOTE-045 trial: pembrolizumab (Pembro) versus investigator's choice (paclitaxel, docetaxel, or vinflunine) in recurrent, advanced urothelial cancer. Ann Oncol 2019;30(suppl_5):v356–402.

57. Wang C, Thudium KB, Han M, et al. In vitro characterization of the anti-PD-1 antibody Nivolumab, BMS-936558, and in vivo toxicology in non-human Primates. Cancer Immunol Res 2014;2:846–56.

58. Sharma P, Retz M, Siefker-Radtke A, et al. Nivolumab in metastatic urothelial carcinoma after platinum therapy (CheckMate 275): a multicentre, single-arm, phase 2 trial. Lancet Oncol 2017;18:312–22.

59. U.S.FDA: nivolumab for treatment of urothelial carcinoma. Available at: https://www.fda.gov/drugs/resources-information-approved-drugs/nivolumab-treatment-urothelial-carcinoma.

60. Galsky MD, Saci A, Szabo PM, et al. Nivolumab in patients with advanced platinum-resistant urothelial carcinoma: efficacy, safety, and biomarker analyses with extended follow-up from checkmate 275. Clin Cancer Res 2020;26(19):5120–8.

61. Sharma P, Callahan MK, Bono P, et al. Nivolumab monotherapy in recurrent metastatic urothelial carcinoma (CheckMate 032): a multicentre, open-label, two-stage, multi-arm, phase 1/2 trial. Lancet Oncol 2016;17:1590–8.

62. U.S. FDA: durvalumab (Imfinzi). Available at: https://www.fda.gov/drugs/resources-information-approved-drugs/durvalumab-imfinzi.

63. Powles T, O'Donnell PH, Massard C, et al. Efficacy and safety of durvalumab in locally advanced or metastatic urothelial carcinoma: updated results from a phase 1/2 Open-label Study. JAMA Oncol 2017;3:e172411.

64. Boyerinas B, Jochems C, Fantini M, et al. Antibody-dependent cellular cytotoxicity activity of a novel anti-PD-L1 antibody avelumab (MSB0010718C) on human tumor cells. Cancer Immunol Res 2015;3:1148–57.

65. U.S. FDA: FDA grants accelerated approval to avelumab for urothelial carcinoma. Available at: https://www.fda.gov/drugs/resources-information-approved-drugs/fda-grants-accelerated-approval-avelumab-urothelial-carcinoma.

66. Apolo AB, Infante JR, Balmanoukian A, et al. Avelumab, an anti-programmed death-ligand 1 antibody, in patients with refractory metastatic urothelial carcinoma: results from a multicenter, phase Ib study. J Clin Oncol 2017;35:2117–24.

67. Patel MR, Ellerton J, Infante JR, et al. Avelumab in metastatic urothelial carcinoma after platinum failure (JAVELIN solid tumor): pooled results from two expansion cohorts of an open-label, phase 1 trial. Lancet Oncol 2018;19:51–64.
68. Maughan BL, Bailey E, Gill DM, et al. Incidence of immune-related adverse events with program death receptor-1- and program death receptor-1 ligand-directed therapies in genitourinary cancers. Front Oncol 2017;7:56.
69. Powles T, Park SH, Voog E, et al. Avelumab maintenance therapy for advanced or metastatic urothelial carcinoma. N Engl J Med 2020;383(13):1218–30.
70. U.S. FDA: FDA approves avelumab for urothelial carcinoma maintenance treatment. Available at: https://www.fda.gov/drugs/drug-approvals-and-databases/fda-approves-avelumab-urothelial-carcinoma-maintenance-treatment.
71. Siefker-Radtke AO, Millikan RE, Tu SM, et al. Phase III trial of fluorouracil, interferon alpha-2b, and cisplatin versus methotrexate, vinblastine, doxorubicin, and cisplatin in metastatic or unresectable urothelial cancer. J Clin Oncol 2002;20:1361–7.
72. Galsky MD, Wang H, Hahn NM, et al. Phase 2 trial of gemcitabine, cisplatin, plus ipilimumab in patients with metastatic urothelial cancer and impact of DNA damage response gene mutations on outcomes. Eur Urol 2018;73:751–9.
73. Galsky MD, Arranz Arija JÁ, Bamias A, et al. Atezolizumab with or without chemotherapy in metastatic urothelial cancer (IMvigor130): a multicentre, randomised, placebo-controlled phase 3 trial. Lancet 2020;395:1547–57.
74. Alva A, Csőszi T, Ozguroglu M, et al. Pembrolizumab (P) combined with chemotherapy (C) vs C alone as first-line (1L) therapy for advanced urothelial carcinoma (UC): KEYNOTE-361. Ann Oncol 2020;31(suppl_4):S1142–215.
75. Powles TB, van der Heijden MS, Castellano Gauna D. A phase III, randomized, open-label study of first-line durvalumab (D) with or without tremelimumab (T) vs standard of care chemotherapy in patients with unresectable, locally advanced or metastatic urothelial carcinoma (DANUBE). Ann Oncol 2020;31(suppl_4):S550.
76. Sharma P, Siefker-Radtke A, Braud Fd, et al. Nivolumab (N) alone or in combination with ipilimumab (I) in patients (pts) with platinum-pretreated metastatic urothelial carcinoma (mUC): extended follow-up from CheckMate 032. Ann Oncol 2020;31(suppl_4):S550.
77. Siefker-Radtke AO, Fishman MN, Balar AV, et al. NKTR-214 + nivolumab in first-line advanced/metastatic urothelial carcinoma (mUC): updated results from PIVOT-02. J Clin Oncol 2019;37(suppl 7S) [abstact: 388].
78. Petrylak DP, Arkenau H-T, Perez-Gracia JL, et al. A multicohort phase I study of ramucirumab (R) plus pembrolizumab (P): interim safety and clinical activity in patients with urothelial carcinoma. J Clin Oncol 2017;35(suppl 6S) [abstract: 349].
79. Apolo AB, Nadal R, Girardi DM, et al. Phase I study of cabozantinib and nivolumab alone or with ipilimumab for advanced or metastatic urothelial carcinoma and other genitourinary tumors. J Clin Oncol 2020;38(31):3672–84.
80. Msaouel P, Siefker-Radtke AO, Sweis R, et al. Sitravatinib (sitra) in combination with nivolumab (nivo) demonstrates clinical activity in checkpoint inhibitor (CPI) naïve, platinum-experienced patients (pts) with advanced or metastatic urothelial carcinoma (UC). Ann Oncol 2020;34(suppl_4):S550.
81. Volgelzang NJ, Encarnacion CA, Cohn AL, et al. Phase Ib/II trial of lenvatinib plus pembrolizumab in urothelial cancer. J Clin Oncol 2019;37(8):11.

82. Powles TB, Balar A, Gravis G, et al. An adaptive, biomarker directed platform study in metastatic urothelial cancer (BISCAY) with durvalumab in combination with targeted therapies. Ann Oncol 2019;30(suppl_5) [abstract: 9020].

83. Haugsten EM, Wiedlocha A, Olsnes S, et al. Roles of fibroblast growth factor receptors in carcinogenesis. Mol Cancer Res 2010;8:1439–52.

84. McConkey DJ, Choi W, Shen Y, et al. A Prognostic gene expression signature in the molecular classification of chemotherapy-naive urothelial cancer is predictive of clinical outcomes from neoadjuvant chemotherapy. A phase 2 trial of dose-dense methotrexate, vinblastine, doxorubicin, and cisplatin with bevacizumab in urothelial cancer. Eur Urol 2016;69:855–62.

85. Knowles MA, Hurst CD. Molecular biology of bladder cancer: new insights into pathogenesis and clinical diversity. Nat Rev Cancer 2015;15:25–41.

86. Perera TPS, Jovcheva E, Mevellec L, et al. Discovery and pharmacological characterization of JNJ-42756493 (Erdafitinib), a functionally selective small-molecule FGFR family inhibitor. Mol Cancer Ther 2017;16:1010–20.

87. Tabernero J, Bahleda R, Dienstmann R, et al. Phase I dose-escalation study of JNJ-42756493, an oral pan-fibroblast growth factor receptor inhibitor, in patients with advanced solid tumors. J Clin Oncol 2015;33:3401–8.

88. Loriot Y, Necchi A, Park SH, et al. Erdafitinib (ERDA; JNJ-42756493), a pan-fibroblast growth factor receptor (FGFR) inhibitor, in patients (pts) with metastatic or unresectable urothelial carcinoma (mUC) and FGFR alterations (FGFRa): phase 2 continuous versus intermittent dosing. J Clin Oncol 2018;36:411.

89. Wang L, Gong Y, Saci A, et al. Fibroblast growth factor receptor 3 alterations and response to PD-1/PD-L1 blockade in patients with metastatic urothelial cancer. Eur Urol 2019;76:599–603.

90. Loriot Y, Necchi A, Park SH, et al. Erdafitinib in locally advanced or metastatic urothelial carcinoma. N Engl J Med 2019;381:338–48.

91. U.S. FDA: FDA grants accelerated approval to erdafitinib for metastatic urothelial carcinoma. Available at: https://www.fda.gov/drugs/resources-information-approved-drugs/fda-grants-accelerated-approval-erdafitinib-metastatic-urothelial-carcinoma.

92. Siefker-Radtke AO, Necchi A, Park SH, et al. Erdafitinib in locally advanced or metastatic urothelial carcinoma (mUC): long-term outcomes in BLC2001. J Clin Oncol 2020;38(suppl) [abstract: 5015].

93. Schuler M, Cho BC, Sayehli CM, et al. Rogaratinib in patients with advanced cancers selected by FGFR mRNA expression: a phase 1 dose-escalation and dose-expansion study. Lancet Oncol 2019;20:1454–66.

94. Pal SK, Rosenberg JE, Hoffman-Censits JH, et al. Efficacy of BGJ398, a fibroblast growth factor receptor 1-3 inhibitor, in patients with previously treated advanced urothelial carcinoma with FGFR3 alterations. Cancer Discov 2018; 8(7):812–21.

95. Necchi A, Pouessel D, Leibowitz-Amit R, et al. Interim results of fight-201, a phase 2, open-label, multicenter study of INCB054828 in patients (pts) with metastatic or surgically unresectable urothelial carcinoma (UC) harboring fibroblast growth factor (FGF)/FGF receptor (FGFR) genetic alterations (GA). Ann Oncol 2018;29(suppl_8):viii3030–331.

96. Necchi A, Castellano DE, Mellado B, et al. Fierce-21: phase II study of vofatamab (B-701), a selective inhibitor of FGFR3, as salvage therapy in metastatic urothelial carcinoma (mUC). J Clin Oncol 2019;37(suppl) [abstract: 409].

97. Siefker-Radtke AO, Currie G, Abella E, et al. FIERCE-22: Clinical activity of vofatamab (V) a FGFR3 selective inhibitor in combination with pembrolizumab

(P) in WT metastatic urothelial carcinoma, preliminary analysis. J Clin Oncol 2019;37(suppl) [abstract: 4511].

98. Doronina SO, Toki BE, Torgov MY, et al. Development of potent monoclonal antibody auristatin conjugates for cancer therapy. Nat Biotechnol 2003;21:778–84.

99. Rosenberg JE, Sridhar SS, Zhang J, et al. EV-101: a phase i study of single-agent enfortumab vedotin in patients with nectin-4-positive solid tumors, including metastatic urothelial carcinoma. J Clin Oncol 2020;38:1041–9.

100. Rosenberg JE, O'Donnell PH, Balar AV, et al. Pivotal trial of enfortumab vedotin in urothelial carcinoma after platinum and anti-programmed death 1/programmed death ligand 1 therapy. J Clin Oncol 2019;37:2592–600.

101. U.S. FDA: FDA grants accelerated approval to enfortumab vedotin-EJFV for metastatic urothelial cancer. Available at: https://www.fda.gov/drugs/resources-information-approved-drugs/fda-grants-accelerated-approval-enfortumab-vedotin-ejfv-metastatic-urothelial-cancer.

102. Rosenberg JE, Flaig TW, Friedlander TW, et al. Study EV-103: preliminary durability results of enfortumab vedotin plus pembrolizumab for locally advanced or metastatic urothelial carcinoma. J Clin Oncol 2020;38(suppl 6) [abstract: 441].

103. FDA grants fast track designation to sacituzumab govitecan in locally advanced mUC. Available at: https://www.targetedonc.com/view/fda-grants-fast-track-designation-to-sacituzumab-govitecan-in-locally-advanced-muc.

104. Tagawa ST, Faltas BM, Lam ET, et al. Sacituzumab govitecan (IMMU-132) in patients with previously treated metastatic urothelial cancer (mUC): results from a phase I/II study. J Clin Oncol 2019;37(suppl 7S) [abstract: 354].

105. Loriot Y, Balar AV, Petrylak DP, et al. TROPHY-U-01 cohort 1 final results: a phase II study of sacituzumab govitecan (SG) in metastatic urothelial cancer (mUC) that has progressed after platinum (PLT) and checkpoint inhibitors (CPI). Ann Oncol 2020;31(suppl_4):S1142–215.

106. Sheng X, Zhou A-P, Yao X, et al. A phase II study of RC48-ADC in HER2-positive patients with locally advanced or metastatic urothelial carcinoma. J Clin Oncol 2019;37(suppl) [abstract: 4509].

107. Sonpavde G, Bellmunt J. Bladder cancer: angiogenesis as a therapeutic target in urothelial carcinoma. Nat Rev Urol 2016;13:306–7.

108. Sridhar SS, Winquist E, Eisen A, et al. A phase II trial of sorafenib in first-line metastatic urothelial cancer: a study of the PMH phase II consortium. Invest New Drugs 2011;29:1045–9.

109. Necchi A, Mariani L, Zaffaroni N, et al. Pazopanib in advanced and platinum-resistant urothelial cancer: an open-label, single group, phase 2 trial. Lancet Oncol 2012;13:810–6.

110. Bellmunt J, González-Larriba JL, Prior C, et al. Phase II study of sunitinib as first-line treatment of urothelial cancer patients ineligible to receive cisplatin-based chemotherapy: baseline interleukin-8 and tumor contrast enhancement as potential predictive factors of activity. Ann Oncol 2011;22:2646–53.

111. Apolo AB, Nadal R, Tomita Y, et al. Cabozantinib in patients with platinum-refractory metastatic urothelial carcinoma: an open-label, single-centre, phase 2 trial. Lancet Oncol 2020;21:1099–109.

112. Galsky MD, Hahn NM, Powles T, et al. Gemcitabine, Cisplatin, and sunitinib for metastatic urothelial carcinoma and as preoperative therapy for muscle-invasive bladder cancer. Clin Genitourin Cancer 2013;11:175–81.

113. Hurwitz ME, Markowski P, Yao X, et al. Multicenter phase 2 trial of gemcitabine, carboplatin, and sorafenib in patients with metastatic or unresectable transitional-cell carcinoma. Clin Genitourin Cancer 2018;16:437–44.e6.

114. Choueiri TK, Ross RW, Jacobus S, et al. Double-blind, randomized trial of doce-taxel plus vandetanib versus docetaxel plus placebo in platinum-pretreated metastatic urothelial cancer. J Clin Oncol 2012;30:507–12.

115. Jones RJ, Hussain SA, Protheroe AS, et al. Randomized phase II study investi-gating pazopanib versus weekly paclitaxel in relapsed or progressive urothelial cancer. J Clin Oncol 2017;35:1770–7.

116. Petrylak DP, de Wit R, Chi KN, et al. Ramucirumab plus docetaxel versus pla-cebo plus docetaxel in patients with locally advanced or metastatic urothelial carcinoma after platinum-based therapy (RANGE): a randomised, double-blind, phase 3 trial. Lancet 2017;390:2266–77.

117. Rosenberg JE, Ballman KV, Halabi S, et al. CALGB 90601 (Alliance): random-ized, double-blind, placebo-controlled phase III trial comparing gemcitabine and cisplatin with bevacizumab or placebo in patients with metastatic urothelial carcinoma. J Clin Oncol 2019;37(suppl) [abstract: 4503].

118. Iyer G, Al-Ahmadie H, Schultz N, et al. Prevalence and co-occurrence of action-able genomic alterations in high-grade bladder cancer. J Clin Oncol 2013;31: 3133–40.

119. Wülfing C, Machiels J-PH, Richel DJ, et al. A single-arm, multicenter, open-label phase 2 study of lapatinib as the second-line treatment of patients with locally advanced or metastatic transitional cell carcinoma. Cancer 2009;115:2881–90.

120. Powles T, Huddart RA, Elliott T, et al. Phase III, double-blind, randomized trial that compared maintenance lapatinib versus placebo after first-line chemo-therapy in patients with human epidermal growth factor receptor 1/2-positive metastatic bladder cancer. J Clin Oncol 2017 Jan;35:48–55.

121. Choudhury NJ, Campanile A, Antic T, et al. Afatinib activity in platinum-refractory metastatic urothelial carcinoma in patients with ERBB alterations. J Clin Oncol 2016;34:2165–71.

122. Hussain M, Daignault S, Agarwal N, et al. A randomized phase 2 trial of gemci-tabine/cisplatin with or without cetuximab in patients with advanced urothelial carcinoma. Cancer 2014;120:2684–93.

123. Wong YN, Litwin S, Vaughn D, et al. Phase II trial of cetuximab with or without paclitaxel in patients with advanced urothelial tract carcinoma. J Clin Oncol 2012;30:3545–51.

124. Philips GK, Halabi S, Sanford BL, et al. A phase II trial of cisplatin (C), gemcita-bine (G) and gefitinib for advanced urothelial tract carcinoma: results of Cancer and Leukemia Group B (CALGB) 90102. Ann Oncol 2009;20:1074–9.

125. Culine S, Flechon A, Gravis G, et al. Results of the GETUG-AFU 19 trial: a ran-domized phase II study of dose dense methotrexate, vinblastine, doxorubicin, and cisplatin (dd-MVAC) with or without anti-epidermal growth factor receptor (EGF-R) monoclonal antibody panitumumab (PANI) in advanced transitional cell carcinoma (ATCC). J Clin Oncol 2017;(suppl_5) [abstact: r307].

126. Milowsky MI, Iyer G, Regazzi AM, et al. Phase II study of everolimus in metasta-tic urothelial cancer. BJU Int 2013;112:462–70.

127. Pulido M, Roubaud G, Cazeau AL, et al. Safety and efficacy of temsirolimus as second line treatment for patients with recurrent bladder cancer. BMC Cancer 2018;18:194.

128. Rose TL, Chism DD, Alva AS, et al. Phase II trial of palbociclib in patients with metastatic urothelial cancer after failure of first-line chemotherapyBr. J Cancer 2018;119(7):801–7.

129. Bellmunt J, Eigl BJ, Senkus E, et al. Borealis-1: a randomized, first-line, placebo-controlled, phase II study evaluating apatorsen and chemotherapy for patients with advanced urothelial cancer. Ann Oncol 2017;28:2481–8.
130. Rosenberg JE, Hahn NM, Regan MM, et al. Apatorsen plus docetaxel versus docetaxel alone in platinum-resistant metastatic urothelial carcinoma (Borealis-2). Br J Cancer 2018;118:1434–41.

Current Perioperative Therapy for Muscle Invasive Bladder Cancer

Joshua Ma, Peter C. Black, MD*

KEYWORDS

- Urinary bladder neoplasm • Carcinoma • Transitional cell • Drug therapy
- Chemotherapy • Adjuvant • Neoadjuvant • Immunotherapy

KEY POINTS

- Patients with muscle-invasive bladder cancer are susceptible to high rates of local recurrence and distant metastasis, thought to be due to the presence of micrometastasis at diagnosis.
- Neoadjuvant cisplatin-based chemotherapy can be used to eliminate occult metastasis and should be prioritized over adjuvant therapy due to more robust evidence.
- Molecular subtypes, the coexpression extrapolation model, and specific genomic alterations are being tested for their ability to predict response to neoadjuvant chemotherapy.
- Perioperative radiotherapy has been tested to improve locoregional disease control but has not been studied adequately to allow widespread adoption into practice.
- Immune checkpoint inhibitors have demonstrated promising results in early phase clinical trials, but the results of phase 3 randomized controlled trials are awaited to determine the benefit of perioperative immunotherapy, and further biomarker development will be critical for selection of optimal treatment options for muscle-invasive bladder cancer.

INTRODUCTION

Muscle-invasive bladder cancer (MIBC) is treated most commonly with radical cystectomy (RC). A subset of patients also is suitable for trimodal therapy (TMT), which is composed of maximal transurethral bladder tumor resection followed by external beam radiation with concurrent systemic chemotherapy.[1] Despite local treatment with curative intent, approximately half of patients subsequently progress with local or distant recurrence.[2] Perioperative radiotherapy has been evaluated in an effort to enhance locoregional disease control after RC. At the same time, neoadjuvant and adjuvant cisplatin-based chemotherapy can be used to eliminate occult micrometastasis and have been shown to induce a modest survival benefit.[3,4] Especially in the

Funding: None.
Vancouver Prostate Centre, University of British Columbia, Vancouver, Canada
* Corresponding author. Level 6, 2775 Laurel Street, Vancouver, British Columbia V5Z 1M9, Canada.
E-mail address: pblack@mail.ubc.ca

Hematol Oncol Clin N Am 35 (2021) 495–511
https://doi.org/10.1016/j.hoc.2021.02.002
0889-8588/21/© 2021 Elsevier Inc. All rights reserved.

context of RC, however, 2 major barriers have mitigated the potential impact of perioperative chemotherapy: a high rate of cisplatin-ineligibility and the underutilization of perioperative chemotherapy even in cisplatin-eligible patients. Advances in this domain include the advent of immune checkpoint blockade and the potential for introduction of other novel targeted therapies in the near future. This article reviews the current state of perioperative management of bladder cancer and highlights some of the newest regimens and clinical trials that are being conducted.

PERIOPERATIVE RADIOTHERAPY

Urothelial carcinoma (UC) is considered radiosensitive. Perioperative radiation in conjunction with RC has been explored in multiple trials in an effort to reduce the rate of recurrences in the pelvis, which are observed in up to half of cases after RC.[2] In contrast with perioperative chemotherapy, which targets occult metastatic disease, perioperative radiation is administered with the intention of improving local control.

Neoadjuvant Radiotherapy

The key randomized controlled trials (RCTs) related to neoadjuvant radiotherapy (RT) prior to RC are summarized in **Table 1**. Most trials are small, some focused predominantly on squamous cell carcinoma, and several trials were fraught with design flaws. Furthermore, RT techniques and technologies would not meet current standards. The largest and most rigorous trial was a SWOG trial that randomized 140 patients to RT followed by RC versus RC alone.[5] RT had no discernible impact on overall survival (OS). As a result, the investigators in this trial speculated that OS is more dependent on control of systemic micrometastasis than on more definitive local control. The overall clinical trial experience is reflected in 1 meta-analysis of 5 trials that included 796 patients.[6] There was no improvement in 3-year OS (odds ratio [OR] 0.91 [95% CI, 0.64, 1.30]) or 5-year OS (OR 0.71 [95% CI, 0.48, 1.06]) with the addition of RT prior to RC. The sample size does not allow adequate delineation of a possible benefit in higher-stage disease. Most of these trials predate adoption of neoadjuvant chemotherapy (NAC) into treatment guidelines, and there is no consideration of incorporating radiation into a paradigm of combined NAC and RC. Preoperative RT rarely is used in practice.

Adjuvant Radiotherapy

The potential advantage of adjuvant RT is that it can be tailored to pathologic parameters, such as high T stage (pT3b-4) and/or positive surgical margins. A common limitation to adjuvant RT, however, is the localization of small bowel in the radiation field after removal of the bladder, with resultant risk of toxicity. Unfortunately, the clinical trial evidence for adjuvant RT is limited.

Zaghloul and colleagues[7] randomized 236 patients with pT3-4a bilharzial bladder cancer in Egypt into 3 groups: observation versus conventional RT fractionation versus multiple daily fractionation RT. The 5-year disease-free survival was only 25% with RC alone, but 44% and 49% in the 2 adjuvant RT arms. The 5-year local control rate similarly improved from 50% after RC alone to 87% and 93% after RT. Late complications were observed with RT, but the rate was reduced with multiple daily fractionations. Only 20.7% of patients in this trial had UC, with the majority having squamous cell carcinoma. A similar trial was conducted by the same Egyptian group, with the addition of AC in all patients.[8] Local control and disease-free survival again were improved with adjuvant RT. In this second trial, 53% of patients had UC. No

Table 1
Prospective randomized trials investigating perioperative radiotherapy

Authors, Year	Trial Population (all M0)	Control Number	Radiotherapy Number (sample size in radiotherapy group)	Total Number	Radiation Dose (Gy)	Number of Fractions	Endpoint	Control	Radiotherapy (% of the endpoint)	P Value	Hazard Ratio (95% CI)
Neoadjuvant											
Prout et al,[59] 1971	Not specified	92	69	161	45	28–32 d	5-y OS (%)	67[a]	68[a]	>.05	—
Blackard and Byar,[60] 1972		22	23	45	45	4–5 wk	3-y OS (%)	40	40	—	—
Ghoneim et al,[61] 1985	Not specified	49	43	92	20	5	5-y OS (%)	32	39	>.05	—
Anderström et al,[62] 1983	Stage 2/3	22	22	44	—	—	5-y OS (%)	61	75	—	—
Smith et al,[5] 1997	Tis-3 N0-2	72	68	140	20	5	5-y OS (%)	53	43	.23	—
Adjuvant											
Zaghloul et al,[63] 1992	T3	83	75, 78	236	37.5 50	—	5-y DFS (%)	25	49, 44	—	—
Zaghloul et al,[8] 2018	T3b-4a and/ or G3 and/ or N+	45[b]	75[b]	120	45	30	2-y OS (%)	60	71	.11	0.61 (0.33, 1.11)
Neoadjuvant vs adjuvant											
El-Monim et al,[64] 2013	T2-4a	50[c]	50	100	50	25	3-y OS (%)	53.4	51.8	.689	—

Abbreviation: DFS, disease-free survival.
[a] Values estimated from Kaplan-Meier curves.
[b] All patients received adjuvant GC.
[c] Control patients received preoperative RT.

patients in either trial received NAC. The results of these trials are not considered generalizable to patients with UC.

These trial results are encouraging enough that several additional, international, single-arm trials are under way to study the effects of adjuvant RT with modern RT techniques (NCT03718741, NCT02951325, and NCT02397434). Unfortunately, a cooperative group RCT in North America was terminated due to slow accrual (NCT02316548).

PERIOPERATIVE CHEMOTHERAPY
Neoadjuvant Chemotherapy

Cisplatin-based, multiagent NAC is the standard of care for treatment of MIBC. Multiple clinical trials and meta-analyses have demonstrated an absolute survival benefit of 5% to 8% at 5 years with NAC over RC alone,[4,9,10] as summarized in **Table 2**. SWOG 8710 was a pivotal trial that showed that the relative risk of death in patients receiving methotrexate, vinblastine, doxorubicin, and cisplatin (MVAC) prior to RC was reduced by 33% compared with patients undergoing RC alone.[9] The median survival was extended from 46 months to 77 months with NAC in this trial. This and subsequent trials, as well as real-world evidence, have suggested that pathologic response after NAC is a potential surrogate measure of OS, with excellent outcomes observed in patients with no residual disease (ypT0N0) or only residual nonmuscle invasive (≤ypT1N0) disease.[11,12]

The BA06 30894 trial, with 976 patients, was the largest trial testing NAC. This trial also was noteworthy because approximately half of patients received radiation to the bladder and the other half underwent RC. Neoadjuvant cisplatin, methotrexate, and vinblastine (CMV) reduced the risk of death by 16% compared with local therapy alone, with a corresponding 6% survival benefit at 10 years. There was no differential benefit between patients treated with RT or RC. Based on this compelling evidence in a large number of patients, numerous guidelines strongly recommend cisplatin-based NAC in patients with cT2-4aN0M0 bladder cancer.[13,14]

Although the best evidence for NAC is derived from the 2 trials described using MVAC and CMV, the most commonly used regimen is gemcitabine in combination with cisplatin (GC). GC has not been tested adequately in the NAC setting,[15,16] and its use is based on better tolerability with similar disease control in the metastatic setting.[17] Dose-dense MVAC (ddMVAC) mostly has replaced standard MVAC due to better tolerability with at least equivalent disease control[18] and because the shortened treatment duration allows patients to proceed to definitive local therapy sooner.[19] The V05 VESPER trial provided the first evidence in a head-to-head comparison that neoadjuvant ddMVAC yields a higher rate of pathologic response (≤ypT1N0) than GC at the cost of increased toxicity.[20] The pathologic complete response (cPR) (ypT0N0) rate, however, was not improved with ddMVAC, and the comparison of 6 cycles of ddMVAC versus 4 cycles GC (both administered over 12 weeks) may have confounded the results in favor of ddMVAC. Results for progression-free survival and OS have not yet been reported.

Patients who are cisplatin-ineligible are recommended to proceed directly to definitive local therapy. Carboplatin-based NAC should not be administered because of the absence of evidence supporting its use in the neoadjuvant setting.[13,14] Because the benefit of neoadjuvant cisplatin is considered modest and carboplatin has been demonstrated to be inferior to cisplatin in advanced disease,[21] it is possible that the delay in definitive local therapy caused by ineffective carboplatin-based NAC ultimately could harm patients.[22]

The role of NAC in patients with variant histology remains controversial. Variants, such as plasmacytoid, micropapillary, and sarcomatoid carcinoma, all portend a higher risk of extravesical extension, nodal involvement, and distant metastasis,

Table 2
Prospective randomized trials investigating neoadjuvant cisplatin-based combination chemotherapy

Authors, Year	Trial Population (all M0)	Control Number	Neoadjuvant Chemotherapy Number	Total	Chemotherapy Regimen	Median Follow-up (mo)	Control, 5-y Overall Survival (%)	Neoadjuvant Chemotherapy, 5-y Overall Survival (%)	P Value	Hazard Ratio (95% CI)
Bassi et al,[65] 1999	T2-T4 N0	104	102	206	Cisplatin, methotrexate, vinblastine, doxorubicin	—	—	—	—	0.93 (0.64, 1.35)
Sengelov et al,[66] 2002 (RC arm only)	T2-4b Nx-3	16	17	33	Cisplatin, methotrexate	—	46	83	.76	
Grossman et al,[9] 2003	T2-4a N0	154	153	307	Cisplatin, methotrexate, vinblastine, doxorubicin	100.8, 104.4	43	57	.06	1.33 (1.00, 1.76)
Sherif et al,[67] 2004	T1G3-T4a Nx	314	306	620	Cisplatin + methotrexate or doxorubicin	56.4	48	56	.045	0.80 (0.64, 0.99)
Griffiths et al,[10] 2011	T2-4a Nx-0	485	491	976	CMV	96	43	49	.037	0.84 (0.72, 0.99)
Khaled et al,[68] 2014	T2-4a N0-2	55	59	114	GC	37.4	51.2 yr)	51.9 (3 y)	.399	0.75 (0.39, 1.46)
Kitamura et al,[69] 2014	T2-4a N0	66	64	130	Cisplatin, methotrexate, vinblastine, doxorubicin	55	62.4	72.3	.07	0.65 (0.26, 1.65)
Osman et al,[70] 2014	T2-4a N0	30	30	60	GC	—	50 (3 y)	60 (3 y)	.05	0.80 (0.35, 1.83)
Cortesi, unpublished, 2020	T2-4 N0	71	82	153	Cisplatin, methotrexate, vinblastine, epirubicin	37	—	—	—	0.91 (0.60, 1.39)
Advanced Bladder Cancer Meta-analysis Collaboration,[a4] 2005	T1G3-T4b Nx-N3	1213	1220	2433	Meta-analysis	—	—	—	.003	0.86 (0.77, 0.95)

[a] Data provided for platinum-based combination chemotherapy.
data compiled from original studies and updated individual patient data reported in advanced badder cancer meta-analysis.

suggesting that treatment intensification would be desirable, but their response to NAC is poorly characterized, and the delay in definitive local therapy may be harmful if NAC is ineffective.[23] On the other hand, there is consensus that small cell/neuroendocrine carcinoma should be treated with cisplatin/etoposide if possible, even for T1 disease,[24,25] and primary squamous cell carcinoma and adenocarcinoma should not be treated with NAC.[25] UC with glandular or squamous differentiation must be distinguished from the corresponding pure variants, and there is evidence from the SWOG 8710 trial that patients with these variants may fare better than conventional UC with NAC,[26] which is consistent with what is known about molecular subtyping.[27]

NAC continues to be underutilized despite strong endorsement in treatment guidelines. In preliminary results of the SWOG S1011 trial, which was designed to compare outcomes between standard and extended pelvic lymph node dissection at the time of RC, 56% of patients received NAC.[28] This trial required that all participating sites go through a credentialing process, and it was conducted primarily at academic sites in the United States and Canada, so this level of utilization may represent a benchmark for reasonable use of NAC. Reports on contemporary practice patterns in the broader community practice indicate that NAC utilization rates have increased steadily in the past decade and now are approximately 30%.[29,30] A survey among members of the Society of Urologic Oncology showed that the major barriers to adoption of NAC included patient age and comorbidities, potential delay in surgery, and perceived marginal benefit of NAC.[31] The usage rate in this cohort was between 30% and 57%.

These barriers to delivery of NAC could be overcome with predictive clinical models or biomarkers that identify which patients are most likely to benefit from NAC and which patients should forego NAC, with its associated risk of adverse effects and delay in definitive local therapy, due to a low likelihood of response. The group at MD Anderson Cancer Center (MDACC) has suggested a clinical model for determining which patients need NAC most, although it does not integrate any prediction of response to NAC.[32] In this model, patients are considered at high risk of progression after cystectomy based on the following features: presence of hydroureteronephrosis, clinical (c)T3b-4a disease (based on examination under anesthesia and cross-sectional imaging), lymphovascular invasion, micropapillary features, or neuroendocrine features. Patients were considered low risk if they lacked these features and had less than or equal to cT2 disease. In a retrospective series of 297 patients who underwent RC without NAC, OS, disease-specific survival, and progression-free survival all clearly were greater in low-risk patients compared with high-risk patients. Low-risk patients had a 5-year disease-specific survival of 82.7% after RC, implying that NAC was unlikely to add relevant benefit in these patients. It was shown in low-risk patients that disease-specific survival was comparable between patients who were found on RC to have organ-confined disease and those with higher-stage disease at RC. The latter frequently underwent AC, which likely contributed to the favorable outcome.

Three biomarkers have received some attention for their potential to predict response to NAC: molecular subtypes, the coexpression extrapolation (COXEN) model, and specific genomic alterations. Choi and colleagues[33] originally proposed that the p53 subtype was least responsive to NAC, which was linked to a gene signature of senescence and high fibroblast infiltration. Further studies augmented this with the finding that tumors of the basal subtype may derive the greatest benefit from NAC.[27] Luminal papillary tumors, on the other hand, have a low risk of upstaging at RC and appear to derive less benefit from NAC.[34] These findings are preliminary and require validation in clinical trials. The COXEN model is similarly dependent on RNA expression, but here tumor gene expression is compared with established signatures that correlate with response to specific drug combinations. The SWOG S1314 trial attempted to validate the COXEN model prospectively for both MVAC and GC, but the primary endpoint was not met for either regimen.[35] Loss-of-function alterations in 1 of a panel of DNA damage repair genes appears to sensitize to DNA-damaging cisplatin-based NAC, which in turn is associated with high pathologic response rates and excellent OS. The best characterized alterations are mutations in ERCC2[36,37] or in 1 of ATM, FANNC, or RB1.[38] These and other DNA damage repair gene alterations are being tested in 3 different nonrandomized, phase 2 trials to see if they can be used to preserve the bladder after NAC with or without concomitant immunotherapy (NCT03609216, NCT02710734, and NCT03558087). In these trials, patients with tumors harboring specific DNA damage repair gene alterations will retain their bladders after neoadjuvant therapy if they have no evidence of residual invasive disease on clinical restaging. A positive signal in these trials will require subsequent validation in larger RCTs.

Adjuvant Chemotherapy

The role of AC after RC remains controversial. Several RCTs have compared AC to salvage or no chemotherapy, but all have suffered from poor accrual or small sample size (**Table 3**). For instance, the European Organisation for Research and Treatment of Cancer (EORTC) 30994 trial was going to be the definitive large trial to determine the value of AC, but it accrued only 284 of a planned 660 patients, and therefore it was underpowered.[39] A German trial closed early when a significant survival benefit was observed with cisplatin-based combination AC after enrolling only 49 patients.[40] The trial has not had an impact on routine clinical practice, however, due to the very small sample size.

The most recent meta-analysis demonstrated a significant benefit of AC with respect to OS.[3] This benefit was comparable to NAC (23% reduced relative risk of death from all causes and 34% reduced relative risk of death from bladder cancer), but the meta-analysis included only 945 patients from 9 trials. This low overall sample size and some faults in the design of the original trials leave inadequate evidence to provide a strong recommendation for broad implementation of AC in patients with extravesical extension (pT3-4) or nodal involvement (pN1-3). Given the stronger evidence in support of NAC, its use should be prioritized in eligible patients, and AC should be considered for patients with adverse pathologic features on RC who did not receive NAC. An additional advantage of NAC over AC is the increased likelihood that patients will receive both therapies if the chemotherapy is administered first.[41] Furthermore, as with NAC, there is no evidence to support routine use of adjuvant carboplatin-based chemotherapy. Different from the neoadjuvant context, however, in the adjuvant setting, the chemotherapy is not delaying definitive local therapy, so the potential harm of carboplatin-based AC may be mitigated.

Biomarkers to predict response to AC have not yet been identified. Preliminary retrospective reports suggested that p53 alterations may indicate a poor prognosis after RC[42] but also an increased likelihood of responding to chemotherapy.[43] This led to a phase 3 trial that randomized patients with p53-altered (based on immunohistochemistry) pT1-2N0M0 bladder cancer to adjuvant MVAC versus observation after RC.[44] The trial was powered to detect a reduction in the 3-year recurrence rate from 50% without AC to 30% with AC. In the final analysis, however, the 5-year recurrence rate was only 20%, with no difference on the basis of p53 status and no difference in p53-altered tumors randomized to chemotherapy versus observation. The value of p53 as a prognostic marker also has been refuted since this trial was designed.[45]

Table 3
Prospective randomized trials investigating adjuvant cisplatin-based chemotherapy

Authors, Year	Trial Population (all M0)	Control	Adjuvant Chemo-therapy	Total	Chemotherapy Regimen	Median Follow-up (mo)	Control, 5-y Overall Survival (%)	Adjuvant Chemotherapy, 5-y Overall Survival (%)	P Value	Hazard Ratio (95% CI)
Skinner et al,[71] 1991	T3-4 and/or N1-3	52	50	102	Cisplatin, doxorubicin, cyclophosphamide	32	29	52	.0062	0.75 (0.48, 1.19)
Studer et al,[72] 1994	T1-4a N0-1	45	46	91	Cisplatin	69	54	57	.65	1.02 (0.57, 1.84)
Freiha et al,[73] 1996	T3b-4 N0-3	27	28	55	CMV	62	36	63	.32	0.74 (0.36, 1.53)
Bono,[74] 1997	T2-T4a N0	47	43	90	Cisplatin, methotrexate	69	—	—	—	0.65 (0.34, 1.25)
Otto et al,[75] 2003	T3 N0-3	53	55	108	Cisplatin, methotrexate, vinblastine, epirubicin	—	—	—	—	0.82 (0.48, 1.38)
Lehmann et al,[76] 2006	T3-4a and/or N1-3	23	26	49	Cisplatin, methotrexate, vinblastine, doxorubicin or epirubicin		17.4	38.5	.069	0.57 (0.31, 1.05)
Paz-Ares et al,[77] 2010	T3-4 and/or N1-3	74	68	142	Cisplatin, paclitaxel, gemcitabine	30	31	60	.0009	0.38 (0.22, 0.65)
Stadler et al,[44] 2011[a]	p53+ pT1/T2N0	56	58	114	Cisplatin, methotrexate, vinblastine, doxorubicin	65	NR	>100	—	1.11 (0.45, 2.72)
Cognetti et al,[78] 2012	T2G3 or T3-T4 and/or N1-2	92	102	194	GC	35	53.7	43.4	.24	1.29 (0.84, 1.99)
Sternberg et al,[39] 2014	T3-4 and/or N1-3	143	141	284	Cisplatin, methotrexate, vinblastine, doxorubicin; or GC	84	53.6	47.7	.13	0.78 (0.56, 1.08)
Leow et al,[3] 2014	T1-T4 N0-3	470	475	945	Meta-analysis of patients treated with cisplatin-based chemotherapy				.049	0.77 (0.59, 0.99)

[a] p53+ = greater than or equal to 10% nuclear reactivity on p53 immunohistochemistry.

data compiled from original studies and updated individual patient data reported in advanced bladder cancer meta-analysis.

The p53 trial, as with most AC trials, struggled with slow accrual. The clinical trial landscape now has shifted toward testing immunotherapy (discussed later), and early indicators of patient accrual suggest that there is more enthusiasm for these trials. The IMvigor010 trial, for example, accrued 809 patients,[46] which compares with 945 patients from 9 trials included in the most recent meta-analysis of AC.[3] The future of AC itself is uncertain, because additional clinical trials testing AC seem unlikely.

PERIOPERATIVE IMMUNOTHERAPY

Clinical trials testing perioperative immunotherapy have been gaining momentum as an alternative to cisplatin-based chemotherapy. The potential value is even greater for the large portion of cisplatin-ineligible patients who otherwise would undergo RC alone. Currently approved immunotherapy is restricted to immune checkpoint inhibitors targeting programmed cell death protein 1 (PD-1) and programmed death ligand 1 (PD-L1). Inhibitors of cytotoxic T-lymphocyte–associated protein 4 (CTLA-4) have been tested in trials but have not been approved for UC. These agents have been adopted for routine use in platinum-refractory locally advanced or metastatic UC and in some countries for first-line therapy for cisplatin-ineligible patients with the same disease. Although only approximately 20% of patients demonstrate an objective response to therapy, the response often is durable.

It is natural that immune checkpoint inhibitors have migrated from the metastatic to the perioperative setting and are being evaluated in multiple large RCTs as both neoadjuvant and adjuvant therapies. Neoadjuvant therapy has the theoretic advantage of treating in the presence of abundant tumor antigen, whereas this exposure is dramatically decreased in the adjuvant setting. On the other hand, ineffective therapy in the neoadjuvant context can delay definitive local therapy and lead to worse outcomes in individual patients. There also is the potential for an increased risk of perioperative complications with neoadjuvant therapy, although this has not been observed to date with anti–PD-L1 immunotherapy.[47] These risks are mitigated with adjuvant therapy, which also can be administered in a more precise, risk-adapted manner. On the other hand, surgical complications can prevent the administration of adjuvant therapy.[41]

Neoadjuvant Immunotherapy

Two key single-arm phase 2 trials testing neoadjuvant single-agent immune checkpoint inhibition have been published: PURE-01[48] and ABACUS.[49] In the PURE-01 trial, 114 patients with cT2-4aN0M0 bladder cancer, regardless of cisplatin eligibility, received 3 cycles of 200-mg pembrolizumab every 3 weeks prior to RC. The pCR rate was 37%, and downstaging to non–muscle-invasive tumors ($\leq$ypT1N0M0) was observed in 55% of patients. These numbers are comparable to RCTs testing NAC[9] but reflect a much higher response rate than observed in patients with metastatic disease. In this trial, positive PD-L1 immunohistochemical staining (combined positive score [CPS] $\geq$10%) and high tumor mutational burden were associated with improved outcome. There was some evidence of differential responses based on the presence of different histologic variants.

The ABACUS trial enrolled 95 patients with cT2-4aN0M0 disease who were ineligible for or declined cisplatin-based NAC. After receiving 2 cycles of 1200-mg atezolizumab every 3 weeks prior to RC the pCR rate was 31%.[49] Notably, 8 patients in this trial did not proceed to RC, and in 3 cases this was due to treatment-related adverse events. Extensive exploratory biomarker analysis was conducted in the ABACUS trial, revealing that the presence of preexisting T-cell immunity correlated with increased response rates, but PD-L1 expression and tumor mutational burden were not predictive of response as they were in the PURE-01 trial.

Four additional noncomparative phase 2 trials have reported early results from combination immunotherapy in the neoadjuvant context: NABUCCO,[50] a trial from MDACC,[51] BLASST-1,[52] and Hoosier Cancer Research Network GU14-188.[53] In the NABUCCO trial, 24 patients with either cT3-4aN0-3M0 or cT1-2N1-3M0 UC of the bladder or upper tract who were ineligible for or declined cisplatin-based NAC received 3 cycles of ipilimumab (CTLA-4 inhibitor) and nivolumab (PD-1 inhibitor) prior to RC or nephroureterectomy. To maximize safety, ipilimumab was administered alone in the first cycle and nivolumab was administered alone in the third cycle. The primary endpoint of this trial was feasibility, to ensure that the addition of the CTLA-4 inhibitor ipilimumab did not have a negative impact on delivery of definitive local therapy. Only 1 patient experienced a delay in RC due to a treatment-related adverse event. The pCR rate was 46% and downstaging to non–muscle-invasive disease was observed in 58%. In line with the results of the PURE-01 trial, responses were more common in patients with high PD-L1 expression (CPS $\geq$10%). Furthermore, the appearance of tertiary lymphoid structures by immunofluorescence in the RC specimen after neoadjuvant treatment proved to be a marker of response. These are promising results, especially considering that this was a higher-risk population than either of the 2 preceding trials with single-agent immunotherapy.

The MDACC trial tested a similar neoadjuvant combination of dual checkpoint blockade with tremelimumab (CTLA-4 inhibitor) and durvalumab (PD-L1 inhibitor). The 28 cisplatin-ineligible patients (including 3 patients who declined cisplatin-based chemotherapy) in this trial demonstrated high-risk MIBC features, defined as stage cT3-4, variant histology, lymphovascular invasion and/or hydronephrosis, or high-grade upper tract UC. In the intention-to-treat analysis, the rate of pCR was 31.5% and downstaging to less than or equal to pT1N0 occurred in 50%. Four patients did not undergo RC and 3 experienced a minor delay in surgery, including 2 due to adverse effects of systemic immunotherapy. The response rate in this trial did not correlate to PD-L1 status by immunohistochemistry. In contrast to the NABUCCO trial, tertiary lymphoid structures in pretreatment tumor tissue correlated to response to dual-agent immunotherapy in this trial.

In the BLASST-1 trial, 41 patients with cT2-4aN0-1M0 bladder cancer received 4 cycles of GC and nivolumab every 3 weeks prior to RC.[52] Down-staging to organ confined, non–muscle-invasive disease ($\leq$ypT1N0M0) was the primary endpoint of this trial and was observed in 66% of patients. A pCR defined as pT0 or pTIS occurred in 49%, and no patient experienced a delay in RC due to adverse events. Similar to the BLASST-1 trial, 43 patients in the cisplatin-eligible arm of the GU14-188 trial received 4 cycles of neoadjuvant GC plus 5 cycles of pembrolizumab every 3 weeks prior to RC.[54] Four patients did not undergo RC (3 due to patient choice and 1 due to grade 4 thrombocytopenic purpura, all of whom were alive and free of recurrence after a median of 32 months), and 3 others were not included in the final analysis. Of the 36 who underwent RC, the response was less than or equal to ypT1N0 in 61% and ypT0N0 in 44%.[54] Another similar trial testing GC plus pembrolizumab in cisplatin-eligible patients has finished accrual but has not yet been reported (NCT02690558). In the cisplatin-ineligible arm of GU14-188, gemcitabine (3 weekly doses per 4-week cycle for 3 cycles) plus pembrolizumab (every 3 weeks for 5 cycles) caused downstaging to less than or equal to pT1N0M0 disease in 52% of patients with cT2-4aN0M0 bladder cancer prior to RC.[53] The pCR rate was 45% and 3 patients did not proceed to RC due to disease progression. It is noteworthy that 90% of patients in BLASST-1 but only 46% in both cohorts of GU14-188 had cT2N0M0 disease entering the trial. It is important also in these trials to note the variable proportion of patients who did not proceed to RC.

There are numerous other early-phase trials under way testing neoadjuvant immunotherapy as well as larger prospective RCTs, as reviewed by Sonpavde and colleagues.[55] This field is evolving rapidly and significant shifts in the standard of care can be anticipated in the near future. The trials cited in this article differ with respect to cisplatin eligibility, tumor stage studied, and trial endpoints, which together prevent any meaningful cross-trial comparison. Furthermore, the trials all use pathologic response as an endpoint, which is recognized as a surrogate for OS or disease-specific survival after NAC,[12] but it is not clear if it also is a surrogate after immunotherapy. It, therefore, is impossible to delineate the added benefit of dual immunotherapy or combined chemotherapy and immunotherapy compared with respective monotherapies. Two large phase 3 RCTs testing combined platinum chemotherapy and immunotherapy and 1 phase 3 RCT testing dual immunotherapy in patients with locally advanced or metastatic UC in the first-line setting have reported no benefit of combined therapy,[56–58] suggesting that this combination might not lead to the desired additive or synergistic effects, and perhaps the same patients respond to both treatments. The path forward in the metastatic and perioperative settings, therefore, may be individualized use of 1 or the other based on predictive biomarkers. The trials discussed in this article highlight how important it will be to identify predictive biomarkers for neoadjuvant treatment to enable rational selection of chemotherapy, immunotherapy, or immediate RC or TMT, because use of ineffective treatment could affect curability, and adverse effects could make definitive local therapy impossible.

Adjuvant Immunotherapy

Three large phase 3 RCTs are assessing the efficacy of adjuvant immune checkpoint inhibitors versus placebo or observation after RC in patients with adverse pathologic features, including either pT3-4 and/or nodal involvement in any patient or ypT2 disease in patients who received NAC. The results of CheckMate 274 (NCT02632409), testing nivolumab versus placebo, have been announced as a press release but have not yet been made public. The trial met its coprimary endpoints of progression-free survival in the overall population and in the PD-L1-positive subgroup. The AMBASSADOR trial (NCT03244384), testing pembrolizumab, still is ongoing. IMvigor010 (NCT02450331) has reported no improvement in disease-free survival (final analysis) or OS (interim analysis) in patients receiving atezolizumab compared with those under observation after RC.[46] There are subtle differences in patient inclusion criteria and trial design, so that a verdict on the efficacy of adjuvant immunotherapy will need to await final results of all 3 trials.

An evolving paradigm is the use of combination neoadjuvant chemoimmunotherapy in the sense of induction therapy before RC, followed by adjuvant immunotherapy after RC as maintenance therapy. For instance, the NIAGARA trial is testing the use of neoadjuvant GC plus durvalumab followed by adjuvant durvalumab compared with neoadjuvant GC alone (NCT03732677). Keynote-866 (NCT03924856) is a similar trial with pembrolizumab, and the ENERGIZE trial is evaluating the combination of nivolumab or both nivolumab and linrodostat with GC (NCT03661320). For cisplatin-ineligible patients, 1 trial is comparing neoadjuvant and adjuvant nivolumab with or without bempegaldesleukin (NKTR-214), an interleukin-2 agonist, to RC alone (NCT04209114). Similarly, Keynote-905 is testing the combination of perioperative pembrolizumab plus or minus enfortumab vedotin, an antibody-drug conjugate targeting nectin-4, in cisplatin-ineligible patients undergoing RC. These are just examples of the numerous novel combinations being tested perioperatively in patients with MIBC.

SUMMARY

The ability to define optimal management of MIBC has suffered from a lack of rigorous clinical trial evidence to drive treatment decisions, and adoption of existing evidence into clinical practice has been poor. TMT is rightly experiencing some degree of a renaissance as an alternative to RC in appropriately selected patients, but a randomized trial comparing RC to TMT seems unlikely at this point. The evidence for NAC is clear, and it has been recommended by the guidelines for more than a decade, but its uptake has been slow and incomplete. Treatment of MIBC, however, appears to be on the brink of a major paradigm shift, with unprecedented clinical trial activity in the neoadjuvant and adjuvant disease states. Multiple large phase 3 trials are under way, in addition to numerous smaller trials exploring novel combinations, so that the number of patients currently enrolled in clinical trials vastly supersedes the sum of all clinical trial activity prior to the advent of immunotherapy. This activity has the potential to benefit patients greatly, but recent results from the first-line metastatic setting give grounds for pause, because not all monotherapy and combination therapies have achieved the desired improvement in patient outcomes. Nonetheless, further rigorous testing of established and novel therapies, along with development and testing of predictive biomarkers, is likely to revolutionize the perioperative care of patients with MIBC in the near future.

CLINICS CARE POINTS

- Evidence does not support routine use of perioperative radiation in the treatment of MIBC.
- Neoadjuvant cisplatin-based chemotherapy should be offered to all eligible patients with MIBC.
- Adjuvant cisplatin-based chemotherapy should be considered in eligible patients with adverse pathologic features (pT3/4 and/or pN1-3) after RC.
- There is no role for carboplatin-based chemotherapy in the neoadjuvant or adjuvant setting
- Patients should be offered enrollment in clinical trials whenever possible, especially with combination immunotherapy having demonstrated promising results in early-phase trials.

REFERENCES

1. Kulkarni GS, Hermanns T, Wei Y, et al. Propensity score analysis of radical cystectomy versus bladder-sparing trimodal therapy in the setting of a multidisciplinary bladder cancer clinic. J Clin Oncol 2017;35(20):2299–305.
2. Mari A, Campi R, Tellini R, et al. Patterns and predictors of recurrence after open radical cystectomy for bladder cancer: a comprehensive review of the literature. World J Urol 2018;36(2):157–70.
3. Leow JJ, Martin-Doyle W, Rajagopal PS, et al. Adjuvant chemotherapy for invasive bladder cancer: a 2013 updated systematic review and meta-analysis of randomized trials. Eur Urol 2014;66(1):42–54.
4. Advanced Bladder Cancer Meta-analysis Collaboration. Neoadjuvant chemotherapy in invasive bladder cancer: update of a systematic review and meta-analysis of individual patient data advanced bladder cancer (ABC) meta-analysis collaboration. Eur Urol 2005;48(2):202–5 [discussion 5–6].
5. Smith JA Jr, Crawford ED, Paradelo JC, et al. Treatment of advanced bladder cancer with combined preoperative irradiation and radical cystectomy versus

radical cystectomy alone: a phase III intergroup study. J Urol 1997;157(3):805–7 [discussion: 7–8].

6. Huncharek M, Muscat J, Geschwind JF. Planned preoperative radiation therapy in muscle invasive bladder cancer; results of a meta-analysis. Anticancer Res 1998;18(3B):1931–4.

7. Zaghloul MS, Awwad HK, Akoush HH, et al. Postoperative radiotherapy of carcinoma in bilharzial bladder: improved disease free survival through improving local control. Int J Radiat Oncol Biol Phys 1992;23(3):511–7.

8. Zaghloul MS, Christodouleas JP, Smith A, et al. Adjuvant sandwich chemotherapy plus radiotherapy vs adjuvant chemotherapy alone for locally advanced bladder cancer after radical cystectomy: a randomized phase 2 trial. JAMA Surg 2018; 153(1):e174591.

9. Grossman HB, Natale RB, Tangen CM, et al. Neoadjuvant chemotherapy plus cystectomy compared with cystectomy alone for locally advanced bladder cancer. N Engl J Med 2003;349(9):859–66.

10. Griffiths G, Hall R, Sylvester R, et al. International phase III trial assessing neoadjuvant cisplatin, methotrexate, and vinblastine chemotherapy for muscle-invasive bladder cancer: long-term results of the BA06 30894 trial. J Clin Oncol 2011; 29(16):2171–7.

11. Sonpavde G, Goldman BH, Speights VO, et al. Quality of pathologic response and surgery correlate with survival for patients with completely resected bladder cancer after neoadjuvant chemotherapy. Cancer 2009;115(18):4104–9.

12. Zargar H, Zargar-Shoshtari K, Lotan Y, et al. Final Pathological Stage after Neoadjuvant Chemotherapy and Radical Cystectomy for Bladder Cancer-Does pT0 Predict Better Survival than pTa/Tis/T1? J Urol 2016;195(4 Pt 1):886–93.

13. Kulkarni GS, Black PC, Sridhar SS, et al. Canadian Urological Association guideline: Muscle-invasive bladder cancer. Can Urol Assoc J 2019;13:230–8.

14. Witjes JA, Bruins HM, Cathomas R, et al. European Association of Urology guidelines on muscle-invasive and metastatic bladder cancer: summary of the 2020 guidelines. Eur Urol 2020;79(1):82–104.

15. Zargar H, Shah JB, van Rhijn BW, et al. Neoadjuvant Dose Dense MVAC versus Gemcitabine and Cisplatin in Patients with cT3-4aN0M0 bladder cancer treated with radical cystectomy. J Urol 2018;199(6):1452–8.

16. Galsky MD, Pal SK, Chowdhury S, et al. Comparative effectiveness of gemcitabine plus cisplatin versus methotrexate, vinblastine, doxorubicin, plus cisplatin as neoadjuvant therapy for muscle-invasive bladder cancer. Cancer 2015; 121(15):2586–93.

17. von der Maase H, Sengelov L, Roberts JT, et al. Long-term survival results of a randomized trial comparing gemcitabine plus cisplatin, with methotrexate, vinblastine, doxorubicin, plus cisplatin in patients with bladder cancer. J Clin Oncol 2005;23(21):4602–8.

18. Sternberg CN, de Mulder PH, Schornagel JH, et al. Randomized phase III trial of high-dose-intensity methotrexate, vinblastine, doxorubicin, and cisplatin (MVAC) chemotherapy and recombinant human granulocyte colony-stimulating factor versus classic MVAC in advanced urothelial tract tumors: European Organization for Research and Treatment of Cancer Protocol no. 30924. J Clin Oncol 2001; 19(10):2638–46.

19. Zargar H, Shah JB, van de Putte EEF, et al. Dose dense MVAC prior to radical cystectomy: a real-world experience. World J Urol 2017;35(11):1729–36.

20. Culine S, Gravis G, Flechon A, et al. Randomized phase III trial of dose-dense methotrexate, vinblastine, doxorubicin, and cisplatin (dd-MVAC) or gemcitabine

and cisplatin (GC) as perioperative chemotherapy for muscle invasive urothelial bladder cancer (MIUBC): Preliminary results of the GETUG/AFU V05 VESPER trial on toxicity and pathological responses. J Clin Oncol 2020;38(6_suppl):437.

21. Galsky MD, Chen GJ, Oh WK, et al. Comparative effectiveness of cisplatin-based and carboplatin-based chemotherapy for treatment of advanced urothelial carcinoma. Ann Oncol 2012;23(2):406–10.

22. Zargar H, Espiritu PN, Fairey AS, et al. Multicenter assessment of neoadjuvant chemotherapy for muscle-invasive bladder cancer. Eur Urol 2015;67(2):241–9.

23. Black AJ, Black PC. Variant histology in bladder cancer: diagnostic and clinical implications. Translational Cancer Res 2020;9(10):6565–657.

24. Moretto P, Wood L, Emmenegger U, et al. Management of small cell carcinoma of the bladder: Consensus guidelines from the Canadian Association of Genitourinary Medical Oncologists (CAGMO). Can Urol Assoc J 2013;7(1–2):E44–56.

25. Witjes JA, Babjuk M, Bellmunt J, et al. EAU-ESMO consensus statements on the management of advanced and variant bladder cancer-an international collaborative multistakeholder effort(dagger): under the auspices of the EAU-ESMO Guidelines Committees. Eur Urol 2020;77(2):223–50.

26. Scosyrev E, Ely BW, Messing EM, et al. Do mixed histological features affect survival benefit from neoadjuvant platinum-based combination chemotherapy in patients with locally advanced bladder cancer? A secondary analysis of Southwest Oncology Group-Directed Intergroup Study (S8710). BJU Int 2011;108(5):693–9.

27. Seiler R, Ashab HAD, Erho N, et al. Impact of molecular subtypes in muscle-invasive bladder cancer on predicting response and survival after neoadjuvant chemotherapy. Eur Urol 2017;72(4):544–54.

28. Lerner SP, Svatek RS. What is the standard of care for pelvic lymphadenectomy performed at the time of radical cystectomy? Eur Urol 2019;75(4):612–4.

29. Karim S, Mackillop WJ, Brennan K, et al. Estimating the optimal perioperative chemotherapy utilization rate for muscle-invasive bladder cancer. Cancer Med 2019;8(14):6258–71.

30. Duplisea JJ, Mason RJ, Reichard CA, et al. Trends and disparities in the use of neoadjuvant chemotherapy for muscle-invasive urothelial carcinoma. Can Urol Assoc J 2019;13(2):24–8.

31. Cowan NG, Chen Y, Downs TM, et al. Neoadjuvant chemotherapy use in bladder cancer: a survey of current practice and opinions. Adv Urol 2014;2014:746298.

32. Culp SH, Dickstein RJ, Grossman HB, et al. Refining patient selection for neoadjuvant chemotherapy before radical cystectomy. J Urol 2014;191(1):40–7.

33. Choi W, Porten S, Kim S, et al. Identification of distinct basal and luminal subtypes of muscle-invasive bladder cancer with different sensitivities to frontline chemotherapy. Cancer Cell 2014;25(2):152–65.

34. Lotan Y, Boorjian SA, Zhang J, et al. Molecular subtyping of clinically localized urothelial carcinoma reveals lower rates of pathological upstaging at radical cystectomy among luminal tumors. Eur Urol 2019;76(2):200–6.

35. Flaig TW, Tangen CM, Daneshmand S, et al. SWOG S1314: A randomized phase II study of co-expression extrapolation (COXEN) with neoadjuvant chemotherapy for localized, muscle-invasive bladder cancer. J Clin Oncol 2019;37(15_suppl):4506.

36. Van Allen EM, Mouw KW, Kim P, et al. Somatic ERCC2 mutations correlate with cisplatin sensitivity in muscle-invasive urothelial carcinoma. Cancer Discov 2014;4(10):1140–53.

37. Liu D, Plimack ER, Hoffman-Censits J, et al. Clinical Validation of Chemotherapy Response Biomarker ERCC2 in Muscle-Invasive Urothelial Bladder Carcinoma. JAMA Oncol 2016;2(8):1094–6.
38. Plimack ER, Dunbrack RL, Brennan TA, et al. Defects in DNA repair genes predict response to neoadjuvant cisplatin-based chemotherapy in muscle-invasive bladder cancer. Eur Urol 2015;68(6):959–67.
39. Sternberg CN, Skoneczna I, Kerst JM, et al. Immediate versus deferred chemotherapy after radical cystectomy in patients with pT3-pT4 or N+ M0 urothelial carcinoma of the bladder (EORTC 30994): an intergroup, open-label, randomised phase 3 trial. Lancet Oncol 2015;16(1):76–86.
40. Stockle M, Meyenburg W, Wellek S, et al. Adjuvant polychemotherapy of nonorgan-confined bladder cancer after radical cystectomy revisited: long-term results of a controlled prospective study and further clinical experience. J Urol 1995;153(1):47–52.
41. Millikan R, Dinney C, Swanson D, et al. Integrated therapy for locally advanced bladder cancer: final report of a randomized trial of cystectomy plus adjuvant M-VAC versus cystectomy with both preoperative and postoperative M-VAC. J Clin Oncol 2001;19(20):4005–13.
42. Esrig D, Elmajian D, Groshen S, et al. Accumulation of Nuclear p53 and Tumor Progression in Bladder Cancer. N Engl J Med 1994;331(19):1259–64.
43. Cote RJ, Esrig D, Groshen S, et al. p53 and treatment of bladder cancer. Nature 1997;385(6612):123–5.
44. Stadler WM, Lerner SP, Groshen S, et al. Phase III study of molecularly targeted adjuvant therapy in locally advanced urothelial cancer of the bladder based on p53 status. J Clin Oncol 2011;29(25):3443–9.
45. Malats N, Bustos A, Nascimento CM, et al. P53 as a prognostic marker for bladder cancer: a meta-analysis and review. Lancet Oncol 2005;6(9):678–86.
46. Hussain MHA, Powles T, Albers P, et al. IMvigor010: Primary analysis from a phase III randomized study of adjuvant atezolizumab (atezo) versus observation (obs) in high-risk muscle-invasive urothelial carcinoma (MIUC). J Clin Oncol 2020;38(15_suppl):5000.
47. Briganti A, Gandaglia G, Scuderi S, et al. Surgical safety of radical cystectomy and pelvic lymph node dissection following neoadjuvant pembrolizumab in patients with bladder cancer: prospective assessment of perioperative outcomes from the PURE-01 Trial. Eur Urol 2020;77(5):576–80.
48. Necchi A, Raggi D, Gallina A, et al. Updated Results of PURE-01 with Preliminary Activity of Neoadjuvant Pembrolizumab in Patients with Muscle-invasive Bladder Carcinoma with Variant Histologies. Eur Urol 2020;77(4):439–46.
49. Powles T, Kockx M, Rodriguez-Vida A, et al. Clinical efficacy and biomarker analysis of neoadjuvant atezolizumab in operable urothelial carcinoma in the ABACUS trial. Nat Med 2019;25(11):1706–14.
50. van Dijk N, Gil-Jimenez A, Silina K, et al. Preoperative ipilimumab plus nivolumab in locoregionally advanced urothelial cancer: the NABUCCO trial. Nat Med 2020;26(12):1839–44.
51. Gao J, Navai N, Alhalabi O, et al. Neoadjuvant PD-L1 plus CTLA-4 blockade in patients with cisplatin-ineligible operable high-risk urothelial carcinoma. Nat Med 2020;26(12):1845–51.
52. Gupta S, Sonpavde G, Weight CJ, et al. Results from BLASST-1 (Bladder Cancer Signal Seeking Trial) of nivolumab, gemcitabine, and cisplatin in muscle invasive bladder cancer (MIBC) undergoing cystectomy. J Clin Oncol 2020;38(6_suppl):439.

53. Kaimakliotis HZ, Adra N, Kelly WK, et al. Phase II neoadjuvant (N-) gemcitabine (G) and pembrolizumab (P) for locally advanced urothelial cancer (laUC): Interim results from the cisplatin (C)-ineligible cohort of GU14-188. J Clin Oncol 2020; 38(15_suppl):5019.
54. Hoimes CJ, Adra N, Fleming MT, et al. Phase Ib/II neoadjuvant (N-) pembrolizumab (P) and chemotherapy for locally advanced urothelial cancer (laUC): Final results from the cisplatin (C)- eligible cohort of HCRN GU14-188. J Clin Oncol 2020;38(15_suppl):5047.
55. Sonpavde G, Necchi A, Gupta S, et al. ENERGIZE: a Phase III study of neoadjuvant chemotherapy alone or with nivolumab with/without linrodostat mesylate for muscle-invasive bladder cancer. Future Oncol 2020;16(2):4359–68.
56. Galsky MD, Arija JÁ A, Bamias A, et al. Atezolizumab with or without chemotherapy in metastatic urothelial cancer (IMvigor130): a multicentre, randomised, placebo-controlled phase 3 trial. Lancet 2020;395(10236):1547–57.
57. Available at: https://www.astrazeneca.com/media-centre/press-releases/2020/update-on-phase-iii-danube-trial-for-imfinzi-and-tremelimumab-in-unresectable-stage-iv-bladder-cancer-06032020.html. Accessed July 1, 2020.
58. Available at: https://www.merck.com/news/merck-provides-update-on-phase-3-keynote-361-trial-evaluating-keytruda-pembrolizumab-as-monotherapy-and-in-combination-with-chemotherapy-in-patients-with-advanced-or-metastatic-urothelial-carc/. Accessed July 1, 2020.
59. Prout GR Jr, Slack NH, Bross ID. Preoperative irradiation as an adjuvant in the surgical management of invasive bladder carcinoma. J Urol 1971;105(2):223–31.
60. Blackard CE, Byar DP. Results of a clinical trial of surgery and radiation in stages II and 3 carcinoma of the bladder. J Urol 1972;108(6):875–8.
61. Ghoneim MA, Ashamallah AK, Awaad HK, et al. Randomized trial of cystectomy with or without preoperative radiotherapy for carcinoma of the bilharzial bladder. J Urol 1985;134(2):266–8.
62. Anderström C, Johansson S, Nilsson S, et al. A prospective randomized study of preoperative irradiation with cystectomy or cystectomy alone for invasive bladder carcinoma. Eur Urol 1983;9(3):142–7.
63. Zaghloul MS, Awwad HK, Akoush H, et al. Postoperative radiotherapy of carcinoma in bilharzial bladder. Improved disease-free survival through improving local control. Int J Radiat Oncol Biol Phys 1992;19:200.
64. El-Monim HA, El-Baradie MM, Younis A, et al. A prospective randomized trial for postoperative vs. preoperative adjuvant radiotherapy for muscle-invasive bladder cancer. Urol Oncol 2013;31(3):359–65.
65. Bassi P, Pappagallo GL, Sperandio P, et al. Neoadjuvant M-VAC chemotherapy of invasive bladder cancer: results of a multicenter phase III trial. J Urol 1999; 161(4S).
66. Sengeløv L, Maase HVD, Lundbeck F, et al. Neoadjuvant chemotherapy with cisplatin and methotrexate in patients with muscle-invasive bladder tumours. Acta Oncologica 2002;41(5):447–56.
67. Sherif A, Holmberg L, Rintala E, et al. Neoadjuvant cisplatinum based combination chemotherapy in patients with invasive bladder cancer: a combined analysis of two nordic studies. Eur Urol 2004;45(3):297–303.
68. Khaled HM, Shafik HE, Zabhloul MS, et al. Gemcitabine and cisplatin as neoadjuvant chemotherapy for invasive transitional and squamous cell carcinoma of the bladder: effect on survival and bladder preservation. Clin Genitourinary Cancer 2014;12(5):e233–40.

69. Kitamura H, Tsukamoto T, Shibata T, et al. Randomised phase III study of neoadjuvant chemotherapy with methotrexate, doxorubicin, vinblastine and cisplatin followed by radical cystectomy compared with radical cystectomy alone for muscle-invasive bladder cancer: Japan Clinical Oncology Group Study JCOG0209. Ann Oncol 2014;25(6):1192–8.
70. Osman MA, Gabr AM, Elkady MS. Neoadjuvant chemotherapy versus cystectomy in management of stages II, and III urinary bladder cancer. Arch Ital Urol Androl 2014;86(4):278–83.
71. Skinner DG, Daniels JR, Russell CA, et al. The role of adjuvant chemotherapy following cystectomy for invasive bladder cancer: a prospective comparative trial. J Urol 1991;145(3):459–64.
72. Studer UE, Bacchi M, Biedermann C, et al. Adjuvant cisplatin chemotherapy following cystectomy for bladder cancer: results of a prospective randomized trial. J Urol 1994;152(1):81–4.
73. Freiha F, Reese J, Torti FM. A randomized trial of radical cystectomy versus radical cystectomy plus cisplatin, vinblastine and methotrexate chemotherapy for muscle invasive bladder cancer. J Urol 1996;155(2):495–500.
74. Bono A. Adjuvant chemotherapy in locally advanced bladder cancer: final analysis of a controlled multicentre study. Acta Urol Ital 1997;11:5–8.
75. Otto T, Goebell PJ, Rübben H. Perioperative chemotherapy in advanced bladder cancer - part ii: adjuvant treatment. Onkologie 2003;26(5):484–8.
76. Lehmann J, Franzaring L, Thüroff J, et al. Complete long-term survival data from a trial of adjuvant chemotherapy vs control after radical cystectomy for locally advanced bladder cancer. BJU Int 2006;97(1):42–7.
77. Paz-Ares L, Solsona E, Esteban E, et al. Randomized phase III trial comparing adjuvant paclitaxel/gemcitabine/cisplatin (PGC) to observation in patients with resected invasive bladder cancer: Results of the Spanish Oncology Genitourinary Group (SOGUG) 99/01 study. J Clin Oncol 2010;28(18_suppl):LBA4518.
78. Cognetti F, Ruggeri EM, Felici A, et al. Adjuvant chemotherapy with cisplatin and gemcitabine versus chemotherapy at relapse in patients with muscle-invasive bladder cancer submitted to radical cystectomy: an Italian, multicenter, randomized phase III trial. Ann Oncol 2012;23(3):695–700.

Current Therapy and Emerging Intravesical Agents to Treat Non–Muscle Invasive Bladder Cancer

Kelly K. Bree, MD, Nathan A. Brooks, MD, Ashish M. Kamat, MD*

KEYWORDS

- Non–muscle invasive bladder cancer • BCG naive • BCG failure
- Intravesical therapy

KEY POINTS

- A well-performed transurethral resection of bladder tumor (TURBT), ideally with optical enhanced cystoscopy, and diligent evaluation of pathology is the key first step in appropriate management of patients with non–muscle invasive bladder cancer (NMIBC).
- Intravesical treatment of NMIBC should be based on risk stratification; patients with low-grade tumors should receive a single postoperative intravesical chemotherapy, patients with high-grade, high-risk disease should undergo intravesical immunotherapy with BCG induction and maintenance.
- In patients who develop high-grade recurrence following BCG therapy who qualify as having BCG unresponsive disease, radical cystectomy has long remained the gold standard.
- Pembrolizumab was approved by the FDA in 2020 for BCG unresponsive CIS with or without papillary disease in those patients who refuse or are ineligible for radical cystectomy. Valrubicin is also approved in the BCG failure setting, and other agents, such as nadofaragene firadenovec, vicinium, and hyperthermic chemotherapy, are in various phases of the registration/approval process.
- Off-label combination intravesical chemotherapy (eg, with gemcitabine/docetaxel) is a viable alternative for some patients.

INTRODUCTION
Diagnosis

Non–muscle invasive bladder cancer (NMIBC) comprises approximately 75% of new bladder cancer cases diagnosed in the United States annually.[1] The most common presenting symptom of NMIBC is hematuria, either gross or microscopic. Irritative voiding symptoms in the absence of urinary tract infection may be seen with

Department of Urology, The University of Texas MD Anderson Cancer Center, 1515 Holcombe Boulevard, Houston, TX 77030, USA
* Corresponding author.
E-mail address: AKamat@MDAnderson.org

Hematol Oncol Clin N Am 35 (2021) 513–529
https://doi.org/10.1016/j.hoc.2021.02.003
0889-8588/21/© 2021 Elsevier Inc. All rights reserved.

carcinoma *in situ* (CIS). Diagnosis is confirmed via direct visualization with cystoscopy and endoscopic excision via transurethral resection of bladder tumor (TURBT). The entire bladder and urethra must be examined with careful documentation of size, location, and number of lesions or mucosal abnormalities. Initial evaluation should also include imaging of the upper urinary tract. If pathology demonstrates T1 disease and/or there was incomplete initial resection, repeat TURBT should be performed of the primary tumor site. Repeat resection should also be considered in those with high-risk, high-grade Ta tumors (>3 cm or multifocal).

Risk Stratification

Current guidelines recommend risk stratification at the time of each occurrence or recurrence. Both the American Urologic Association (AUA) and the European Association of Urology (EAU) have included risk stratification paradigms in their current guidelines (**Table 1**). Although there are some similarities between the two risk stratification systems, the EAU system is the more widely used given the clear demarcation of high-grade tumors as high risk and all low-grade tumors as low risk. The EAU intermediate-risk category is comprised of any tumors not meeting high- or low-risk criteria; conversely, the AUA intermediate-risk guidelines includes high-grade Ta

Table 1
NMIBC risk stratification

	Low Risk	Intermediate Risk	High Risk
AUA	LG solitary Ta ≤3 cm PUNLMP	Recurrence within 1 y, LG Ta LG solitary Ta >3 cm LG multifocal Ta HG Ta ≤3 cm LG T1	HG T1 Any recurrent, HG Ta HG Ta >3 cm or multifocal Any CIS Any BCG failure in HG case Any variant histology Any LVI Any HG prostatic urethral involvement
EAU	Primary, solitary tumor TaG1 (PUNLMP, LG) Tumor <3 cm No CIS	All tumors not meeting criteria for low or high risk	T1 tumor G3 (HG) tumor Any CIS Multiple, recurrent, and large (>3 cm) Ta (G1 or G2); all features must be present Highest risk tumors: HG T1 with concurrent CIS Multiple and/or large HG T1 Recurrent HG T1 HG T1 with CIS in prostatic urethra Some forms of variant histology LVI

Abbreviations: BCG, bacillus Calmette-Guérin; HG, high grade; LG, low grade; LVI, lymphovascular invasion; PUNLMP, papillary urothelial neoplasm of low malignant potential.

Adapted from Chang SS, Boorjian SA, Chou R et al. Diagnosis and treatment of non-muscle invasive bladder cancer: AUA/SUO guideline. J Urol 2016;196(4): 1021 to 1029 and Babjuk M, Burger M, Compérat EM, et al. European Association of Urology Guidelines on Non-muscle invasive bladder cancer (Ta T1 and carcinoma in situ) – 2019 update. Eur Urol 2019;76(5):639 to 657; with permission.

tumors. Primary high-grade Ta tumors are rare and demonstrate marked heterogenicity; however, they have a significant risk of recurrence, with increased progression if this occurs within the first year, irrespective of tumor size or multifocality.[2] This risk is mitigated with the administration of bacillus Calmette-Guérin (BCG) and highlights that this subset of high-grade tumors may best be categorized with their other high-grade counterparts as in the EAU guidelines.

RISK-ADOPTED INTRAVESICAL THERAPY (BACILLUS CALMETTE-GUÉRIN NAIVE)
Low-Risk Non–Muscle Invasive Bladder Cancer

The AUA/Society of Urologic Oncology, EAU, and the National Comprehensive Cancer Network advocate for the use of a single postoperative dose of intravesical chemotherapy within 24 hours of TURBT to prevent tumor cell implantation and early recurrence.[3,4] This installation is contraindicated in patients in whom overt or suspected bladder perforation is present. Single-dose adjuvant chemotherapy provides an absolute risk reduction in tumor recurrence of 15%, however without altering time to progression or death.[5] Phase III randomized trials have reported reduced recurrence rates in patients with suspected NMIBC receiving gemcitabine and mitomycin C,[6,7] and as such these two agents remain the most widely used in the United States. Per National Comprehensive Cancer Network guidelines, gemcitabine is currently the preferred agent for single-dose postoperative intravesical therapy given its more favorable side effect profile and lower cost. Decision for further adjuvant therapy should be individualized based on patient prognosis. For those at low risk of recurrence, single postoperative intravesical therapy is likely satisfactory. Single installation of epirubicin after transurethral resection has also been shown in a randomized trial by Gudjonsson and colleagues[8] to reduce the likelihood of tumor recurrence, primarily in patients with small, low-risk tumors; however, this agent is not currently available in the United States. In addition to the standard adjuvant intravesical therapy, mitomycin C is also being explored as a chemoablative agent in a phase IV trial (NCT03348969) and results are forthcoming.

Intermediate-Risk Non–Muscle Invasive Bladder Cancer

Intermediate-risk disease comprises a heterogenous group of patients with NMIBC. To simplify the cumbersome criteria of other risk-stratification symptoms, the International Bladder Cancer Group (IBCG) defines intermediate-risk disease as those with multiple and/or recurrent low-grade Ta tumors.[9] Furthermore, the IBCG created an algorithm to assist in selection of adjuvant intravesical therapy and duration based on four risk factors: (1) tumor multifocality, (2) tumor size greater than 3 cm, (3) early recurrence (<1 year), and (4) frequent recurrences (>1 per year). In patients with intermediate-risk NMIBC, clinicians should consider administration of a 6-week course of induction intravesical chemotherapy or immunotherapy. Intravesical therapy with BCG, mitomycin C, doxorubicin, or epirubicin has been shown to be more effective at reducing bladder cancer recurrence than no intravesical therapy, with BCG and mitomycin C being superior to the other agents.[10] Additionally, among intermediate-risk patients, a systematic review found gemcitabine to be equally efficacious to BCG in prevention of recurrence and progression.[11] Given the heterogenicity of the intermediate-risk NMIBC population, clinicians should consider the adverse events associated with BCG when selecting between BCG and intravesical chemotherapy. In those patients who completely respond to induction chemotherapy therapy (defined as a normal cystoscopy and cytology and negative biopsy if performed), maintenance therapy is considered but the frequency and benefit remain controversial. Commonly used regimens include monthly maintenance treatment for 6 to 12 months. In patients who completely respond to induction BCG, clinicians can consider 1 year of maintenance therapy, as tolerated.

High-Risk Non–Muscle Invasive Bladder Cancer

Unlike low- and intermediate-risk NMIBC, progression (but not necessarily recurrence) rates are much higher in the high-risk population. Multiple meta-analyses have documented the superiority of BCG to TURBT alone or TURBT and intravesical chemotherapy.[10] Initial induction BCG therapy is typically given once a week for 6 weeks with reassessment performed 12 weeks after initiation of treatment.[12] Several meta-analyses demonstrate superiority of BCG to intravesical chemotherapy in preventing recurrence and progression in those receiving maintenance therapy.[13,14] All guidelines recommend the use of maintenance therapy in high-risk patients with the Southwest Oncology Group (SWOG) 8507 dose schedule being the most widely used.[15] The regimen consists of weekly BCG induction for 6 weeks followed by 3 weekly instillations at months 3 and 6, and then every 6 months for up to 3 years. The efficacy of this regimen has been confirmed by the EORTC randomized trial, which demonstrated reduced recurrence (hazard ratio [HR], 1.61; 95% confidence interval [CI], 1.13–2.30, $P = .009$) when full dose maintenance was administered for 3 years.[16] These data are further corroborated by meta-analyses demonstrating the superiority of BCG to intravesical chemotherapy when maintenance therapy was administered.[17,18] Especially considering the global BCG shortage, alternative treatments options are of paramount importance. A phase III trial (NCT03031660) of an alternate strain of BCG (Tokyo-172) with and without intradermal priming is currently being investigated.

Select patients with highest risk features may benefit from initial radical cystectomy (RC) rather than delayed treatment with intravesical agents. The EAU guidelines clearly delineate selected patients at highest risk and most likely to benefit from RC including: high-grade T1 with concurrent CIS, multiple and/or large high-grade T1, recurrent high-grade T1, high-grade T1 with CIS in the prostatic urethra, some forms of variant histology, and the presence of lymphovascular invasion.[4] Pathologic upstaging can occur in up to 50% of T1 patients at the time of cystectomy[19] and it remains unclear if intravesical therapy alters progression in these highest risk patients. Thus, despite the significant morbidity associated with RC it remains an important treatment option for select patients.

For a summary of suggested risk-stratified intravesical therapies see **Table 2**.

Future Directions

There are a multitude of clinical trials currently exploring alternative treatments for BCG-naive disease (**Table 3**).

Table 2			
Summary of suggested intravesical treatments according to risk category			
	Risk Category		
Treatments	Low	Intermediate	High
Single postoperative intravesical instillation of chemotherapeutic	Yes Agent: gemcitabine or mitomycin C	Yes Agent: gemcitabine or mitomycin C	No benefit
Induction intravesical therapy		Yes Agent: BCG or chemotherapy	Yes Agent: BCG
Maintenance intravesical therapy		Can be considered Duration: 6–12 mo	Yes Duration: 3 y

Table 3
Current clinical trials for patients with BCG-naive NMIBC registered on clinicaltrials.gov

Agent	Study Type	Study Design	Prior Intravesical Therapy	Study Population	Investigator	Study ID
Alt-803	Ib	Randomized Arm A: ALT-803 + BCG Arm B: BCG	No prior BCG	HG Ta/T1 or CIS	Altor BioScience	NCT02138734
eRapa	II	Randomized Arm A: eRapa Arm B: placebo	No prior BCG	Ta, Tis, or T1	Rapamycin Holdings, Inc	NCT04375813
Pembrolizumab	II	Nonrandomized, single arm	No prior BCG	HG T1	Memorial Sloan Kettering	NCT03504163
Gemcitabine/docetaxel	II	Nonrandomized, single arm	No prior BCG	Intermediate or high risk	Sidney Kimmel Comprehensive Cancer Center at Johns Hopkins	NCT04386746
Atezolizumab	III	Randomized Arm A: BCG Arm B: BCG + atezolizumab	No prior BCG	High risk	UNICANCER	NCT03799835
Mitomycin C	III	Randomized Arm A: mitomycin C + BCG Arm B: BCG	No prior BCG	HG Ta or any T1 disease	University of Sydney	NCT02948543
Apaziquone	III	Randomized Arm A: apaziquone+ placebo Arm B: apaziquone x2 Arm C: placebo x2	No prior BCG	Ta, G1-2	Spectrum Pharmaceuticals, Inc	NCT02563561
Tokyo-172 strain BCG ± priming	III	Randomized Arm A: TICE BCG Arm B: Tokyo-172 BCG Arm C: Tokyo-172 BCG + priming	No prior BCG	HG Ta, T1, or CIS	Southwest Oncology Group	NCT03091660
Atezolizumab	Ib	Nonrandomized, single arm Arm A: atezolizumab + BCG	BCG-naive or no BCG within last 3 y	High risk	Fundacion Oncosur	NCT04134000

(continued on next page)

Table 3
(continued)

Agent	Study Type	Study Design	Study Population	Prior Intravesical Therapy	Investigator	Study ID
Durvalumab	III	Randomized Arm A: durvalumab + BCG (induction + maintenance) Arm B: durvalumab + BCG (induction only) Arm C: BCG	High risk	BCG-naive or no BCG within last 3 y	AstraZeneca	NCT03528694
UGN-102	IIb	Nonrandomized, single arm	LG Ta at intermediate risk for recurrence	BCG-naive or no BCG within last 2 y	UrogGen Pharma, Ltd	NCT03358503
PF-06801591	III	Randomized Arm A: PF-06801591 + BCG (induction + maintenance) Arm B: PF-06801591 + BCG (induction only) Arm C: BCG (induction + maintenance)	High risk	BCG-naive or no BCG within last 2 y	Pfizer	NCT04165317
Chemoresection with mitomycin C	IV	Randomized Arm A: neoadjuvant mitomycin C Arm B: adjuvant mitomycin C	LG or HG Ta	BCG-naive or no BCG within last 2 y	Jorgen Bjerggard Jensen	NCT03348969
Ty21	I	Nonrandomized, single arm	Low or intermediate risk	Not discussed	University of Lausanne Hospitals	NCT03421236
Pemigatinib	II	Nonrandomized, single arm	Recurrent low or intermediate risk	Not discussed	Sidney Kimmel Comprehensive Cancer Center at Johns Hopkins	NCT03914794
TMX-101	II	Nonrandomized, single arm	CIS	Not discussed	Telormedix SA	NCT01731652
Epirubicin	IV	Randomized Arm A: epirubicin Arm B: control	Intermediate and high risk	Not discussed	Mansoura University	NCT02214602

Abbreviations: Alt-803, interleukin-15 superagonist; eRapa, encapsulated rapamycin; PF-06801591, sasanlimab; TMX-101, vesimune; Ty21, typhoid vaccine; UGN-102, mitomycin.

INTRAVESICAL THERAPIES FOR NON–MUSCLE INVASIVE BLADDER CANCER FOLLOWING BACILLUS CALMETTE-GUÉRIN FAILURE
Background

Although a significant proportion of patients with CIS (more than 80%) achieve a complete response (CR) with BCG,[15] only about 50% maintain a durable response.[20] In general, most advocate for RC in such patients; however, the usage rates for RC in this patient population in the United States remains low, such that only about 6% of patients with NMIBC undergo RC every year.[21] Because the rate of failure for BCG far outpaces the rate of RC, there is a large demand for alternative therapies to prevent recurrence and progression for patients with NMIBC. Early research in this area has been conducted in largely retrospective or phase I/II trials with small patient cohorts and has been plagued by varying definitions of disease risk and recurrence. Multiple agents have been evaluated for which a complete summary is beyond the scope of this article outlining current and emerging intravesical therapies. A list of historic intravesical therapies for NMIBC after BCG failure is provided in **Table 4**.

Definitions

To address issues of heterogeneity in the BCG lexicon, in 2016, the IBCG proposed a standard classification system for recurrence after BCG (BCG failure) to guide clinical trial enrollment and to allow for intertrial comparison. This system encompasses four domains including BCG intolerant, relapsing, refractory, and unresponsive disease[26] and has been adopted by the EAU in their most recent guidelines (summarized in **Table 5**). The AUA/Society of Urologic Oncology and EAU have adopted guidelines for recurrence after BCG therapy (see **Table 5**).[3,4] The Food and Drug Administration (FDA) has also adapted the BCG-unresponsive definition (from the IBCG and the GU ASCO Groups[27]) for the purposes of inclusion into single-arm clinical trials.[28] In addition, FDA guidance has allowed for these single-arm trials to investigate novel therapies for patient with NMIBC and BCG-failure for which CR to therapy may be selected as the primary end point. CR is defined as either negative cystoscopy and cytology or biopsy-confirmed low-grade or benign recurrence.[27] This standardized system has allowed for a surge in ongoing trials to address the unmet needs in this field.

Repeat Bacillus Calmette-Guérin Therapy

The response rate of patients with CIS to induction BCG is in the range of 50%. However, 60% respond to an additional maintenance course, which is why the BCG unresponsive definition involves assessment after adequate BCG, defined as at least

Table 4	
Historic intravesical therapies for NMIBC after BCG failure	
Agent Name	
Mitomycin C	Docetaxel
Thermo or electromotive chemotherapy	Paclitaxel-hyaluronic acid
Valrubicin[a]	Gemcitabine with mitomycin C
Vicinium	Mycobacterium cell wall
Gemcitabine	BCG with interferon
Nab-paclitaxel	Photodynamic therapy

[a] Valrubicin is FDA approved for the treatment of CIS after BCG failure with a 2-year CR rate of 4%. For a more detailed discussion of these agents, see References[22-25].

Table 5
Comparison of AUA and EAU guidelines for the classification and management of BCG failure

	AUA	EAU
Immediate cystectomy	Initial therapy for patients with persistent T1HG on resection TUR, CIS, LVI, or variant histology Offer to a patient fit for surgery with T1HG after a single course of intravesical BCG	Initial therapy for those at high risk of progression Any BCG unresponsive tumor
Bladder sparing	Options for patients with intermediate or high risk NMIBC after completion of adequate BCG who are unfit or unwilling to undergo cystectomy: Clinical trial Intravesical therapy Systemic immunotherapy	Option for patients with BCG unresponsive tumors who are not candidates for RC and includes: Intravesical therapy Systemic therapy Clinical trial
Additional BCG course	Offer second BCG course for patients with CIS or TaHG after a single intravesical course of BCG Do not offer a third BCG course for: BCG intolerance Recurrent HG disease within 6 mo of adequate BCG[a]	N/A
BCG after chemotherapy failure	N/A	Use BCG for BCG-naive patients failing intravesical chemotherapy
Completely resected, recurrence Ta disease	N/A	Second course of BCG
BCG refractory	N/A	T1HG tumor present 3 mo after last BCG TaHG present after 3 mo or at 6 mo after reinduction or mBCG If CIS alone is present at 3 mo and persists at 6 mo after either reinduction or mBCG Any HG tumor recurrent during mBCG
BCG relapsing	N/A	Recurrence of any HG tumor after completion of mBCG therapy after an initial response
BCG unresponsive	N/A	BCG refractory of HG recurrence within 6 mo of completion of adequate BCG (Ta or T1) or within 12 mo of adequate BCG (CIS)
BCG intolerant	N/A	Adverse reaction to BCG precluding treatment completion

Abbreviations: HG, high grade; LVI, lymphovascular invasion; mBCG, maintenance BCG; N/A, not applicable; TUR, transurethral resection.
[a] Adequate BCG defined as completion of 1 induction course (5 or 6 doses) of BCG plus either a second induction course or a maintenance course (2 or 3 doses).

induction and one maintenance course. Beyond this period, further response to BCG is so low as to not be justified except in rare cases.

Food and Drug Administration–Approved Options

Valrubicin is a lipid soluble semisynthetic analogue of doxorubicin and was the first FDA-approved treatment option for BCG-refractory patients with CIS who are not candidates for RC. Although the initial trials demonstrated a CR of 41%,[29] long-term outcomes data published by Dinney and colleagues[30] demonstrated only 18% CR and 4% recurrence-free survival (RFS) at 2 years.

Immune checkpoint inhibitor (ICI) therapy functions to recover the antitumor immune response by inhibiting the inhibitor of this response, namely Programmed Death-1 (PD-1) and Programmed Death Ligand-1 (PDL-1) in regard to bladder cancer therapy.[31] Currently, pembrolizumab, an anti-PD-1 antibody, is the only other FDA-approved therapy besides valrubicin for patients with BCG-unresponsive NMIBC. Outcomes for 97 patients in cohort A (patients with CIS) in the Keynote-057 trial (NCT02625961) have been reported and were presented to the FDA. For this cohort of patients, the CR rate was 41% at 3 months with median duration of response being 16.2 months. Thus, the extrapolated 12-month RFS was 21% with no treatment-related deaths. Treatment-related adverse events occurred in 63.1% of patients and were grade 3 or 4 in 12.6% of patients.[32] Currently, clinical trials are underway with single-agent ICI therapy and combination of systemic ICI therapy with radiation, intravesical BCG, intravesical chemotherapy, novel intravesical agents, and even intravesical ICI therapy alone (**Tables 6** and **7**).

Other Treatment Options

Nadofaragene firadenovec

Nadofaragene firadenovec (Instiladrin) is a gene therapy transfected via a nonreplicating adenovirus vector harboring the human interferon-α2b gene, which is instilled into the bladder. Nadofaragene firadenovec is instilled into the bladder once every 3 months.[33] Similar to pembrolizumab, data for nadofaragene firadenovec have only been presented in abstract form. In the multicenter, phase 3, single-arm clinical trial (NCT02773849) of 157 patients, nadofaragene firadenovec was well tolerated with up to 33% of patients experiencing local, limited treatment-related events, including two grade 4 events (not related to the study medication) and no deaths. One-hundred three patients had CIS with a 3-month CR rate of 53.4% and a 12-month RFS of 24% for the overall cohort. For the 48 patients with high-grade Ta or T1 tumors, RFS at 12 months was 44%.[34,35] Overall, nadofaragene firadenovec has demonstrated promise in terms of tolerability and RFS.

Continued evaluation of overall and progression-free survival and cost/benefit analysis are needed for nadofaragene firadenovec, pembrolizumab, and other emerging therapies.

Intravesical gemcitabine/docetaxel

An additional treatment modality with promise is intravesical therapy with sequentially administered gemcitabine and docetaxel, which has demonstrated tolerability and efficacy in the BCG failure population, although only through retrospective series.[36] The largest of such was a multi-institutional series recently published by Steinberg and colleagues.[36] The authors evaluated 276 patients with a median follow-up of 22.9 months who received intravesical gemcitabine (1 g in 50 mL sterile water, dwell time 60–90 minutes) followed by docetaxel (37.5 mg in 50 mL saline, dwell time after catheter removal 60–120 minutes) after BCG failure. At 2 years, recurrence-free, high-grade

Table 6
Current clinical trials of systemic therapy for BCG failure in NMIBC as of review of the National Clinical Trials database (NCT) on August 2, 2020

Agent	Phase	Study Population	Investigator	Study ID
PANVAC with BCG vs BCG alone	II	1 prior BCG failure	NCI	NCT02015104
Erdafitinib vs intravesical chemotherapy	II	Recurrence after BCG therapy	Janssen Research & Development	NCT04172675
Avelumab with whole-bladder radiotherapy	II	BCG unresponsive	Institut Paoli-Calmettes	NCT03950362
Durvalumab + radiation therapy + BCG	I/II	BCG unresponsive	Hoosier Cancer Research Network	NCT03317158
Nivolumab vs nivolumab + BMS- 986205 vs Nivolumab + BMS- 986205 + BCG	II	BCG unresponsive	Bristol-Myers Squibb	NCT03519256
IV ALT-801 with IV gemcitabine	I/II	BCG failure	Altor BioScience	NCT01625260
Pembrolizumab with G0070 + DDM	II	BCG unresponsive	CG Oncology, Inc	NCT04387461
IV durvalumab with intravesical vicinium	I	BCG failure	NCI	NCT03258593
IV pembrolizumab with intravesical gemcitabine	II	BCG unresponsive	NCI	NCT04164082
Dovitinib	II	BCG refectory	Hoosier Cancer Research Network	NCT01732107
Durvalumab	II	BCG refectory CIS	H. Lee Moffitt Cancer Center and Research Institute	NCT02901548
Atezolizumab	II	BCG unresponsive	NCI	NCT02844816
Everolimus with intravesical gemcitabine	I/II	BCG refectory CIS	Memorial Sloan Kettering Cancer Center	NCT01259063
Sunitinib malate	II	BCG refectory	Case Comprehensive Cancer Center	NCT01118351

Abbreviations: ALT- 801, recombinant interleukin-2; BMS-986205, linrodostat mesylate; DDM, n-dodecyl-B-D-maltoside; G0070, vicinium; IV, intravenous; NCI, National Cancer Institute.

Table 7
Current clinical trials for intravesical therapy registered in ClinicalTrials.gov

Agent	Phase	Study Population	Investigator	Study ID
Abraxane (nanoparticle albumin bound paclitaxel)	I/II	Recurrent HG NMIBC	Columbia University	NCT00583349
Mycobacterium wall	I	BCG refractory NMIBC	Cadila Pharmaceuticals	NCT00694798
ALT-803 with BCG vs ALT-803 alone	II	BCG unresponsive HG NMIBC	Altor BioScience	
BCG + gemcitabine	I/II	BCG relapsing HG NMIBC	Memorial Sloan Kettering Cancer Center	NCT04179162
Photodynamic therapy	II	BCG unresponsive or intolerant	University Health Network, Toronto	NCT03945162
VPM1002BC	I/II	Recurrence after BCG	Swiss Group for Clinical Cancer Research	NCT02371447
Oral APL-1202 + BCG vs APL-1202 alone	Ib	Recurrence after BCG	Asieris Pharmaceutical Technologies Co, Ltd	NCT03672240
CG0070 CG0070 with DDM	II III	BCG failure	CG Oncology, Inc	NCT02365818 NCT04452591
SCH 72105 + SCH 209702	Ib	BCG refractory	M.D. Anderson Cancer Center	NCT01162785
Intravesical pembrolizumab with BCG	I	BCG refractory	Northwestern University	NCT02808143
Vicinium	III	BCG failure	Viventia Bio	NCT02449239
E7766	I/Ib	BCG unresponsive	Eisai Inc	NCT04109092
Electromotive MMC	II	BCG failure	University of Rome Tor Vergata	NCT04311580
Thermochemotherapy vs best therapy	III	BCG failure	Cancer Research Campaign Clinical Trials Center	NCT01094964
sEphB4-has	I	BCG unresponsive	University of Southern California	NCT03352796
Docetaxel-PM vs MMC	III	BCG refractory	Samyang Biopharmaceuticals Corporation	NCT02282395
Inodiftagene vixteplasmid	II	BCG unresponsive	Anchiano Therapeutics Israel Ltd	NCT03719300
EN3348 vs MMC	III	BCG unresponsive	Bioniche Life Sciences Inc	NCT01200992

Abbreviations: ALT-803, interleukin-15 superagonist; APL-1202, oral methionine aminopeptidase II inhibitor; DDM, n-dodecyl-B-D-maltoside; docetaxel-PM, docetaxel in polymeric micelles; E7766, STING agonist; EN3348, mycobacterial cell wall complex; G0070, vicinium; MMC, mitomycin C; SCH 209702, Syn3; SCH 72105, gene therapy with interferon-α-2b; sEphB4-HAS, decoy receptor for the membrane-bound ligand Ephrin-B2; VPM1002BC, modified BCG.

recurrence-free, and cancer-specific survival were 46%, 52%, and 96%, respectively. The rate of progression to muscle-invasive or metastatic disease was 7%. A multivariable analysis demonstrated that BCG failure category, including BCG-unresponsive disease, was not associated with RFS and that providing maintenance therapy improved RFS. In addition, RFS was not associated with disease stage or the presence of CIS. Thus, although retrospective, intravesical gemcitabine/docetaxel is a reasonable option for patients with BCG failure with the caveat that prospective trials are warranted to confirm these findings. A comparison for each of the four discussed therapies is presented in **Table 8**.

Novel immune checkpoint inhibitors
In addition to pembrolizumab, other novel ICI therapies targeting the PD-1/PD-L1 axis are currently under evaluation including avelumab and durvalumab, with or without additional agents including BCG.

Vicinium
Vicinium is a protein consisting of fused epithelial cell adhesion molecule antibody to *Pseudomonas* exotoxin A, which inhibits protein synthesis. Publicly available data are limited but intravesical installation demonstrated promising tolerability and 3-month CR rates of up to 40%.[37] The treatment regimen is intense because it entails intravesical instillation of 30-mg vicinium (2-hour dwell time) with induction with twice weekly instillations for 6 weeks followed by weekly instillations for 6 weeks. After 3 months, patients are reassessed and those who remain disease free receive maintenance therapy every other week for 2 years.

Device-delivered therapy
Device-delivered therapy including photodynamic therapy and device-assisted electromotive or heated chemotherapy represent other promising therapies for NMIBC. The mechanism of action of photodynamic therapy is dependent on light activation of photosensitized target tissues, with the 5-aminolevulinic acid derivative hexaminolevulinate currently under investigation. Bader and colleagues[38] reported on phase I results of 17 patients treated with hexaminolevulinate-based photodynamic therapy demonstrating an acceptable safety profile; however, only two patients remained

Table 8
Comparison of intravesical therapies for BCG-failure

Agent	12-mo RFS	24-mo RFS	PFS	G5 Toxicity	N	Manuscript Available
Valrubicin	20% (Ta/T1) 80% (CIS)	15% (Ta/T1) 80% (CIS)	22.4 mo (Ta/T1) 8.7 mo (CIS)	0	42	Yes
Pembrolizumab[a]	20% (CIS)	N/A	Pending	1	97	No
Nadofaragene firadenovec[b]	24% (CIS) 44% (Ta/T1)	N/A	Pending	0	158 CIS = 103 Ta/T1 = 48	No
Gem/Doce	60%	46%	93% @ 24 mo	0	276	Yes

Abbreviations: G5, grade 5; N/A, not applicable; PFS, progression-free survival.
[a] Keynote 057 arm A reporting on 97 patients for FDA approval.
[b] Multicenter, open-label phase 3 trial results from meeting abstract presentations.

recurrence-free at 21 months. Additional photosensitizing agents including TLD1433 are also currently being explored (NCT03945162).

Electromotive drug administration uses electrokinetic forces to accelerate drug delivery across the urothelium. This modality has previously been prospectively evaluated in 108 patients with CIS with or without concomitant T1 tumors; intravesical electromotive drug administration delivered mitomycin C provided superior CR compared with mitomycin C alone and similar CR rates to BCG.[39]

Radiofrequency-induced thermochemotherapy with the delivery of hyperthermia to the urothelium, thereby potentiating the cytotoxic effects of chemotherapy, has previously been shown in randomized control trials to show benefit in the BCG-naive setting and it may offer another potential therapeutic avenue for patients in the BCG failure space. In the phase III, randomized control HYMN trial (NCT01094964), 104 patients were randomized to six weekly instillations of two cycles of 20-mg mitomycin C (50 mL sterile water) at 42°C versus six weekly instillations of BCG. Patients in both groups who were disease-free at 3 months were continued on maintenance therapy with their respective treatment. Disease-free survival rates were similar between the two groups (HR, 1.33; 95% CI, 0.84–2.10; $P = .23$); however, subgroup analysis demonstrated that disease-free survival was significantly lower in the thermochemotherapy group among patients with CIS (HR, 2.06; 95% CI, 1.17–3.62; $P = .01$).[40]

Other Agents

Other agents under investigation include ALT-803, linrodostat mesylate (BMS-986205), and albumin-bound rapamycin nanoparticles. ALT-803 is a complex of an interleukin-15 receptor and an interleukin-15 superagonist protein that has demonstrated antitumor activity across a spectrum of diseases and is a potent stimulator of CD8 T cells and natural killer cells.[41] Linrodostat mesylate is a selective, oral inhibitor of indoleamine 2,3-dioxygenase 1 with some promise for NMIBC and MIBC when given in conjunction with other therapies.[42]

SUMMARY

A single postoperative dose of intravesical chemotherapy remains the recommended treatment of those with low-risk NMIBC; however, patients with intermediate- or high-risk disease should be offered induction intravesical therapy. Additional maintenance therapy should be considered in both populations but is mandatory in those with high-risk disease. Despite this treatment, a significant proportion of patients have disease recurrence or persistence. Although RC with urinary diversion remains the gold standard for improving RFS, progression-free survival, overall survival, and cancer-specific survival after BCG failure for patients with high-risk NMIBC both fit and willing to undergo surgery, utilization rates remain low.[43,44] Practical alternatives are thus greatly needed.

Recent FDA approval for pembrolizumab and ongoing review of nadofaragene firadenovec represent the most robust and promising advances made in the last 20 years. Although not supported by high-quality, prospective evidence, intravesical gemcitabine/docetaxel has demonstrated promise in this setting with reduced cost likely when compared with nadofaragene firadenovec and pembrolizumab and without the immune-mediated toxicity when compared with pembrolizumab. Multiple promising local and systemic agents are currently in phase II or III trials. The future for salvage therapy after BCG failure is bright and strengthened by the standardization of defined failure and recurrence classification.

CLINICS CARE POINTS

- Risk stratification of NMIBC can aid in selection of optimal intravesical treatment regimen.
- BCG failure includes various subcategories. One classification recommended by the IBCG includes: BCG intolerant, BCG relapsing, BCG refractory, and BCG unresponsive categories.
- For many patients after BCG failure, especially those who are in the BCG unresponsive category, radical cystectomy remains the standard of care; however, it remains significantly underused and undesired by patients.
- Pembrolizumab and valrubicin (CIS only) remain the only FDA-approved therapies for patients in the BCG unresponsive category.
- Nadofaragene firadenovec represents a promising intravesical therapy option currently under FDA review.
- Intravesically administered sequential chemotherapy (eg, with gemcitabine and docetaxel) is a viable alternative for patients, based on large multicenter retrospective analysis.
- Multiple systemic, intravesical, and combination therapies are currently under evaluation for patients with NMIBC in the BCG-naive and BCG-failure spaces, providing hope for alternative options to radical cystectomy in this underserved patient population.

DISCLOSURE

A.M. Kamat has served as a consultant or sat on the advisory board of the following: Abbott Molecular, Arquer, ArTara, Asieris, Astra Zeneca, BioClin Therapeutics, BMS, Cepheid, Cold Genesys, Eisai, Engene, Inc, Ferring, FerGene, Imagin, Janssen, MDxHealth, Medac, Merck, Pfizer, Photocure, ProTara, Roviant, Seattle Genetics, Sessen Bio, Theralase, TMC Innovation, and US Biotest. He has received grant funding or research support from: Adolor, BMS, FKD Industries, Heat Biologics, Merck, Photocure, SWOG/NIH, SPORE, and AIBCCR.

REFERENCES

1. Kamat AM, Hahn NM, Efstathiou JA, et al. Bladder cancer. Lancet 2016;388: 2796–810.
2. Quhal F, D'Andra D, Soria F, et al. Primary Ta high grade bladder tumors: determination of the risk of progression. Urol Oncol 2020;00:1–5.
3. Chang SS, Boorjian SA, Chou R, et al. Diagnosis and treatment of non-muscle invasive bladder cancer: AUA/SUO guideline. J Urol 2016;196(4):1021–9.
4. Babjuk M, Burger M, Compérat EM, et al. European Association of Urology guidelines on non-muscle invasive bladder cancer (Ta T1 and carcinoma in situ): 2019 update. Eur Urol 2019;76(5):639–57.
5. Sylvester RJ, Oosterlinck W, Holman S, et al. Systematic review and individual patient data meta-analysis of randomized trials comparing a single immediate instillation of chemotherapy after transurethral resection with transurethral resection alone in patients with stage pTa-pT1 urothelial carcinoma of the bladder: which patients benefit from installation? Eur Urol 2016;69:231–44.
6. Messing EM, Tangen CM, Lerner SP, et al. Effect of intravesical instillation of gemcitabine vs saline immediately following resection of suspected low-grade non-muscle-invasive bladder cancer on tumor recurrence: SWOG S0337 randomized clinical trial. JAMA 2018;319:1880–8.

7. Bosschiter J, Nieuwenhuijzen JA, van Ginkel T, et al. Value of an immediate intra-vesical instillation of mitomycin C in patients with non-muscle-invasive bladder cancer: a prospective multicenter randomized study of 2243 patients. Eur Urol 2018;73:226–32.

8. Gudjónsson S, Adell L, Merdasa F, et al. Should all patients with non–muscle-invasive bladder cancer receive early intravesical chemotherapy after transure-thral resection? The results of a prospective randomised multicentre study. Eur Urol 2009;55(4):773–80.

9. Kamat AM, Witjes JA, Brausi M, et al. Defining and treating the spectrum of intermediate-risk NMIBC. J Urol 2014;192(2):305–15.

10. Chou R, Buckley D, Fu R, et al. Emerging approaches to diagnosis and treatment of non–muscle-invasive bladder cancer [Internet] (Comparative Effectiveness Reviews, No. 153.). Rockville (MD): Agency for Healthcare Research and Quality (US); 2015. Available at: https://www.ncbi.nlm.nih.gov/books/NBK330472/.

11. Jones G, Cleves A, Wilt TJ, et al. Intravesical gemcitabine for non-muscle inva-sive bladder cancer. Cochrane Database Syst Rev 2012;1:CD009294.

12. Morales A, Eidinger D, Bruce AW. Intracavitary bacillus Calmette-Guerin in the treatment of superficial bladder tumors. J Urol 1976;116:180–3.

13. Malmstrom PU, Sylvester RJ, Crawford DE, et al. An individual patient data meta-analysis of the long-term outcome of randomised studies comparing intravesical mitomycin C versus bacillus Calmette-Guerin for non-muscle-invasive bladder cancer. Eur Urol 2009;56:247.

14. Sylvester RJ, van der Meijden AP, Lamm DL. Intravesical bacillus Calmette-Guerin reduces the risk of progression in patients with superficial bladder cancer: a meta-analysis of the published results of randomized clinical trials. J Urol 2002; 168(5):1964–70.

15. Lamm DL, Blumentein BA, Crissman JD, et al. Maintenance bacillus Calmette-Guerin immunotherapy for recurrent Ta, T1, and carcinoma in situ transitional cell carcinoma of the bladder: a randomized southwest oncology group study. J Urol 2000;163(4):1124–9.

16. Oddens J, Brausi M, Sylvester R, et al. Final results of an EORTC-GU cancers group randomized study of maintenance bacillus Calmette–Guerin in intermedi-ate- and high-risk Ta, T1 papillary carcinoma of the urinary bladder: one-third dose versus full dose and 1 year versus 3 years of maintenance. Eur Urol 2013;63(3):462–72.

17. Sylvester RJ, Van der Meijden APM, Witjes JA, et al. Bacillus Calmette-Guerin versus chemotherapy for the intravesical treatment of patients with carcinoma in situ of the bladder; a meta-analysis of the published results of randomized clin-ical trials. J Urol 2005;174:86–92.

18. Bohle A, Bock PR. Intravesical bacille Calmette-Guerin versus mitomycin C in su-perficial bladder cancer: formal meta-analysis of comparative studies on tumor progression. Urology 2004;63:682–7.

19. Chalasani V, Kassouf W, Chin JL, et al. Radical cystectomy for the treatment of T1 bladder cancer: the Canadian Bladder Cancer Network experience. Can Urol As-soc J 2011;5(2):83–7.

20. Witjes JA. Management of BCG failures in superficial bladder cancer: a review. Eur Urol 2006;49:790–7.

21. Parker WP, Smelser W, Lee EK, et al. Utilization and outcomes of radical cystec-tomy for high-grade non–muscle-invasive bladder cancer in elderly patients. Clin Genitourin Cancer 2018;16:e79.

22. Kamat AM, Lerner SP, O'Donnell M, et al. Evidence-based assessment of current and emerging bladder-sparing therapies for non–muscle-invasive bladder cancer after bacillus Calmette-Guerin therapy: a systematic review and meta-analysis. Eur Urol Oncol 2020;3:318.

23. Brooks NA, O'Donnell M. Treatment options in non-muscle-invasive bladder cancer after BCG failure. Indian J Urol 2015;31(4):312–9.

24. Hassler MR, Shariat SF, Soria F. Salvage therapeutic strategies for bacillus Calmette–Guerin failure. Curr Opin Urol 2019;29(3):239–46.

25. Yates DR, Brausi MA, Catto JWF, et al. Treatment options available for bacillus Calmette-Guérin failure in non–muscle-invasive bladder cancer. Eur Urol 2012; 62:1088–96.

26. Kamat AM, Colombel M, Sundi D, et al. BCG-unresponsive non-muscle-invasive bladder cancer: recommendations from the IBCG. Nat Rev Urol 2017;14(4): 244–55.

27. Lerner SP, Bajorin DF, Dinney CP, et al. Summary and recommendations from the National Cancer Institute's clinical trials planning meeting on novel therapeutics for non-muscle invasive bladder cancer. Bladder Cancer 2016;2(2):165–202.

28. Li R, Tabayoyong WB, Guo CC, et al. Prognostic implication of the United States Food and Drug Administration-defined BCG-unresponsive disease. Eur Urol 2019;75(1):8–10.

29. Greenberg RE, Bahnson RR, Wood D, et al. Initial report on intravesical administration of N-trifluoroacetyladreiamycin-14-valerate (AD 32) to patients with refractory superficial transitional cell carcinoma of the urinary bladder. Urology 1997; 49:471–5.

30. Dinney CP, Greenberg RE, Steinberg GD. Intravesical valrubicin in patients with bladder carcinoma in situ and contraindication to or failure after bacillus Calmette-Guerin. Urol Oncol 2013;31:1635–42.

31. Vaddepally RK, Kharel P, Pandey R, et al. Review of indications of FDA-approved immune checkpoint inhibitors per NCCN guidelines with the level of evidence. Cancers 2020;12(3):738.

32. Balar AV, Kamat AM, Kulkarni GS, et al. Pembrolizumab (pembro) for the treatment of patients with Bacillus Calmette-Guérin (BCG) unresponsive, high-risk (HR) non–muscle-invasive bladder cancer (NMIBC): over two years follow-up of KEYNOTE-057. J Clin Oncol 2020;38(supplemental 15):5041.

33. Duplisea JJ, Mokkapati S, Plote D, et al. The development of interferon-based gene therapy for BCG unresponsive bladder cancer: from bench to bedside. World J Urol 2019;37(10):2041–9.

34. Boorjian SA, Dinney CPN, SUO Clinical Trials Consortium. Safety and efficacy of intravesical nadofaragene firadenovec for patients with high-grade, BCG unresponsive nonmuscle invasive bladder cancer (NMIBC): results from a phase III trial. J Clin Oncol 2020;38(6):442.

35. Boorjian S, Dinney CP, SUO Clinical Trials Consortium. PD12-07: A phase III study to evaluate the safety and efficacy of intravesical nadofaragene firadenovec for patients with high-grade, BCG unresponsive non-muscle invasive bladder cancer: papillary disease cohort results. J Urol 2020;203(supplemental 4):e261–2.

36. Steinberg RL, Thomas LJ, Brooks N, et al. Multi-institution evaluation of sequential gemcitabine and docetaxel as rescue therapy for nonmuscle invasive bladder cancer. J Urol 2020;203(5):902–9.

37. Shore N, O'Donnell M, Keane T, et al. PD03-02: phase 3 results of vicinium in BCG-unresponsive non-muscle invasive bladder cancer. J Urol 2020; 203(supplemental 4):e72.

38. Bader MJ, Stepp H, Beyer W, et al. Photodynamic therapy of bladder cancer: a phase I study using hexaminolevulinate (HAL). Urol Oncol 2013;31(7):1178–83.
39. Di Stasi SM, Giannatoni A, Stephen RL, et al. Intravesical electromotive mitomycin C versus passive transport mitomycin C for high risk superficial bladder cancer: a prospective randomized study. J Urol 2003;170:777–82.
40. Tan WS, Panchal A, Buckley L, et al. Radiofrequency-induced thermo-chemotherapy effect versus a second course of bacillus Calmette-Guerin or institutional standard in patients with recurrence of non-muscle invasive bladder cancer following induction or maintenance bacillus Calmette-Guerin therapy (HYMN): a phase III, open-label, randomised controlled trial. Eur Urol 2019;75(1):63–71.
41. Rhode PR, Egan JO, Xu W, et al. Comparison of the superagonist complex, ALT-803, to IL15 as cancer immunotherapeutics in animal models. Cancer Immunol Res 2016;4:49–60.
42. Hahn NM, Chang S, Meng M, et al. A phase II, randomized study of nivolumab (NIVO), NIVO plus linrodostat mesylate, or NIVO plus intravesical bacillus Calmette-Guerin (BCG) in BCG-unresponsive, high-risk, nonmuscle invasive bladder cancer (NMIBC): CheckMate 9UT. J Clin Oncol 2020;38(supplemental 15):TPS5090.
43. Denzinger S, Fritsche HM, Otto W, et al. Early versus deferred cystectomy for initial high-risk pT1G3 urothelial carcinoma of the bladder: do risk factors define feasibility of bladder-sparing approach? Eur Urol 2008;53(1):146–52.
44. Jäger W, Thomas C, Haag S, et al. Early vs delayed radical cystectomy for 'high-risk' carcinoma not invading bladder muscle: delay of cystectomy reduces cancer-specific survival. BJU Int 2011;108(8 Pt 2):E284–8.

Diagnosis and Staging of Bladder Cancer

Hamed Ahmadi, MD[a], Vinay Duddalwar, MD[b], Siamak Daneshmand, MD[a,c],*

KEYWORDS

- Bladder cancer • Staging • Diagnosis • Imaging • Enhanced cystoscopy
- Transurethral resection of bladder tumor

KEY POINTS

- Cystoscopy remains the gold standard procedure for initial diagnosis of bladder cancer (BCa). Some emerging evidence suggests the possibility of replacing cystoscopy with Cxbladder at the initial work-up of patients at low risk of BCa.
- Transurethral resection of bladder tumor is the mainstay of clinical staging of BCa to assess depth, grade, variant histology, and extent of invasion. When available, enhanced endoscopic technologies should be used to increase detection rate of additional papillary and/or flat lesions and ensure complete tumor resection.
- Multiparametric MRI is an alternative option for local staging of BCa.
- Molecular subtyping could be an integral part of initial staging in the near future in order to tailor an individualized, optimal course of treatment of each patient in the era of immunotherapy and targeted treatments.

INTRODUCTION

Bladder cancer (BCa) is the second most common genitourinary and fourth most common cancer overall in the United States, with an estimated 81,400 newly diagnosed cases (62,100 men and 19,300 women) and approximately 17,980 new deaths in 2020.[1] Urothelial carcinoma (UC) is the predominant histologic type in Western countries, accounting for 90% of all BCa cases. However, non-UCs are more common in other parts of the world. Much less commonly, UCs can originate from the urothelial lining of renal pelvis, ureter, or urethra. Most patients (70%) present with non–muscle-invasive bladder cancer (NMIBC), which carries a high risk of recurrence (50%–70%) and can progress to muscle-invasive bladder cancer (MIBC) in about 10% to 20% of cases.[2] Despite some evidence suggesting a role for screening in population

[a] Department of Urology, University of Southern California/Norris Comprehensive Cancer Center, 1441 Eastlake Avenue, Suite 7416, Los Angeles, CA 90089, USA; [b] Department of Radiology, University of Southern California, 1441 Eastlake Avenue, Los Angeles, CA 90089, USA; [c] USC/Norris Comprehensive Cancer Center, USC Institute of Urology, 1441 Eastlake Avenue, Suite 7416, Los Angeles, CA 90089, USA
* Corresponding author. USC/Norris Comprehensive Cancer Center, USC Institute of Urology, 1441 Eastlake Avenue, Suite 7416, Los Angeles, CA 90089,
E-mail address: daneshma@med.usc.edu

Hematol Oncol Clin N Am 35 (2021) 531–541
https://doi.org/10.1016/j.hoc.2021.02.004
0889-8588/21/© 2021 Elsevier Inc. All rights reserved.

hemonc.theclinics.com

at high risk of developing BCa,[3] BCa screening is currently not recommended, mostly because of a lack of a standardized definition for high-risk group, which would lead to overdiagnosis and overtreatment if implemented in routine clinical practice.[4]

DISCUSSION
Presentation

The classic presentation for patients with BCa is painless hematuria (macroscopic or microscopic). However, irritative voiding symptoms, such as frequency, urgency, and dysuria, could also be the initial manifestation, especially in patients with carcinoma in situ (CIS). Pain and constitutional symptoms are usually present in patients with locally advanced or metastatic disease and is generally associated with poor prognosis. The prevalence of BCa ranges between 10% and 20% in patients presenting with gross hematuria and between 3% and 5% in patients presenting with microscopic hematuria (MH).[5,6] Given the much lower incidence of BCa in patients with MH and that approximately 18% of all cases of MH have completely benign causes, there are some controversies regarding the optimal group that would benefit from a full work-up for possible BCa. The American Urological Association (AUA) currently recommends full diagnostic work-up in all patients 35 years or older with MH, defined as 3 or greater red blood cells (RBCs) per high-power field (HPF), in the absence of known benign cause.[7] However, other organizations recommend against diagnostic work-up in nonsmoking women aged between 35 and 50 year with fewer than 25 RBCs per HPF.[8]

Diagnostic Work-up

Currently recommended work-up in patients with gross hematuria or significant MH includes cystoscopy, urine cytology, and upper tract imaging.

Cystoscopic Examination

White light cystoscopy (WLC) is the standard of care during the initial diagnostic work-up of BCa in the office using a flexible cystoscope. The sensitivity and specificity of WLC for detection of papillary bladder tumor range from 62% to 84% and 43% to 98%, respectively. Its sensitivity decreases for small papillary lesions and CIS.[9] Almost all abnormal bladder lesions detected on office cystoscopy need to be resected in the operating room using a rigid cystoscope to determine the histology and depth of invasion. Similar to flexible WLC, rigid WLC is also operator dependent, has a low sensitivity for detecting small papillary and flat lesions, and shows suboptimal ability to determine the margins of resection.[10]

Enhanced Cystoscopy Technologies

Several enhanced imaging technologies have been introduced in recent years in order to improve the detection rate of bladder tumors. They are generally categorized into 3 categories: (1) macroscopic technologies such as blue light cystoscopy (BLC) and narrow band imaging (NBI), microscopic imaging that has similar overall field of view and spatial resolutions compared with WLC; (2) microscopic imaging technologies such as optical coherence tomography and confocal laser endomicroscopy that could provide cellular resolutions as well as subsurface imaging that could theoretically provide histologic cancer characterization, including grading and staging; and (3) molecular imaging in which fluorescently labeled binding agents such as antibodies, peptides, or small molecules are being captured using macroscopic enhanced imaging technologies.[11] Out of all these intriguing technologies, the largest and strongest body of evidence belongs to BLC, which is currently recommended as an adjunct procedure to WLC in initial staging work-up of BCa in both American and European guidelines.[12,13]

Blue light cystoscopy

This technology was first developed in Europe but was later approved in the United States for use in conjunction with rigid WLC at the time of transurethral resection of bladder tumor (TURBT) in 2010 and for surveillance of patients at high risk of recurrence in outpatient settings using flexible cystoscopy in 2018. Hexaminolevulinate (HAL; known as Cysview in the United States and Hexvix in Europe) is the agent used in this technology. HAL is a heme precursor that preferentially accumulates protoporphyrin IX and other photoactive porphyrins in the mitochondria of neoplastic tissue and emits fluorescence when exposed to blue light. A phase III prospective trial, conducted in 17 centers in the United States, showed similar improvements in cancer detection for flexible BLC.[14] Flexible BLC is typically not used for initial work-up of bladder lesions before any pathologic proof of BCa and is currently only recommended for surveillance in patients at high risk of recurrence following initial TURBT and/or after intravesical treatment. Another significant advantage of BLC at time of TURBT, compared with WLC, is the improved ability to determine the margins of resection. The need for preoperative or pre–office visit catheterization and cost associated with purchase of the endoscopic equipment are some of the potential drawbacks of this technology.[15]

Urine Cytology and Other Urine-based Tumor Markers

Cytology remains the most common adjunct procedure to cystoscopy for detection of high-grade (HG) BCa, including CIS and HG upper tract urothelial cancer, because of its exceptionally high specificity (<2% false-positive rate). However, it has low sensitivity overall for detection of BCa, ranging from 12% for low-grade to 64% for HG tumors.[16] There are several US Food and Drug Administration (FDA)–approved urine-based tumor markers available, designed to overcome the drawbacks of cytology (**Table 1**). These markers are mainly based on differential expression of tumor-related materials such as RNA, proteins, tumor-related DNA methylation changes, or cellular markers.[17] Despite the improved sensitivity compared with cytology, they remain inferior to cytology for diagnosis of BCa. Despite of some evidence suggesting a potential role for fluorescence in situ hybridization in early detection of BCa recurrence after bacillus

---

Table 1
Diagnostic performances of US Food and Drug Administration–approved urinary markers for the detection and surveillance of bladder cancer

		Sensitivity (%)	Specificity (%)
BTA stat	Single step office based	57–83	60–92
BTA TRAK	Sandwich immunoassay	66	65
Cxbladder	qPCR of 5 mRNA	81	85
NMP 22 ELISA	ELISA (laboratory based)	47–100	78
NMP 22 BladderCheck	Point-of-care office test	47–100	78
uCyst	Cytology plus immunofluorescence	50–100	69–79
UroVysion	Fluorescence in situ	41–70	80

Abbreviations: BTA, bladder tumor–associated antigen; ELISA, enzyme-linked immunosorbent assay; mRNA, messenger RNA; NMP, nuclear matrix protein; PCR, polymerase chain reaction; qPCR, quantitative polymerase chain reaction.

Calmette-Guérin treatment,[18] none of these markers are currently recommended to replace cytology for initial diagnosis of BCa.[12,19] However, early studies on Cxbladder as a screening tool have shown promising results. A large-scale, community-based study in New Zealand showed that 32% of cystoscopies could be avoided by using Cxbladder to screen patients with hematuria, and the Cxbladder test has been incorporated into the local health care screening algorithm for patients with microhematuria in some counties within the country.[20] A multi-institutional trial in North America is currently underway to address the same question (NCT03988309) in order to avoid cystoscopy in patients who are otherwise at low risk of harboring UC.

Imaging

Imaging is an essential part of both initial diagnosis and staging of BCa. Computed tomography (CT) urogram has completely replaced intravenous urography as the most common cross-sectional imaging for BCa diagnosis and staging. CT urogram not only allows the assessment of renal parenchyma and upper tract urothelium, it can also evaluate other genitourinary conditions that may cause hematuria, such as urolithiasis and renal masses.[21]

Absence of ionizing radiation, high degree of soft tissue contrast, and multiplanar imaging capability have made multiparametric MRI a potential alternative option for staging of BCa (**Fig. 1**). Earlier studies suggested acceptable sensitivity for MRI in differentiating organ-confined from locally advanced BCa. However, it had poor sensitivity in detecting nodal disease, and interobserver agreement for both local and nodal staging was suboptimal.[22] Similar to prostate imaging-reporting and data system (PI-RADS) for prostate cancer, a vesical imaging-reporting and data system (VI-RADS) protocol was developed in 2018 as a way to standardize reporting format for BCa staging to, at the least, improve interobserver agreement. This reporting system incorporates T2-weighted (T2W), diffusion-weighted, and dynamic contrast-enhanced images to assess risk of tumor invasion. The overall score ranges from 1 to 5, with VI-RADS 1 indicating no muscularis propria invasion and no tumor infiltration and VI-RADS 5 indicating extravesical extension of tumor. VI-RADS 1 and 2 are more indicative of non–muscle-invasive BCa, whereas VI-RADS 4 and 5 suggest either muscle-invasive disease or

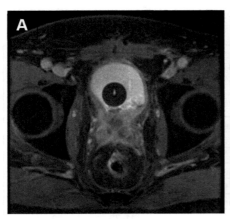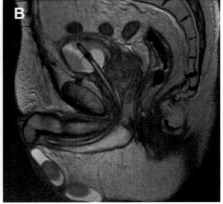

Fig. 1. MRI of a patient with history of prostate cancer after radiation treatment and muscle-invasive bladder cancer on TURBT. (*A*) Axial postcontrast fat-suppressed T2-weighted image and (*B*) sagittal postcontrast spoiled gradient recalled echo sequence showing local invasion to prostate and seminal vesicles (clinical T4a).

extravesical extension. VI-RADS 3, like PI-RADS 3, is indeterminate for muscle invasion (**Fig. 2**).[23] Several validation studies have shown a sensitivity between 76% and 95%, and specificity between 44% and 93% for differentiating NMIBC from MIBC, with inter-observer agreement between 0.73 and 0.92.[24] As opposed to the encouraging results for staging of organ-confined disease, MRI seems to underperform for nodal staging. Lymphadenopathy is mainly defined by size in BCa staging and is less dependent on nodal tissue characteristics on imaging. Therefore, MRI has shown low sensitivity and only moderate specificity in detecting abnormal lymph nodes.[22,25,26] PET with ^{18}F-fluoro-D-glucose is not currently recommended for local staging of BCa because of the excretion of radiotracer into the bladder. However, evidence supports its potential role in other settings: PET/CT could improve detection of involved nodes that are still not considered abnormal by size criteria.[27] Also, it could potentially be used to assess any other sites of metastasis when surgical resection is being considered for oligometastatic disease.[28] PET may also play a role in assessing response to neoadjuvant chemotherapy. A recent study showed that PET/CT could identify complete responders to neoadjuvant chemotherapy (pathologic T0 at time of cystectomy) with a sensitivity of 75% and specificity of 90%.[29] In addition, PET/CT might be superior to

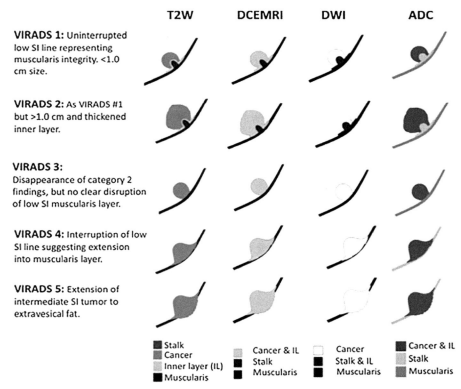

Fig. 2. Multiparametric MRI appearances of VI-RADS scores 1 to 5 using T2. ADC, apparent diffusion coefficient; DCEMRI, dynamic contrast enhancement MRI; DWI, diffusion-weighted imaging; SI, signal intensity. (*From* Panebianco, V., Narumi, Y., Altun, E. et al, 2018. Multiparametric Magnetic Resonance Imaging for Bladder Cancer: Development of VI-RADS (Vesical Imaging-Reporting And Data System). *European Urology*, [online] 74(3), pp.294-306. Available at: <http://www.sciencedirect.com/science/article/pii/S030228381830335X>; with permission.) Figure 3 in original

conventional CT imaging in detecting recurrence of disease after intent-to-cure treatment. One meta-analysis showed pooled sensitivity and specificity of 94% and 92% in detecting recurrent or residual BCa.[30] Bone scans are only recommended if there is an increased alkaline phosphatase level or in the presence of signs or symptoms of bone involvement, such as new-onset bone pain.[31]

Radiomics

Over the last few years, there has been increasing interest and published literature on the role of radiomics evaluation and treatment of BCa.[32] It uses high-throughput extraction of quantitative metrics from clinical imaging and subsequent analysis by various artificial intelligence techniques (**Fig. 3**). It has been applied to both CT and MRI studies for diagnosis, grading, subtype classification, treatment response evaluation, and prediction, as well as in multiomic analysis to find correlates to molecular analysis.[33–36] Multiomic analysis is of increasing interest because it is a method of translating knowledge gained from translational and experimental studies from biomarker and molecular characterization studies directly into clinical applications.[37,38] Although this is currently mostly limited to retrospective, single-center studies, the increasing experience in this technique, along with an understanding of its strengths and limitations, will lead to a maturation and clinical use of this technique.[39]

Transurethral Resection of Bladder Tumor

After the initial work-up suggests the possibility of bladder tumor, TURBT is the primary method of diagnosis and staging of BCa. It can be performed under local, spinal, or general anesthesia, depending on factors such as preoperative risk assessment and tumor characteristics, including size and location. Most tumors are resected using a loop resectoscope, especially at the time of initial diagnosis. In small, superficial papillary lesions, cold cup biopsy can be used to obtain the specimen and the rest

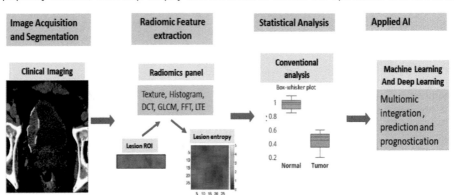

Fig. 3. Typical workflow for radiomics. A representative image from a contrast-enhanced CT scan in a 75-year-old male patient with T3a tumor along the right lateral wall of the urinary bladder. The tumor may be segmented (*yellow outline*) by an expert reviewer or may be semiautomated. The segmented image is then processed using various radiomic extraction algorithms and software programs. The extracted results can be analyzed using conventional analytical techniques or, for further applied analysis, can be analyzed using various artificial intelligence techniques, include machine and deep learning. This process can include integration with other genomic, molecular, as well as clinical data. This analysis can then be used to build models for diagnosis, risk stratification, treatment optimization, and outcome analysis. AI, artificial intelligence; DCT, Discrete cosine transform; FFT, fast Fourier transform; GLCM, Gray-level Co-occurrence Matrix; LTE, Laws transform.

of tumor can be fulgurated. For large and sessile lesions, staged resection is usually performed, where the tumor is resected layer by layer until the base of the tumor is reached. This maneuver minimizes the risk of bladder perforation. Deep resection of bladder tumor base is then performed to obtain muscle to assess the depth of invasion and is sent separately. Smaller, more friable tumors that are attached to the bladder wall by a narrow stalk can be resected en bloc to minimize tumor fragmentation and cautery artifact. Both bipolar and monopolar electrocautery can be used successfully for TURBT. However, bipolar TURBT is preferred because it is associated with shorter operative and catheterization time and decreased obturator nerve reflex, incidence of bladder perforation, and a decreased tumor recurrence rate.[10] If available, the use of enhanced endoscopic techniques, especially BLC, is recommended in order to improve detection rate, especially for CIS lesions, and to decrease recurrence and potentially progression rate.[40,41]

Bimanual examination after TURBT could provide essential staging information. For instance, a palpable mass after TURBT indicates extravesical extension (cT3) of tumor until proved otherwise. Also, a fixed palpable mass raises the possibility of pelvic side wall or adjacent organ invasion (cT4b).

Staging

Bladder cancers are staged using the eighth edition of the tumor, node, metastasis/ American Joint Committee on Cancer (AJCC) system and graded using the 2004 World Health Organization/International Society of Urological Pathology (ISUP) grading system.[42,43] Patients with bladder tumors extending into the prostatic stroma are staged T4a regardless of route. However, direct invasion through the bladder wall is associated with a worse prognosis compared with invasion through the prostatic urethra.[44] In situ extension of UC into prostatic glands and ducts, or even extension into the seminal vesicles via mucosal/epithelial extension without stromal invasion, would be considered Tis only. UCs arising from the prostatic urethra alone are staged according the urethral cancer staging system, where prostatic stromal invasion is considered T2.

Given the revolutionary developments in BCa genetics in the past decade, there has been a great emphasis on molecular subtyping of BCa in addition to traditional microscopic staging based on depth of invasion and histologic appearances. Although a few molecular subtype classification systems have been suggested for NMIBC, the focus has been mostly on MIBC, partly because of abundance of tissue available for analysis in postcystectomy patients.[45] Of all proposed classification systems, the most recognized classification system was derived from The Cancer Genome Atlas (TCGA) data, which provided comprehensive molecular and clinicopathologic features of 412 MIBC tumors. Clustering of messenger RNA (mRNA) expression levels in the TCGA study allowed the identification of 5 molecularly distinct MIBC subtypes (luminal-papillary, luminal-infiltrated, luminal, basal-squamous, and neuronal), each with its own distinct prognostic and therapeutic characteristics.[46] For instance, the luminal-papillary subtype (35%) is characterized by a papillary morphology and is associated with the best overall survival rate. It also possesses fibroblast growth factor receptor 3 (FGFR3) alterations, which suggests that tumors belonging to this category could have an impressive response to FGFR inhibitors. It has also been suggested that these tumors might have a limited response to neoadjuvant chemotherapy and are best served with early cystectomy (**Fig. 4**). It is unclear whether the same categorization could be applied to NMIBC, but, given the growing intravesical or systemic treatment options for NMIBC and MIBC, there needs to be more emphasis on exploring molecular subtyping in patients with BCa at early stages of treatment, preferably at the time of diagnosis.

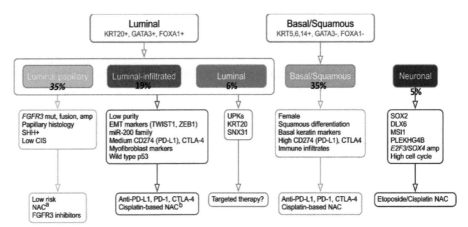

Fig. 4. Different molecular subtypes of MIBC based on mRNA expression and proposed schema for optimal therapeutic approach for each subtype. CTLA-4, cytotoxic T lymphocyte–associated protein 4; EMT, epithelial-mesenchymal transition; NAC, neoadjuvant chemotherapy; PD-1, programmed cell death protein 1; PD-L1, programmed death-ligand 1; SHH, sonic hedgehog. [a] Low predicted likelihood of response, based on preliminary data. [b] Low response rate. (*Adapted from* Panebianco, V., Narumi, Y., Altun, E. and Bochner, B., 2018. Multiparametric Magnetic Resonance Imaging for Bladder Cancer: Development of VI-RADS (Vesical Imaging-Reporting And Data System). *European Urology*, [online] 74(3), pp.294-306. Available at: <http://www.sciencedirect.com/science/article/pii/S030228381830335X>; with permission.) Figure 7 in original.)

SUMMARY

Although cystoscopic examination remains the gold standard technique for initial diagnosis of BCa, the potential role of Cxbladder in reducing the number of cystoscopies in patients who present with microscopic or gross hematuria awaits further evidence. Despite significant progress in enhanced cystoscopic techniques, BLC and, to a lesser degree, NBI are the only 2 modalities that are well supported by evidence, and, if available, should be used during initial staging of BCa. Multiparametric MRI could be an important imaging tool in local staging of BCa. However, it still seems to be highly dependent on technique and interpretation and suffers from nodal understaging. With ever-expanding targeted therapy options in both NMIBC and MIBC, molecular subtyping could become an essential part of initial histologic staging in the near future to help in identifying ideal therapeutic options and directing the clinical course.

CLINICS CARE POINTS

Diagnosis

- Cystoscopy remains the gold standard procedure for initial diagnosis of BCa. Some evidence suggests that cystoscopy could be avoided, at least in a subset of patients with MH who are at low risk for developing BCa using Cxbladder.

- Despite its low sensitivity, cytology remains an important part of initial diagnostic work-up because of its exceptionally high specificity.

- CT urogram is the most commonly used imaging for initial diagnosis of BCa and has widely replaced intravenous urography.

Staging

- TURBT is the mainstay of clinical staging of BCa to assess depth, grade, and extent of the disease as well as presence of variant histology. When available, enhanced endoscopic technologies, especially BLC and NBI, should be applied to increase detection rate of additional papillary and/or flat lesions and ensure complete tumor resection.

- Multiparametric MRI is an alternative option for local staging of BCa. However, it seems to be a suboptimal option to assess nodal involvement.

- Given the expanding list of targeted therapy agents and immunotherapy medications in both MIBC and NMIBC, molecular subtyping will soon become an integral part of initial staging of BCa to tailor an individualized, optimal course of treatment of each patient.

DISCLOSURE

Dr S. Daneshmand serves on the advisory board of Janssen, Ferring, Photocure, Taris, Spectrum, Pacific Edge, QED, Abbvie, Johnson & Johnson, Janssen, Seattle Genetics, Nucleix, Aduro, and Bristol Myer Squibb, and additionally as consultant to Pacific Edge and Photocure, Inc. Dr V. Duddalwar is advisory board member of DeepTek and serves as a consultant for Radmetrix. Dr H. Ahmadi has nothing to disclose.

REFERENCES

1. Siegel RL, Miller KD, Jemal A. Cancer statistics, 2020. CA A Cancer J Clin 2020; 70:7–30.
2. Rubben H, Lutzeyer W, Fischer N, et al. Natural history and treatment of low and high risk superficial bladder tumors. J Urol 1988;139(2):283–5.
3. Vickers AJ, Bennette C, Kibel AS, et al. Who should be included in a clinical trial of screening for bladder cancer?: a decision analysis of data from the Prostate, Lung, Colorectal and Ovarian Cancer Screening Trial. Cancer 2013;119(1): 143–9.
4. Moyer VA, USPST Force. Screening for bladder cancer: U.S. preventive services task force recommendation statement. Ann Intern Med 2011;155(4):246–51.
5. Khadra MH, Pickard RS, Charlton M, et al. A prospective analysis of 1,930 patients with hematuria to evaluate current diagnostic practice. J Urol 2000; 163(2):524–7.
6. Grossfeld GD, Litwin MS, Wolf JS, et al. Evaluation of asymptomatic microscopic hematuria in adults: the American Urological Association best practice policy– part I: definition, detection, prevalence, and etiology. Urology 2001;57(4): 599–603.
7. Davis R, Jones JS, Barocas DA, et al. Diagnosis, evaluation and follow-up of asymptomatic microhematuria (AMH) in adults: AUA guideline. J Urol 2012; 188(6 Suppl):2473–81.
8. Committee on gynecologic practice AUS. committee opinion No.703: asymptomatic microscopic hematuria in women. Obstet Gynecol 2017;129(6):e168–72.
9. Jocham D, Stepp H, Waidelich R. Photodynamic diagnosis in urology: state-of-the-art. Eur Urol 2008;53(6):1138–48.
10. Zainfeld D, Daneshmand S. Transurethral resection of bladder tumors: improving quality through new techniques and technologies. Curr Urol Rep 2017;18(5):34.
11. Pearce S, Daneshmand S. Enhanced endoscopy in bladder cancer. Curr Urol Rep 2018;19(10):84.

12. Chang SS, Boorjian SA, Chou R, et al. Diagnosis and treatment of non-muscle invasive bladder cancer: AUA/SUO guideline. J Urol 2016;196(4):1021–9.

13. Woldu SL, Bagrodia A, Lotan Y. Guideline of guidelines: non-muscle-invasive bladder cancer. BJU Int 2017;119(3):371–80.

14. Daneshmand S, Patel S, Lotan Y, et al. Efficacy and safety of blue light flexible cystoscopy with hexaminolevulinate in the surveillance of bladder cancer: a phase III, comparative, multicenter study. J Urol 2018;199(5):1158–65.

15. Liu JJ, Droller MJ, Liao JC. New optical imaging technologies for bladder cancer: considerations and perspectives. J Urol 2012;188(2):361–8.

16. Lotan Y, Roehrborn CG. Sensitivity and specificity of commonly available bladder tumor markers versus cytology: results of a comprehensive literature review and meta-analyses. Urology 2003;61(1):109–18 [discussion 118].

17. Xylinas E, Kluth LA, Rieken M, et al. Urine markers for detection and surveillance of bladder cancer. Urol Oncol 2014;32(3):222–9.

18. Kamat AM, Li R, O'Donnell MA, et al. Predicting response to intravesical bacillus calmette-guerin immunotherapy: are we there yet? a systematic review. Eur Urol 2018;73(5):738–48.

19. Babjuk M, Bohle A, Burger M, et al. EAU guidelines on non-muscle-invasive uro-thelial carcinoma of the bladder: update 2016. Eur Urol 2017;71(3):447–61.

20. Davidson PJ, McGeoch G, Shand B. Inclusion of a molecular marker of bladder cancer in a clinical pathway for investigation of haematuria may reduce the need for cystoscopy. N Z Med J 2019;132(1497):55–64.

21. Trinh TW, Glazer DI, Sadow CA, et al. Bladder cancer diagnosis with CT urography: test characteristics and reasons for false-positive and false-negative results. Abdom Radiol (NY) 2018;43(3):663–71.

22. Daneshmand S, Ahmadi H, Huynh LN, et al. Preoperative staging of invasive bladder cancer with dynamic gadolinium-enhanced magnetic resonance imaging: results from a prospective study. Urology 2012;80(6):1313–8.

23. Panebianco V, Narumi Y, Altun E, et al. Multiparametric magnetic resonance imaging for bladder cancer: development of vi-rads (vesical imaging-reporting and data system). Eur Urol 2018;74(3):294–306.

24. Pecoraro M, Takeuchi M, Vargas HA, et al. Overview of VI-RADS in bladder cancer. AJR Am J Roentgenol 2020;214(6):1259–68.

25. Galgano SJ, Porter KK, Burgan C, et al. The role of imaging in bladder cancer diagnosis and staging. Diagnostics 2020;10(9):703.

26. Caglic I, Panebianco V, Vargas HA, et al. MRI of bladder cancer: local and nodal staging. J Magn Reson Imaging 2020;52(3):649–67.

27. Pichler R, De Zordo T, Fritz J, et al. Pelvic lymph node staging by combined 18F-FDG-PET/CT imaging in bladder cancer prior to radical cystectomy. Clin Genito-urin Cancer 2017;15(3):e387–95.

28. Lu Y-Y, Chen J-H, Ding H-J, et al. A systematic review and meta-analysis of pre-therapeutic lymph node staging of colorectal cancer by 18F-FDG PET or PET/CT. Nucl Med Commun 2012;33(11):1127–33.

29. Soubra A, Gencturk M, Froelich J, et al. FDG-PET/CT for assessing the response to neoadjuvant chemotherapy in bladder cancer patients. Clin Genitourin Cancer 2018;16(5):360–4.

30. Xue M, Liu L, Du G, et al. Diagnostic evaluation of 18F-FDG PET/CT imaging in recurrent or residual urinary bladder cancer: a meta-analysis. Urol J 2020. https://doi.org/10.22037/uj.v0i0.5538.

31. Braendengen M, Winderen M, Fossa SD. Clinical significance of routine pre-cystectomy bone scans in patients with muscle-invasive bladder cancer. Br J Urol 1996;77(1):36–40.
32. Cacciamani GE, Nassiri N, Varghese B, et al. Radiomics and bladder cancer: current status. Bladder Cancer 2020;6(3):343–62.
33. Wang HJ, Hu DK, Yao HH, et al. Radiomics analysis of multiparametric MRI for the preoperative evaluation of pathological grade in bladder cancer tumors. Eur Radiol 2019;29(11):6182–90.
34. Xu SS, Yao QY, Liu Q, et al. Combining DWI radiomics features with transurethral resection promotes the differentiation between muscle-invasive bladder cancer and non-muscle-invasive bladder cancer. Eur Radiol 2020;30(3):1804–12.
35. Zheng JJ, Kong JQ, Wu SX, et al. Development of a noninvasive tool to preoperatively evaluate the muscular invasiveness of bladder cancer using a radiomics approach. Cancer 2019;125(24):4388–98.
36. Fan TW, Malhi H, Varghese B, et al. Computed tomography-based texture analysis of bladder cancer: differentiating urothelial carcinoma from micropapillary carcinoma. Abdom Radiol (NY) 2019;44(1):201–8.
37. Alessandrino F, Gujrathi R, Nassar AH, et al. Predictive role of computed tomography texture analysis in patients with metastatic urothelial cancer treated with programmed death-1 and programmed death-ligand 1 inhibitors. Eur Urol Oncol 2020;3(5):680–6.
38. Lin P, Wen DY, Chen L, et al. A radiogenomics signature for predicting the clinical outcome of bladder urothelial carcinoma. Eur Radiol 2020;30(1):547–57.
39. Rizzo S, Botta F, Raimondi S, et al. Radiomics: the facts and the challenges of image analysis. Eur Radiol Exp 2018;2(1):36.
40. Kamat AM, Cookson M, Witjes JA, et al. The impact of blue light cystoscopy with hexaminolevulinate (HAL) on progression of bladder cancer - a new analysis. Bladder Cancer 2016;2(2):273–8.
41. Jocham D, Witjes F, Wagner S, et al. Improved detection and treatment of bladder cancer using hexaminolevulinate imaging: a prospective, phase III multicenter study. J Urol 2005;174(3):862–6 [discussion 866].
42. Patrick DJ, Fitzgerald SD, Sesterhenn IA, et al. Classification of canine urinary bladder urothelial tumours based on the World Health Organization/International Society of Urological Pathology consensus classification. J Comp Pathol 2006; 135(4):190–9.
43. Paner GP, Stadler WM, Hansel DE, et al. Updates in the eighth edition of the tumor-node-metastasis staging classification for urologic cancers. Eur Urol 2018;73(4):560–9.
44. Esrig D, Freeman JA, Elmajian DA, et al. Transitional cell carcinoma involving the prostate with a proposed staging classification for stromal invasion. J Urol 1996; 156(3):1071–6.
45. Inamura K. Bladder cancer: new insights into its molecular pathology. Cancers (Basel) 2018;10(4):100.
46. Robertson AG, Kim J, Al-Ahmadie H, et al. Comprehensive molecular characterization of muscle-invasive bladder cancer. Cell 2017;171(3):540–56.e525.

Surgery for Bladder and Upper Tract Urothelial Cancer

Vivek Venkatramani, MS, MCh[a,b,]*,
Dipen Jaysukhlal Parekh, MD, MCh[c]

KEYWORDS

- Bladder cancer • Upper tract urothelial cancer • Radical cystectomy • TURBT
- Nephroureterectomy • Surgical management • Robotic surgery

KEY POINTS

- Surgery is an integral part of the diagnosis and treatment of bladder and upper tract cancer.
- Transurethral resection of bladder tumors forms the basis of the management.
- Radical cystectomy for invasive bladder cancer provides good oncological outcomes; however, efforts to reduce its morbidity, such as minimally invasive surgery and early recovery after surgery protocols, are important.
- Conservative surgical management for low-risk upper tract urothelial cancer provides equivalent oncological outcomes without the need for removal of the affected renal unit; however, intensive follow-up is needed.
- Radical nephroureterectomy remains the gold standard management for high-risk upper tract carcinoma.

INTRODUCTION

Bladder cancer remains a very common urologic cancer and is the fourth most common cancer in American men.[1] It has a high morbidity and mortality and can be associated with upper tract urothelial cancer (UTUC), either preceding or following it, as a result of dysplasia affecting the entire urothelial lining (field change). Surgery remains the mainstay for the diagnosis and staging of bladder cancer, as well as the radical treatment of muscle-invasive disease. Surgery plays an equally important role in the diagnosis and management of UTUC.

[a] Nanavati Super-Specialty Hospital, S.V Road, Vile Parle West, Mumbai 400056, India; [b] Department of Urology, University of Miami Miller School of Medicine; [c] Department of Urology, Member Sylvester Cancer Center, University of Miami Miller School of Medicine, University of Miami Health System, 1120 Northwest 14th Street, Suite 1560B, Miami, FL 33136, USA
* Corresponding author.
E-mail address: docvivek@gmail.com

Hematol Oncol Clin N Am 35 (2021) 543–566
https://doi.org/10.1016/j.hoc.2021.02.005
0889-8588/21/© 2021 Elsevier Inc. All rights reserved.

SURGERY FOR BLADDER CANCER
Transurethral Resection of the Bladder Tumor

Once the initial diagnostic work-up has been completed, all patients with suspected bladder cancer undergo a transurethral resection of the bladder tumor (TURBT). This resection forms the basis for clinical staging and subsequent management, and the importance of a high-quality TURBT cannot be overemphasized.[2]

Procedure

The patient is positioned in dorsal lithotomy at the edge of the bed under spinal or general anesthesia. A single dose of antibiotic prophylaxis is given.[2–4]

A thorough bimanual examination under anesthesia forms the first step. The surgeon feels for a mass or induration in order to obtain a baseline idea of the stage. A rigid cystoscope is introduced and a careful cystoscopic examination is performed documenting the status of the anterior and prostatic urethra; the location, size, and appearance of all tumors; the appearance of both ureteric orifices and the nature of their efflux; and the presence of any suspicious areas of carcinoma in situ (CIS).The anterior wall and bladder neck may require the use of a 70° or 120° cystoscope to obtain complete visualization.[2–4]

The urethra is then gently calibrated and the resectoscope is introduced via a visual obturator. The resection can be performed via a monopolar (using sterile water or 1.5% glycine as irrigant) or bipolar (using normal saline as irrigant) electrocautery with a loop electrode. Bipolar resection eliminates the possibility of electrolyte abnormalities caused by fluid absorption and may provide a better pathologic specimen.[5] Other purported advantages, such as hemostasis and reduction in obturator jerk, remain unproved.[5] En bloc resection has been described, with holmium or thulium lasers as well as electrocautery. It has been shown to provide high-quality specimens with presence of muscle in more than 95% cases. It is generally used in selected cases with papillary exophytic tumors.[6–9]

The aim of TURBT is complete resection of all tumors as well as obtaining a separate, representative sample from the detrusor muscle to detect invasion.[2,10] Detrusor muscle in the specimen represents a surrogate for the quality of TURBT because its absence can be associated with significant understaging and may prompt a repeat TURBT.[10–13]

Once hemostasis is achieved and all chips evacuated, a catheter is placed. A bimanual examination is performed at the end of resection after emptying the bladder to complete evaluation. The catheter is removed anywhere from 1 to 7 days postoperatively at the surgeons' discretion and depending on the extent of resection.[3,4]

Complications

TURBT is a difficult technique to master and carries the risk of significant complications, the most clinically relevant of which are hemorrhage and bladder perforation.[14]

1. Hemorrhage. Hemorrhage can occur in about 2% to 13% of cases and is generally associated with large, infiltrative tumors.[5,14–16] Careful resection to a plan, beginning from one end of a large tumor and progressing to the opposite side, with meticulous hemostasis during resection, can help minimize the risk in large tumors. A complete resection of the tumor also allows better hemostasis. Postoperatively, clot evacuation and continuous bladder irrigation with normal saline may be required, and endoscopic coagulation under anesthesia is needed in persistent bleeding.[14]
2. Bladder perforation. The risk of bladder perforation is generally 2% to 5%, with more than 85% of cases being extraperitoneal.[14–17] Extraperitoneal perforation is

diagnosed by visualization of perivesical fat during resection and requires catheter drainage for 5 to 7 days in order to allow spontaneous healing.[4,14] Intraperitoneal perforations can occur during resection on the dome or high posterior wall. In general, these are managed with open exploration and closure of the bladder; however, they can also be more conservatively managed with peritoneal drain placement and catheterization.[14,18] Tumor seeding has been reported anecdotally following perforation (usually intraperitoneal).[14,17]

3. Adductor muscle jerk. The obturator nerve runs in close proximity to the lateral wall of the bladder, and stimulation of the nerve by electrocautery during resection can lead to adductor muscle contraction. When uncontrolled, this can lead to a deep resection and potential bladder perforation. Steps to minimize this include use of an obturator nerve block, general anesthesia with muscle paralysis, resection with lower settings, avoiding overdistention of the bladder, intermittent or staccato technique of applying energy, and changing the position of the neutral electrode.[3–5,14] Initial studies suggested that the use of bipolar TURBT reduces the risk of adductor muscle jerks; however, a large randomized trial found no difference.[5]

Perioperative chemotherapy
A single immediate intravesical dose of chemotherapy has been proved to reduce recurrences by up to 15% without any effect on progression or survival.[19–22] The most benefit is noted in patients with single, small, low-grade tumors.[2] The instillation should be given within 24 hours of TURBT, and it works by preventing implantation of circulating tumor cells. Mitomycin C and gemcitabine are the most commonly used agents.[20,23] In extensive resections, suspected perforation, invasive tumors, or significant bleeding, this instillation should be avoided because there are significant risks of extravasation.[2,19–21]

Bladder biopsies
Biopsies from any suspicious velvety areas should be taken to detect CIS.[2,4,24] In cases with a positive cytology where no nonpapillary tumors are seen, biopsies from normal-looking mucosa may be needed. These biopsies should be mapped and taken from the trigone, dome, anterior, posterior and lateral bladder walls, and prostatic urethra.[25–27] Prostatic urethral biopsies may also be taken in patients with bladder neck tumors and multiple tumors.[28,29] Mapping biopsies can also be done if partial cystectomy or bladder-preservation protocols are planned.[30]

Indications for repeat transurethral resection of the bladder tumor
There are certain situations where a repeat TURBT is needed 2 to 6 weeks after the initial procedure (**Table 1**).[2,24]

Table 1	
Indications for repeat transurethral resection of the bladder tumor	
Indication	**Rationale**
Incomplete initial resection	Essential for adequate staging and management unless cystectomy is planned[2,11]
High-grade tumors (Ta)	Residual tumor rate of 50%. Risk of upstaging 15%. Especially in larger and multifocal tumors[2,31–34]
T1 disease	Upstaging to muscle-invasive disease in 50% if no muscle in initial specimen and 15%–20% if muscle present.[32,35] Complete resection improves response to further intravesical therapy and improves recurrence-free survival[34,36,37]

Enhanced transurethral resection of the bladder tumor

1. Photodynamic/fluorescent/blue-light cystoscopy. Intravesical instillation of a photosensitizing compound such as 5-aminolevulinic acid or hexaminolevulinic acid followed by intraoperative use of blue light is used to improve tumor detection.[25] In tumor cells, photoactive porphyrins are formed and produce a red color under blue light. Studies have shown reduced recurrence rates (both short and long term).[38–40] An increased detection of non–muscle-invasive tumors and CIS has been shown.[41–44] Most studies show no difference in progression or mortality, but a recent study showed a trend toward lower rates and delayed progression.[38–40,45] False-positive rates can be significant in patients with bladder inflammation, recent TURBT, or bacillus Calmette-Guérin (BCG) instillation.[40]
2. Narrow-band imaging (NBI). Two spectrums of light (415 nm and 540 nm) are used. These spectrums are absorbed by hemoglobin and allow better evaluation of the mucosa and submucosal blood vessels.[25] Initial studies showed improved tumor detection with NBI, and recent trials and reviews have also shown a reduced recurrence rate for low-risk tumors at 3 months and 1 year.[46–48]

Radical Cystectomy with Pelvic Lymphadenectomy and Urinary Diversion

Radical cystectomy (RC) is the standard of care for muscle-invasive bladder cancer (MIBC). Indications for RC are detailed in **Box 1**.[24,25,30]

RC includes removal of the bladder and surrounding organs into which the cancer can invade, followed by urinary diversion. It allows excellent local control of disease along with pathologic tumor and lymph node staging. However, RC can be associated with significant morbidity, and patient performance and comorbid status, along with quality-of-life (QOL) expectations, play an important role in decision making. A delay of more than 12 weeks from the diagnosis of MIBC has been shown to affect survival in multiple retrospective series.[49,50]

Preoperative preparation

Preoperative optimization of patients leading up to RC is important and has been associated with better outcomes.[51,52] Smoking should be stopped and regular exercise and improvements in muscle mass and nutrition are advised. Comorbidities should be well evaluated and controlled. All patients (even those planned for continent diversion) visit a stoma therapist and undergo marking of the site and gain familiarity

---

Box 1
Indications for radical cystectomy

Resectable MIBC: T2-4a, N0/1-x, M0

BCG failure for high-grade T1 disease

High-grade T1 disease with unfavorable pathologic characteristics: multifocal tumors, T1b, tumors within a diverticulum, associated CIS, residual T1 disease on re-TURBT, lymphovascular invasion, micropapillary/plasmacytoid/nested variants

Nonurothelial malignancy such as sarcomas, squamous cell carcinoma, adenocarcinoma, signet ring carcinoma

Extensive non–muscle-invasive disease not controllable by TURBT or intravesical therapies (relative indication)

Salvage cystectomy after failure of bladder-preservation protocols

Palliative cystectomy for recurrent gross hematuria, fistula formation, or intractable pain

with the appliance. Antibiotic and thromboprophylaxis (mechanical and pharmacologic) are recommended. Mechanical bowel preparation is not routinely recommended.[30,53,54]

Surgical principles

Men are generally placed supine with or without mild flexion at the anterior superior iliac spine. If a urethrectomy is planned, lithotomy position is preferable. Women are generally placed in low lithotomy to provide access to the vagina.

A lower midline incision is routine. The urachus is excised in continuity with the bladder. The ureters are carefully mobilized to obtain adequate length and preserve their vascularity. The rectum is freed off the bladder in the midline by blunt or sharp dissection up to the level of the prostate, where the Denonvilliers fascia is incised. The pedicles of the bladder may be tackled with suture ligation, clips, sealing devices, or staplers. The dorsal venous complex is oversewn as in a radical prostatectomy and then divided. The urethra is then dissected circumferentially. Preservation of maximal urethral length is important if a neobladder is planned. A frozen section of the urethral margin is mandatory in patients with neobladder.[30,53,54]

Men

In men, RC involves removal of the bladder, perivesical soft tissue, terminal ureters, prostate, seminal vesicles, and vas deferens.[4,30] With increasing focus on improving functional outcomes, techniques to potentially improve voiding and sexual function after RC have been described.[55–60] These techniques seem to be oncologically safe; however, better trials are needed and patient selection is critical. At present, these cannot be recommended as standard and should only be offered to men with organ-confined MIBC (not multifocal and no CIS) without involvement of bladder neck, prostate, or urethra, who are highly motivated to preserve sexual function. The techniques involve various degrees of neurovascular bundle sparing and prostate or seminal sparing, and there are no data to select one approach rather than another. If prostate preservation is considered, a biopsy from the prostatic urethra is recommended to rule out concomitant disease or local invasion.[30,53,54]

Women

In women, along with the bladder, perivesical tissue, and terminal ureters, the ovaries, fallopian tubes, uterus with cervix, and anterior vaginal wall (anterior exenteration) are also removed.[4,30,53,54] In organ-confined MIBC with no cancer in the bladder base, trigone or bladder neck preservation of the vaginal wall and/or uterus may be considered. This method provides better support to the urethra in case a neobladder is planned, helps in preventing postoperative prolapse, and also maintains sexual function.[61] Preservation of the ovaries in premenopausal women is safe and does not increase bladder cancer recurrence. It can be performed unless the woman has an increased risk of ovarian or breast cancer (eg, BRCA1/2 carrier, Lynch syndrome)[62,63]

Lymphadenectomy

About 25% of patients have lymph node metastases on RC, and lymph node status is a powerful predictor of recurrence and survival following RC.[64–66] A bilateral pelvic lymph node dissection (PLND) is an indispensable part of RC; however, the extent of the dissection and its therapeutic benefit remain debated. PLND may be impossible to perform in patients with prior pelvic surgery or radiation, or vascular disease.[53] Based on bladder lymphatic landing zones, it is generally recommended that the external iliac, internal iliac, obturator, and presacral and common iliac nodes up to the level of the ureter crossing superiorly are removed at the time of PLND. The lateral border is the genitofemoral nerve and the caudal border is up to the lacunar ligament and lymph node of Cloquet. The medial extent is the obturator nerve caudally and the internal iliac artery and ureter superiorly.[67-71] A minimum of 10 to 12 lymph nodes evaluated indicates an adequate dissection, and submission of the lymph nodes in separate packets is associated with increased yield.[53] Extending the cranial boundary of dissection to the aortic bifurcation along with greater dissection of presacral nodes was associated with improved node yield and may also be associated with better survival and lower pelvic recurrence; however, those studies were associated with methodologic limitations, including variation in PLND technique.[65,67-79] Furthermore, a recent randomized trial by Gschwend and colleagues[80] showed no benefit when lymphadenectomy (LDN) was extended to the inferior mesenteric artery.

Continent and incontinent diversions

The urinary diversion (UD) following RC is predominantly responsible for complications and long-term QOL after surgery, and a thorough discussion of all types of UD with the patient is essential. Patient preferences, intrinsic patient factors, and tumor factors are used to determine which UD is appropriate on an individual basis. The most common types of diversion are the ileal conduit and orthotopic neobladder (ONB); however, there are no randomized trials comparing them (**Table 2**). The urethral margin has to be negative on frozen section at the time of RC in order to perform an ONB.[4,30,53] Risk factors for urethral involvement are tumor multifocality, CIS, tumor at bladder neck, prostatic urethra, or stromal involvement (in men) and bladder base or anterior vaginal wall involvement (in women).[81,82] Preoperative prostatic urethral biopsies are not as reliable as intraoperative frozen section.[83] A frozen section of the vaginal margin may additionally be performed in women with bulky disease (≥T3b).[84]

Continent cutaneous diversions are low-pressure detubularized bowel reservoirs connected to skin for self-catheterization, the most commonly performed of which is the Indiana pouch.[4,30,53,54] They can be performed in patients who wish to avoid a stoma but are not candidates or are unwilling for ONB.[89]

Cutaneous ureterostomies are the simplest form of UD; however, they are associated with a significant rate of stenosis and urinary tract infection (UTI), so they are only used in morbid patients in whom the quickest procedure is required.[86,90]

Ureterosigmoidostomy was the oldest UD described and involves connection of the ureters to the rectosigmoid colon (which may or may not be fashioned into a pouch). The high complication rate, including UTI and risk of secondary malignancy at the anastomotic site, meant this has fallen out of favor.[4,30,54]

Special intraoperative situations

1. Unresectable disease. RC should not be performed when there are large, unresectable lymph nodes; fixation of bladder to the pelvic sidewall or invasion of the rectosigmoid; or in patients with extensive periureteral disease.[91,92] If large lymph nodes are seen on preoperative imaging, then a computed tomography (CT)–guided biopsy can be performed and chemotherapy given if it is positive.[30]
2. Frozen section of the ureter margins. The incidence of upper tract recurrence following RC is 2% to 8%, and this usually occurs 2 to 4 years after RC.[30] Ureteral margin status or involvement of the distal ureter with tumor is a predictor of this recurrence.[93,94] Gross involvement of the distal ureters by tumor necessitates resection of the tumor completely and in these cases a frozen section may be used to ensure clearance.
   The use of routine frozen sections remains controversial and this practice has largely been given up because the site of recurrence is rarely at the anastomosis

Table 2
Ileal conduit and orthotopic neobladder

	Ileal Conduit	Orthotopic Neobladder
Principle	Incontinent short segment (15 cm) of ileum opening as a cutaneous ureterostomy	Create a spherical, adequate volume and low-pressure reservoir made from detubularized and folded bowel to the urethra
Contraindications	• Inadequate ileum length (prior surgery or radiation, inflammatory bowel disease) If ileum is unavailable, colon segment can be used	• Positive urethral margin • Insufficient bowel length • Inadequate motor function or psychological issues preventing performance of self-catheterization • eGFR<45 mL/min/m^2 • Uncorrectable urethral stricture • Age>80 y (relative)
Advantages	Simple, easy to maintain, low reoperation rates	Naturally situated reservoir with possible benefit in QOL after 1–2 y
Disadvantages	Stoma on abdominal wall may be associated with potential QOL and psychological effects	Technically demanding and patient counseling regarding conversion to ileal conduit intraoperatively needed, need to be ready for CIC
Potential complications	Early complications UTI, including pyelonephritis Ureteroileal leak Late complications Stoma complications (24%) Upper tract functional damage Ureterointestinal stricture Metabolic disorders	Early complications UTI Ureteroileal leak Late complications Anastomotic strictures Need for CIC (5%–25%, women>men) Incontinence (diurnal 8%–10% and nocturnal 20%–30%) Metabolic disorders Malabsorption especially vitamin B$_{12}$ Upper tract functional damage

Abbreviations: CIC, clean intermittent catheterization; eGFR, estimated glomerular filtration rate; UTI, urinary tract infection.
Data from Refs.[4,25,30,53,54,85–88]

and it generally denotes a field change into dysplastic mucosa. Furthermore, it remains uncertain whether presence of CIS at the margin is associated with a worse outcome.[95,96]

3. Urethrectomy. Risk factors for urethral involvement have been discussed previously. Urethral recurrence occurs in 4% to 8% of men after RC and 1% of women.[97–101] In men, urethrectomy should be considered in patients with diffuse CIS of the prostatic urethra or ducts, stromal invasion of the prostate, and positive

urethral margins.[30,102] Small, low-grade papillary tumors may be resected and the urethra preserved in the absence of the other risk factors.[99,103]

Oncologic outcomes
RC provides excellent local control and good long-term outcomes for bladder cancer (**Table 3**). Most recurrences following RC occur within 7 to 18 months after surgery. Major risk factors for recurrence and survival are T stage, lymph node involvement, and positive margins.[65,66,104–108] There is substantial evidence that high-volume centers and surgeons are associated with better perioperative and mortality outcomes.[109,110]

Morbidity
RC remains a morbid procedure with a real risk of mortality (1.2%–3.2% at 30 days and 2.3%–8% at 90 days).[109,111–114] Early complications can be seen in as many as 60% of patients, with 13% being major complications. Most are gastrointestinal (29%, most commonly paralytic ileus) or infectious (25%, most commonly UTI).[86,115] Surgical complications include anastomotic leaks (bowel, ureterointestinal) and lymphoceles.

Late complications are usually related to the use of the bowel segment and diversion performed. Metabolic complications ensuing from the use of ileum are hyperchloremic metabolic acidosis, and some patients need bicarbonate replacement orally. Renal functional deterioration can occur in about 18% of ileal conduits and about 20% with ONB.[86,116–118] Stoma-related complications such as prolapse or hernia can be seen with conduits, and ONB may be associated with neobladder rupture or calculi in the long term. Incontinence or retention can also occur with ONB (see **Table 2**).

Early recovery after surgery for radical cystectomy
Perioperative optimization of patient recovery after RC using early recovery after surgery (ERAS) protocols is followed at most institutions.[119] Preoperative preparation was described earlier. Carbohydrate loading may improve insulin resistance, hasten bowel recovery, and reduce hospital stay.[120] Intraoperatively, goal directed fluid management, temperature control, prophylaxis of postoperative nausea and vomiting, and the use of minimally invasive surgery are recommended. Early mobilization, no nasogastric tube, early resumption of oral fluids postoperatively, minimal narcotic use, and minimal use of drains and tubes are postoperative components of ERAS.[119,121]

Paralytic ileus can be a significant problem after RC, and a prospective trial showed an advantage with the use of the mu-opioid receptor antagonist alvimopan.[122] The first dose is given just before surgery and it is continued until diet is begun or for 15 doses. Chewing gum and the use of metoclopramide may also help bowel recovery.[123]

ERAS protocols tend to be complicated and may be associated with hidden costs and an increased use of home visits or outpatient visits following discharge; therefore, they need to be tailored to each institution and patient.

Table 3 Five-year disease-specific survival after radical cystectomy depending on pT stage	
≤T1	80%–90%
T2	70%–80%
T3	40%–50%
T4	15%–45%
N+	20%–35%

Minimally invasive approaches for radical cystectomy

Given the perioperative morbidity associated with RC, minimally invasive approaches have been attempted. Laparoscopic RC was described first and is still performed in areas where robotic surgery is not available. However, it is a challenging technique to learn and is associated with long operative times. Over the past decade, robotic RC has emerged as the true minimally invasive alternative to RC. The world's first phase 3 multicenter randomized trial comparing open with robotic surgery for any organ site was performed for bladder cancer (randomized open versus robotic radical cystectomy [RAZOR] trial).[124] It showed noninferiority of the robotic approach for the primary oncologic end point of 2-year progression-free survival. Blood loss, transfusion rates, and length of stay were also significantly better for robotic RC. There was no difference in positive margins or lymph node yield.[124] A 3-year follow-up and overall survival outcomes from the RAZOR trial confirmed no difference.[125] Similar perioperative outcomes have been noted in smaller trials.[126–128] The RAZOR and earlier trials involved the UD being constructed extracorporeally, and some researchers believe intracorporeal UD may unlock further benefits of the robotic approach. However, no clear benefits of intracorporeal diversion have been shown to date, and the iROC (Intracorporeal Urinary Diversion Versus Open Radical Cystectomy) randomized trial hopes to answer this question.[129]

Partial cystectomy

In highly selected patients (<5%) partial cystectomy may be considered if the tumor develops in an area of the bladder where an adequate margin can be obtained, such as the dome.[25] Further selection criteria include tumor size less than 3 cm, absence of CIS, no hydronephrosis, adequate bladder function, and no residual T1 or higher-stage disease. About 40% of these patients ultimately require RC.[130,131] Partial cystectomy is also indicated for patients with urachal adenocarcinoma, and may be performed in very selected patients with carcinoma within a bladder diverticulum.[132,133] PLND is also performed in all these patients.

SURGERY FOR UPPER TRACT UROTHELIAL CANCER
Diagnostic Ureterorenoscopy and Biopsy

A cystoscopy is essential in all patients with suspected UTUC to rule out concomitant bladder tumors; however, ureterorenoscopy (URS) and visualization of the tumor with or without biopsy is only indicated when the diagnosis remains in doubt after imaging studies and cytology.[134,135] Voided urine cytology is less sensitive for UTUC than bladder cancer, and positive cytology in the presence of a normal cystoscopy is suspicious for UTUC.[24,135,136] If cytology is being collected from the upper tracts during URS, it should be done before instillation of contrast during retrograde ureteropyelography (RGP) because the contrast may alter cellular architecture, making interpretation difficult.[137] The presence of a filling defect or goblet sign on RGP may also indicate the presence of a space-occupying lesion (75% detection).[134,138] Cytology following barbotage can detect up to 91% of UTUC.[139]

URS can detect the presence, appearance, and size of tumor, as well as allow biopsies to be obtained, increasing the diagnostic yield to 90%.[134,135] Biopsies may be taken via brush or forceps, and tumor grade has excellent correlation (80%–90%) with final histopathology.[134,135] There remains a small risk of undergrading, which may be important if conservative resection is planned.[140]

Because the biopsy samples may be small and shallow, diagnosis of T stage on a biopsy may be difficult (with >25% risk of understaging). Therefore, it is important to combine grade of the tumor and clinical, radiological, and visual data as well to obtain a more accurate risk assessment for each patient.[134,135]

Although the risk of tumor extravasation and dissemination with URS is low, there are some studies showing that it may be associated with an increase in bladder recurrences, so it should be used only in patients with doubtful diagnosis or when organ-preservation strategies are being considered.[141–143]

Kidney-Sparing Surgical Treatments

Kidney-sparing approaches can be offered to patients with low-risk UTUC, including tumors with all the following characteristics: unifocal disease, tumor size less than 2 cm, low-grade cytology, low-grade URS biopsy, and noninvasive appearance on imaging.[144,145] In these patients, survival is comparable with radical treatment, irrespective of the function of the opposite kidney.[146]

In patients with high-risk disease who have a solitary kidney or impaired renal function, renal conservation may be offered after assessing the individual's oncologic risks.[135]

Stringent follow-up is needed in these patients, with regular cystoscopy and imaging studies (CT urography) at 3 and 6 months, and then annually. A repeat URS at 3 months is also recommended. In patients with high-risk tumors who undergo this approach, the follow-up includes urine cytology as well, along with URS at 3 and 6 months after the initial ablation.[135]

1. Ureteroscopic approach

   The tumor is debulked by a biopsy forceps or basket and then ablated with a laser fiber or electrocautery. A URS resectoscope can also be used with no attempt to resect deeper than the visualized intraluminal tumor. Circumferential fulguration with electrocautery should be avoided to prevent stricture formation.[134] Flexible URS is needed for tumors in the pelvicalyceal system (PCS), and lasers are commonly used in conjunction. Holmium laser is preferred because of its shallow depth of penetration (0.5 mm) and excellent hemostatic properties.[147–149] Complications include ureteral perforation and stricture (11%); however, with newer techniques and smaller scopes, this risk has been reduced.[149]

2. Percutaneous or antegrade access

   This access may be needed in tumors of the PCS that are not approachable via URS; however, advances in flexible URS have made this less common.[149,150] The risk of seeding of the access tract is also a consideration; however, it seems uncommon.[149] This approach may also have a role in cases of bulky renal pelvis tumors in patients with a solitary kidney or renal failure.[134,135] Techniques for tumor resection and ablation are similar to URS.[134]

3. Conservative surgical resections

   Distal ureterectomy with ureteral reimplantation is an option for lower ureteral tumors. It can be performed open or via a minimally invasive approach and has good results.[134,151,152] Segmental ureteral resection with ureteroureterostomy plus or minus regional LDN may be attempted for tumors in the upper two-thirds of the ureter.[134,151,152] Partial nephrectomy or pyelectomy and total ureterectomy with ileal replacement have also been described. All these surgeries are rarely done now given the advances in endoscopic management.[134,135]

4. Chemoablation

   Chemotherapeutic agents instilled either antegrade or retrograde via stent have not shown good activity for ablation of upper tract tumors, either as adjuvant treatment or for complete ablation. The use of BCG for upper tract CIS has also not been effective.[135,153]

However, the Olympus trial recently reported on results of chemoablation with an intracavitary mitomycin C hydrogel that converts to a gel at body temperature, allowing sustained drug delivery in the upper tract. It was instilled in 6-weekly doses in patients with low-grade disease and showed a 59% complete response rate in a cohort of 74 patients.[154]

Radical Nephroureterectomy for Upper Tract Urothelial Cancer

Radical nephroureterectomy (RNU) is the standard treatment of all high-risk disease, whatever the location.[134,135] High-risk disease includes any of the following: tumors larger than 2 cm, high-grade cytology, high-grade biopsy, presence of hydronephrosis, multifocality, previous RC for bladder cancer, and any variant histology.[144,145]

The principles of RNU include complete removal of the kidney, ureter, and bladder cuff (to excise the intramural portion of the ureter), taking care to prevent tumor spillage.[155]

Open RNU involves a large midline incision or a 2-incision approach. The kidney is excised within the Gerota fascia along with the entire ureter.[134] Most of these procedures are now performed by a minimally invasive approach to minimize morbidity. To minimize tumor seeding and metastases along port sites, important principles include avoiding entry into the urinary tract, avoiding direct contact of tumor with the instruments, and en bloc removal maintaining a closed urinary system.[156] Laparoscopic surgery for bulky or non–organ-confined UTUC may be inferior to open surgery; however, the robotic approach seems to have equivalent outcomes.[157–159]

Bladder cuff excision

The excision of bladder cuff is an essential part of the procedure because of the high rate of local recurrence (30%–75%) and the difficulty in surveilling this part.[134] Care must be exercised to prevent injury to the opposite ureter. Several approaches have been described to deal with this part of the procedure.[134,160,161] Transurethral approaches involve resecting the ureteral orifice (UO) (pluck technique), incising around the UO and intramural ureter with the Collins knife, and intussusception (stripping technique).[160–163] A transvesical combined cystoscopic and laparoscopic approach has also been described.[164]

In open surgery, the cuff may be excised via a transvesical anterior cystotomy with a 1-cm margin around the ureteric orifice or a completely extravesical approach to core out the intramural ureter.[134] These approaches can be replicated laparoscopically; however, they are technically challenging, so a combination with endoscopic methods and/or stapling devices may be used. Alternatively, the bladder cuff may be excised through the open incision (modified Gibson/Pfannenstiel) that is planned for removal of the entire specimen.[134]

With the robotic approach, a complete replication of open surgery can be performed and has made management of the bladder cuff more straightforward.[159]

Lymphadenectomy

LND is a recommended component of RNU.[135] The overall risk of lymph node involvement is 12% to 25% and increases with T stage.[134,165] Template-based LND is recommended in all cases and templates are available in **Table 4**.[134,135,166–168] Template-based LND has been shown to reduce local recurrences and improve cancer-specific survival in patients with muscle-invasive disease, even if clinically node negative.[169–171] Although survival is not improved in patients with Ta/T1 disease,

Table 4
Recommended lymphadenectomy templates in radical nephroureterectomy

Location	Right-Sided Template	Left-Sided Template
Renal pelvis	Hilar, paracaval, retrocaval, and interaortocaval up to inferior mesenteric artery	Hilar and para-aortic up to inferior mesenteric artery
Upper two-thirds of ureter	Hilar, paracaval, retrocaval, and interaortocaval up to aortic bifurcation	Hilar and para-aortic up to aortic bifurcation
Distal ureter	Ipsilateral common, external, and internal iliac; obturator and presacral	Ipsilateral common, external, and internal iliac; obturator and presacral

accurate staging information can be obtained with an LND.[135] However, there remains a lack of uniformity in templates used, disparity among surgeons performing LND, and there exists an inconsistent pattern of spread in UTUC (compared with bladder cancer), making the true value difficult to estimate.[134]

Postoperative bladder instillation
The risk of a bladder recurrence following UTUC varies from 15% to 75% depending on the location of the upper tract tumor.[134,145,172] A single intravesical instillation of chemotherapy (mitomycin C, pirarubicin) has been shown to reduce this recurrence rate when given 2 to 10 days following surgery.[173–175] If there is concern regarding healing of the bladder suture line, a cystogram may be performed before instillation.[135]

SUMMARY

Bladder cancer remains very common and associated with a high mortality. Surgery begins with TURBT to reach an accurate diagnosis and staging of disease. Advances such as blue-light cystoscopy and NBI have the potential to reduce recurrence rates following TURBT. RC remains the gold standard for MIBC. It provides excellent local control and good long-term outcomes; however, it is associated with significant perioperative morbidity. The use of minimally invasive approaches such as robotic surgery and adoption of ERAS protocols have helped reduce the early morbidity. Late complications are predominantly related to the UD performed, and patient counseling preoperatively is key. LDN is an essential component of the procedure, but its extent remains debated.

UTUC is a rare disease and can occur before or after bladder carcinoma caused by a field urothelial change. Diagnostic URS is needed if doubt exists following cytology and imaging. Low-risk tumors can be managed by conservative approaches such as ureteroscopy, percutaneous approaches, conservative surgery, and chemoablation without compromising oncologic outcomes; however, strict follow-up is essential. High-risk UTUC necessitates RNU with template LDN and bladder cuff excision. This procedure is now predominantly done using a minimally invasive approach. In patients with solitary kidneys or bilateral disease, decisions for conservative procedures need to be taken on an individual basis after accounting for tumor-related and patient-related factors.

CLINICS CARE POINTS

- Repeat TURBT is recommended in cases of high-grade or T1 tumors because of the significant risk of upstaging.

- Radical cystectomy provides excellent local control and good oncologic outcomes however it has a real risk of mortality (1.2-3.2% at 30 days and 2.3-8% at 90days).
- There is no difference in oncologic outcomes between robotic and open radical cystectomy.
- Lymphadenectomy is an essential component of radical cystectomy however the superior extent remains debated. Template-based lymphadenectomy is also recommended as a component of radical nephro-ureterectomy.
- Bladder cuff excision is essential because of the high rate (30-75%) of local recurrence.

DISCLOSURE

Both authors have no financial conflicts of interests to disclose.

REFERENCES

1. Siegel RL, Miller KD, Jemal A. Cancer statistics, 2020. CA Cancer J Clin 2020; 70(1):7–30.
2. Chang SS, Boorjian SA, Chou R, et al. Diagnosis and treatment of non-muscle invasive bladder cancer: AUA/SUO Guideline. J Urol 2016;196(4):1021–9.
3. Stephen Jones J. Non-muscle-invasive bladder cancer (Ta,T1 and CIS). In: Wein AJ, Kavoussi LR, Partin AW, et al, editors. Campbell-walsh Urology, vol. 3, 11th edition. Philadelphia: Elsevier; 2016. p. 2205–22.
4. Navai N, Dinney CPN. Transurethral and open surgery for bladder cancer. In: Wein AJ, Kavoussi LR, Partin AW, et al, editors. Campbell-walsh Urology, vol. 3, 11th edition. Philadelphia: Elsevier; 2016. p. 2242–53.
5. Venkatramani V, Panda A, Manojkumar R, et al. Monopolar versus bipolar transurethral resection of bladder tumors: a single center, parallel arm, randomized, controlled trial. J Urol 2014;191(6):1703–7.
6. Kramer MW, Altieri V, Hurle R, et al. Current Evidence of Transurethral En-bloc Resection of Nonmuscle Invasive Bladder Cancer. Eur Urol Focus 2017;3(6): 567–76.
7. Kramer MW, Rassweiler JJ, Klein J, et al. En bloc resection of urothelium carcinoma of the bladder (EBRUC): a European multicenter study to compare safety, efficacy, and outcome of laser and electrical en bloc transurethral resection of bladder tumor. World J Urol 2015;33(12):1937–43.
8. Hurle R, Lazzeri M, Colombo P, et al. "En Bloc" Resection of Nonmuscle Invasive Bladder Cancer: A Prospective Single-center Study. Urology 2016;90:126–30.
9. Migliari R, Buffardi A, Ghabin H. Thulium Laser Endoscopic En Bloc Enucleation of Nonmuscle-Invasive Bladder Cancer. J Endourol 2015;29(11):1258–62.
10. Herr HW, Donat SM. Quality control in transurethral resection of bladder tumours. BJU Int 2008;102(9 Pt B):1242–6.
11. Brausi M, Collette L, Kurth K, et al. Variability in the recurrence rate at first follow-up cystoscopy after TUR in stage Ta T1 transitional cell carcinoma of the bladder: a combined analysis of seven EORTC studies. Eur Urol 2002;41(5): 523–31.
12. Richterstetter M, Wullich B, Amann K, et al. The value of extended transurethral resection of bladder tumour (TURBT) in the treatment of bladder cancer. BJU Int 2012;110(2 Pt 2):E76–9.
13. Mariappan P, Zachou A, Grigor KM, Edinburgh Uro-Oncology Group. Detrusor muscle in the first, apparently complete transurethral resection of bladder tumour specimen is a surrogate marker of resection quality, predicts risk of early

recurrence, and is dependent on operator experience. Eur Urol 2010;57(5): 843–9.

14. Collado A, Chéchile GE, Salvador J, et al. Early complications of endoscopic treatment for superficial bladder tumors. J Urol 2000;164(5):1529–32.

15. Dick A, Barnes R, Hadley H, et al. Complications of transurethral resection of bladder tumors: prevention, recognition and treatment. J Urol 1980;124(6): 810–1.

16. Kondás J, Váczi L, Szecsó L, et al. Transurethral resection for muscle-invasive bladder cancer. Int Urol Nephrol 1993;25(6):557–63.

17. Mydlo JH, Weinstein R, Shah S, et al. Long-term consequences from bladder perforation and/or violation in the presence of transitional cell carcinoma: results of a small series and a review of the literature. J Urol 1999;161(4):1128–32.

18. Murshidi MS. Intraperitoneal rupture of the urinary bladder during transurethral resection of transitional cell carcinoma. Acta Urol Belg 1988;56(1):68–73.

19. Sylvester RJ, Oosterlinck W, van der Meijden APM. A single immediate postoperative instillation of chemotherapy decreases the risk of recurrence in patients with stage Ta T1 bladder cancer: a meta-analysis of published results of randomized clinical trials. J Urol 2004;171(6 Pt 1):2186–90 [quiz: 2435].

20. Bosschieter J, Nieuwenhuijzen JA, van Ginkel T, et al. Value of an Immediate Intravesical Instillation of Mitomycin C in Patients with Non-muscle-invasive Bladder Cancer: A Prospective Multicentre Randomised Study in 2243 patients. Eur Urol 2018;73(2):226–32.

21. Abern MR, Owusu RA, Anderson MR, et al. Perioperative intravesical chemotherapy in non-muscle-invasive bladder cancer: a systematic review and meta-analysis. J Natl Compr Canc Netw 2013;11(4):477–84.

22. Perlis N, Zlotta AR, Beyene J, et al. Immediate post-transurethral resection of bladder tumor intravesical chemotherapy prevents non-muscle-invasive bladder cancer recurrences: an updated meta-analysis on 2548 patients and quality-of-evidence review. Eur Urol 2013;64(3):421–30.

23. Messing EM, Tangen CM, Lerner SP, et al. Effect of Intravesical Instillation of Gemcitabine vs Saline Immediately Following Resection of Suspected Low-Grade Non-Muscle-Invasive Bladder Cancer on Tumor Recurrence: SWOG S0337 Randomized Clinical Trial. JAMA 2018;319(18):1880–8.

24. Babjuk M, Burger M, Compérat EM, et al. European Association of Urology Guidelines on Non-muscle-invasive Bladder Cancer (TaT1 and Carcinoma In Situ) - 2019 Update. Eur Urol 2019;76(5):639–57.

25. National Comprehensive Cancer Network. Bladder Cancer (Version 4.2020). Available at: https://www.nccn.org/professionals/physician_gls/pdf/bladder_blocks.pdf. Accessed July 1, 2020.

26. van der Meijden A, Oosterlinck W, Brausi M, et al. Significance of bladder biopsies in Ta,T1 bladder tumors: a report from the EORTC Genito-Urinary Tract Cancer Cooperative Group. EORTC-GU Group Superficial Bladder Committee. Eur Urol 1999;35(4):267–71.

27. Hara T, Takahashi M, Gondo T, et al. Risk of concomitant carcinoma in situ determining biopsy candidates among primary non-muscle-invasive bladder cancer patients: retrospective analysis of 173 Japanese cases. Int J Urol 2009;16(3): 293–8.

28. Palou J, Sylvester RJ, Faba OR, et al. Female gender and carcinoma in situ in the prostatic urethra are prognostic factors for recurrence, progression, and disease-specific mortality in T1G3 bladder cancer patients treated with bacillus Calmette-Guérin. Eur Urol 2012;62(1):118–25.

29. Brant A, Daniels M, Chappidi MR, et al. Prognostic implications of prostatic urethral involvement in non-muscle-invasive bladder cancer. World J Urol 2019; 37(12):2683–9.

30. Guzzo T, Vaughn D. Management of metastatic and invasive bladder cancer. In: Wein AJ, Kavoussi LR, Partin AW, et al, editors. Campbell-walsh Urology, vol. 3, 11th edition. Philadelphia: Elsevier; 2016. p. 2223–41.

31. Herr HW. The value of a second transurethral resection in evaluating patients with bladder tumors. J Urol 1999;162(1):74–6.

32. Herr HW. Role of repeat resection in non-muscle-invasive bladder cancer. J Natl Compr Canc Netw 2015;13(8):1041–6.

33. Vianello A, Costantini E, Del Zingaro M, et al. Repeated white light transurethral resection of the bladder in nonmuscle-invasive urothelial bladder cancers: systematic review and meta-analysis. J Endourol 2011;25(11):1703–12.

34. Divrik RT, Yildirim U, Zorlu F, et al. The effect of repeat transurethral resection on recurrence and progression rates in patients with T1 tumors of the bladder who received intravesical mitomycin: a prospective, randomized clinical trial. J Urol 2006;175(5):1641–4.

35. Cumberbatch MGK, Foerster B, Catto JWF, et al. Repeat Transurethral Resection in Non-muscle-invasive Bladder Cancer: A Systematic Review. Eur Urol 2018;73(6):925–33.

36. Herr HW. Restaging transurethral resection of high risk superficial bladder cancer improves the initial response to bacillus Calmette-Guerin therapy. J Urol 2005;174(6):2134–7.

37. Sfakianos JP, Kim PH, Hakimi AA, et al. The effect of restaging transurethral resection on recurrence and progression rates in patients with nonmuscle invasive bladder cancer treated with intravesical bacillus Calmette-Guérin. J Urol 2014;191(2):341–5.

38. Chou R, Selph S, Buckley DI, et al. Comparative Effectiveness of Fluorescent Versus White Light Cystoscopy for Initial Diagnosis or Surveillance of Bladder Cancer on Clinical Outcomes: Systematic Review and Meta-Analysis. J Urol 2017;197(3 Pt 1):548–58.

39. Burger M, Grossman HB, Droller M, et al. Photodynamic diagnosis of non-muscle-invasive bladder cancer with hexaminolevulinate cystoscopy: a meta-analysis of detection and recurrence based on raw data. Eur Urol 2013;64(5): 846–54.

40. Rink M, Babjuk M, Catto JWF, et al. Hexyl aminolevulinate-guided fluorescence cystoscopy in the diagnosis and follow-up of patients with non-muscle-invasive bladder cancer: a critical review of the current literature. Eur Urol 2013;64(4): 624–38.

41. Schmidbauer J, Witjes F, Schmeller N, et al. Improved detection of urothelial carcinoma in situ with hexaminolevulinate fluorescence cystoscopy. J Urol 2004; 171(1):135–8.

42. Jocham D, Witjes F, Wagner S, et al. Improved detection and treatment of bladder cancer using hexaminolevulinate imaging: a prospective, phase III multicenter study. J Urol 2005;174(3):862–6 [discussion: 866].

43. Fradet Y, Grossman HB, Gomella L, et al. A comparison of hexaminolevulinate fluorescence cystoscopy and white light cystoscopy for the detection of carcinoma in situ in patients with bladder cancer: a phase III, multicenter study. J Urol 2007;178(1):68–73 [discussion: 73].

44. Kausch I, Sommerauer M, Montorsi F, et al. Photodynamic diagnosis in non-muscle-invasive bladder cancer: a systematic review and cumulative analysis of prospective studies. Eur Urol 2010;57(4):595–606.

45. Kamat AM, Cookson M, Witjes JA, et al. The Impact of Blue Light Cystoscopy with Hexaminolevulinate (HAL) on Progression of Bladder Cancer - A New Analysis. Bladder Cancer 2016;2(2):273–8.

46. Naselli A, Introini C, Timossi L, et al. A randomized prospective trial to assess the impact of transurethral resection in narrow band imaging modality on non-muscle-invasive bladder cancer recurrence. Eur Urol 2012;61(5):908–13.

47. Naito S, Algaba F, Babjuk M, et al. The Clinical Research Office of the Endourological Society (CROES) Multicentre Randomised Trial of Narrow Band Imaging-Assisted Transurethral Resection of Bladder Tumour (TURBT) Versus Conventional White Light Imaging-Assisted TURBT in Primary Non-Muscle-invasive Bladder Cancer Patients: Trial Protocol and 1-year Results. Eur Urol 2016;70(3):506–15.

48. Xiong Y, Li J, Ma S, et al. A meta-analysis of narrow band imaging for the diagnosis and therapeutic outcome of non-muscle invasive bladder cancer. PLoS One 2017;12(2):e0170819.

49. Sánchez-Ortiz RF, Huang WC, Mick R, et al. An interval longer than 12 weeks between the diagnosis of muscle invasion and cystectomy is associated with worse outcome in bladder carcinoma. J Urol 2003;169(1):110–5 [discussion: 115].

50. Lee CT, Madii R, Daignault S, et al. Cystectomy delay more than 3 months from initial bladder cancer diagnosis results in decreased disease specific and overall survival. J Urol 2006;175(4):1262–7 [discussion: 1267].

51. Ahmadi H, Montie JE, Weizer AZ, et al. Patient Psoas Muscle Mass as a Predictor of Complications and Survival After Radical Cystectomy. Curr Urol Rep 2015; 16(11):79.

52. Ritch CR, Cookson MS, Clark PE, et al. Perioperative Oral Nutrition Supplementation Reduces Prevalence of Sarcopenia following Radical Cystectomy: Results of a Prospective Randomized Controlled Trial. J Urol 2019;201(3):470–7.

53. Chang SS, Bochner BH, Chou R, et al. Treatment of non-metastatic muscle-invasive bladder cancer: AUA/ASCO/ASTRO/SUO Guideline. J Urol 2017;198(3): 552–9.

54. Witjes JA, Bruins HM, Cathomas R, et al. European Association of Urology Guidelines on Muscle-invasive and Metastatic Bladder Cancer: Summary of the 2020 Guidelines. Eur Urol 2020. https://doi.org/10.1016/j.eururo.2020. 03.055.

55. Colombo R, Pellucchi F, Moschini M, et al. Fifteen-year single-centre experience with three different surgical procedures of nerve-sparing cystectomy in selected organ-confined bladder cancer patients. World J Urol 2015;33(10):1389–95.

56. Jacobs BL, Daignault S, Lee CT, et al. Prostate capsule sparing versus nerve sparing radical cystectomy for bladder cancer: results of a randomized, controlled trial. J Urol 2015;193(1):64–70. https://doi.org/10.1016/j.juro.2014. 07.090.

57. Kessler TM, Burkhard FC, Perimenis P, et al. Attempted nerve sparing surgery and age have a significant effect on urinary continence and erectile function after radical cystoprostatectomy and ileal orthotopic bladder substitution. J Urol 2004;172(4 Pt 1):1323–7. https://doi.org/10.1097/01.ju.0000138249.31644.ec.

58. Mertens LS, Meijer RP, de Vries RR, et al. Prostate sparing cystectomy for bladder cancer: 20-year single center experience. J Urol 2014;191(5):1250–5.

59. Muto G, Collura D, Rosso R, et al. Seminal-sparing cystectomy: technical evolution and results over a 20-year period. Urology 2014;83(4):856–61.

60. Rozet F, Lesur G, Cathelineau X, et al. Oncological evaluation of prostate sparing cystectomy: the Montsouris long-term results. J Urol 2008;179(6):2170–4 [discussion: 2174–5].

61. Hernández V, Espinos EL, Dunn J, et al. Oncological and functional outcomes of sexual function-preserving cystectomy compared with standard radical cystectomy in men: A systematic review. Urol Oncol 2017;35(9):539.e17-29.

62. Ali-El-Dein B, Mosbah A, Osman Y, et al. Preservation of the internal genital organs during radical cystectomy in selected women with bladder cancer: a report on 15 cases with long term follow-up. Eur J Surg Oncol 2013;39(4):358–64.

63. Temkin SM, Bergstrom J, Samimi G, et al. Ovarian Cancer Prevention in High-risk Women. Clin Obstet Gynecol 2017;60(4):738–57.

64. Lerner SP, Skinner DG, Lieskovsky G, et al. The rationale for en bloc pelvic lymph node dissection for bladder cancer patients with nodal metastases: long-term results. J Urol 1993;149(4):758–64 [discussion: 764–5].

65. Herr HW, Faulkner JR, Grossman HB, et al. Surgical factors influence bladder cancer outcomes: a cooperative group report. J Clin Oncol 2004;22(14):2781–9.

66. Stein JP, Lieskovsky G, Cote R, et al. Radical cystectomy in the treatment of invasive bladder cancer: long-term results in 1,054 patients. J Clin Oncol 2001;19(3):666–75.

67. Dhar NB, Klein EA, Reuther AM, et al. Outcome after radical cystectomy with limited or extended pelvic lymph node dissection. J Urol 2008;179(3):873–8 [discussion: 878].

68. Jensen JB, Ulhøi BP, Jensen KM-E. Extended versus limited lymph node dissection in radical cystectomy: impact on recurrence pattern and survival. Int J Urol 2012;19(1):39–47.

69. Poulsen AL, Horn T, Steven K. Radical cystectomy: extending the limits of pelvic lymph node dissection improves survival for patients with bladder cancer confined to the bladder wall. J Urol 1998;160(6 Pt 1):2015–9 [discussion: 2020].

70. Simone G, Papalia R, Ferriero M, et al. Stage-specific impact of extended versus standard pelvic lymph node dissection in radical cystectomy. Int J Urol 2013;20(4):390–7.

71. Holmer M, Bendahl P-O, Davidsson T, et al. Extended lymph node dissection in patients with urothelial cell carcinoma of the bladder: can it make a difference? World J Urol 2009;27(4):521–6.

72. Froehner M, Novotny V, Heberling U, et al. Relationship of the number of removed lymph nodes to bladder cancer and competing mortality after radical cystectomy. Eur Urol 2014;66(6):987–90.

73. Herr HW, Bochner BH, Dalbagni G, et al. Impact of the number of lymph nodes retrieved on outcome in patients with muscle invasive bladder cancer. J Urol 2002;167(3):1295–8.

74. Konety BR, Joslyn SA, O'Donnell MA. Extent of pelvic lymphadenectomy and its impact on outcome in patients diagnosed with bladder cancer: analysis of data from the Surveillance, Epidemiology and End Results Program data base. J Urol 2003;169(3):946–50.

75. Koppie TM, Vickers AJ, Vora K, et al. Standardization of pelvic lymphadenectomy performed at radical cystectomy: can we establish a minimum number of lymph nodes that should be removed? Cancer 2006;107(10):2368–74.

76. Morgan TM, Barocas DA, Penson DF, et al. Lymph node yield at radical cystectomy predicts mortality in node-negative and not node-positive patients. Urology 2012;80(3):632–40.

77. Siemens DR, Mackillop WJ, Peng Y, et al. Lymph node counts are valid indicators of the quality of surgical care in bladder cancer: a population-based study. Urol Oncol 2015;33(10):425.e15-23.

78. Stein JP, Cai J, Groshen S, et al. Risk factors for patients with pelvic lymph node metastases following radical cystectomy with en bloc pelvic lymphadenectomy: concept of lymph node density. J Urol 2003;170(1):35–41.

79. Wright JL, Lin DW, Porter MP. The association between extent of lymphadenectomy and survival among patients with lymph node metastases undergoing radical cystectomy. Cancer 2008;112(11):2401–8.

80. Gschwend JE, Heck MM, Lehmann J, et al. Extended versus limited lymph node dissection in bladder cancer patients undergoing radical cystectomy: survival results from a prospective, randomized trial. Eur Urol 2019;75(4):604–11.

81. Kanaroglou A, Shayegan B. Management of the urethra in urothelial bladder cancer. Can Urol Assoc J 2009;3(6 Suppl 4):S211–4.

82. Stein JP, Penson DF, Wu SD, et al. Pathological guidelines for orthotopic urinary diversion in women with bladder cancer: a review of the literature. J Urol 2007;178(3 Pt 1):756–60.

83. Lebret T, Hervé JM, Barré P, et al. Urethral recurrence of transitional cell carcinoma of the bladder. Predictive value of preoperative latero-montanal biopsies and urethral frozen sections during prostatocystectomy. Eur Urol 1998;33(2):170–4.

84. Chen ME, Pisters LL, Malpica A, et al. Risk of urethral, vaginal and cervical involvement in patients undergoing radical cystectomy for bladder cancer: results of a contemporary cystectomy series from M. D. Anderson Cancer Center. J Urol 1997;157(6):2120–3.

85. Lee RK, Abol-Enein H, Artibani W, et al. Urinary diversion after radical cystectomy for bladder cancer: options, patient selection, and outcomes. BJU Int 2014;113(1):11–23.

86. Nieuwenhuijzen JA, de Vries RR, Bex A, et al. Urinary diversions after cystectomy: the association of clinical factors, complications and functional results of four different diversions. Eur Urol 2008;53(4):834–42 [discussion: 842–4].

87. Gerharz EW, Månsson A, Hunt S, et al. Quality of life after cystectomy and urinary diversion: an evidence based analysis. J Urol 2005;174(5):1729–36.

88. Ghosh A, Somani BK. Recent trends in postcystectomy health-related quality of life (qol) favors neobladder diversion: systematic review of the literature. Urology 2016;93:22–6.

89. Al Hussein Al Awamlh B, Wang LC, Nguyen DP, et al. Is continent cutaneous urinary diversion a suitable alternative to orthotopic bladder substitute and ileal conduit after cystectomy? BJU Int 2015;116(5):805–14.

90. Longo N, Imbimbo C, Fusco F, et al. Complications and quality of life in elderly patients with several comorbidities undergoing cutaneous ureterostomy with single stoma or ileal conduit after radical cystectomy. BJU Int 2016;118(4):521–6.

91. Guzzo TJ, Rogers CG, Deng CY, et al. Outcomes of patients after aborted radical cystectomy for intraoperative findings of metastatic disease. BJU Int 2008;102(11):1539–43.

92. Yafi FA, Duclos M, Correa JA, et al. Contemporary outcome and management of patients who had an aborted cystectomy due to unresectable bladder cancer. Urol Oncol 2011;29(3):309–13.

93. Tran W, Serio AM, Raj GV, et al. Longitudinal risk of upper tract recurrence following radical cystectomy for urothelial cancer and the potential implications for long-term surveillance. J Urol 2008;179(1):96–100.

94. Volkmer BG, Schnoeller T, Kuefer R, et al. Upper urinary tract recurrence after radical cystectomy for bladder cancer–who is at risk? J Urol 2009;182(6): 2632–7.

95. Raj GV, Tal R, Vickers A, et al. Significance of intraoperative ureteral evaluation at radical cystectomy for urothelial cancer. Cancer 2006;107(9):2167–72.

96. Lee SE, Byun S-S, Hong SK, et al. Significance of cancer involvement at the ureteral margin detected on routine frozen section analysis during radical cystectomy. Urol Int 2006;77(1):13–7.

97. Cho KS, Seo JW, Park SJ, et al. The risk factor for urethral recurrence after radical cystectomy in patients with transitional cell carcinoma of the bladder. Urol Int 2009;82(3):306–11.

98. Nieder AM, Sved PD, Gomez P, et al. Urethral recurrence after cystoprostatectomy: implications for urinary diversion and monitoring. Urology 2004;64(5): 950–4.

99. Stein JP, Clark P, Miranda G, et al. Urethral tumor recurrence following cystectomy and urinary diversion: clinical and pathological characteristics in 768 male patients. J Urol 2005;173(4):1163–8.

100. Stein JP, Penson DF, Lee C, et al. Long-term oncological outcomes in women undergoing radical cystectomy and orthotopic diversion for bladder cancer. J Urol 2009;181(5):2052–8 [discussion: 2058–9].

101. Ali-El-Dein B. Oncological outcome after radical cystectomy and orthotopic bladder substitution in women. Eur J Surg Oncol 2009;35(3):320–5.

102. Boorjian SA, Kim SP, Weight CJ, et al. Risk factors and outcomes of urethral recurrence following radical cystectomy. Eur Urol 2011;60(6):1266–72.

103. Roth B, Furrer MA, Giannakis I, et al. Positive Pre-cystectomy Biopsies of the Prostatic Urethra or Bladder Neck Do Not Necessarily Preclude Orthotopic Bladder Substitution. J Urol 2019;201(5):909–15.

104. Madersbacher S, Hochreiter W, Burkhard F, et al. Radical cystectomy for bladder cancer today–a homogeneous series without neoadjuvant therapy. J Clin Oncol 2003;21(4):690–6.

105. Manoharan M, Ayyathurai R, Soloway MS. Radical cystectomy for urothelial carcinoma of the bladder: an analysis of perioperative and survival outcome. BJU Int 2009;104(9):1227–32.

106. Hautmann RE, Gschwend JE, de Petriconi RC, et al. Cystectomy for transitional cell carcinoma of the bladder: results of a surgery only series in the neobladder era. J Urol 2006;176(2):486–92 [discussion: 491–2].

107. Ghoneim MA, Abdel-Latif M, el-Mekresh M, et al. Radical cystectomy for carcinoma of the bladder: 2,720 consecutive cases 5 years later. J Urol 2008;180(1): 121–7.

108. Shariat SF, Karakiewicz PI, Palapattu GS, et al. Outcomes of radical cystectomy for transitional cell carcinoma of the bladder: a contemporary series from the Bladder Cancer Research Consortium. J Urol 2006;176(6 Pt 1):2414–22 [discussion: 2422].

109. Nielsen ME, Mallin K, Weaver MA, et al. Association of hospital volume with conditional 90-day mortality after cystectomy: an analysis of the National Cancer Data Base. BJU Int 2014;114(1):46–55.

110. Morgan TM, Barocas DA, Keegan KA, et al. Volume outcomes of cystectomy–is it the surgeon or the setting? J Urol 2012;188(6):2139–44.

111. Stein JP, Skinner DG. Radical cystectomy for invasive bladder cancer: long-term results of a standard procedure. World J Urol 2006;24(3):296–304.

112. Hautmann RE, de Petriconi RC, Volkmer BG. Lessons learned from 1,000 neobladders: the 90-day complication rate. J Urol 2010;184(3):990–4 [quiz: 1235].

113. Hautmann RE, de Petriconi RC, Pfeiffer C, et al. Radical cystectomy for urothelial carcinoma of the bladder without neoadjuvant or adjuvant therapy: long-term results in 1100 patients. Eur Urol 2012;61(5):1039–47.

114. Porter MP, Gore JL, Wright JL. Hospital volume and 90-day mortality risk after radical cystectomy: a population-based cohort study. World J Urol 2011; 29(1):73–7.

115. Shabsigh A, Korets R, Vora KC, et al. Defining early morbidity of radical cystectomy for patients with bladder cancer using a standardized reporting methodology. Eur Urol 2009;55(1):164–74.

116. Madersbacher S, Schmidt J, Eberle JM, et al. Long-term outcome of ileal conduit diversion. J Urol 2003;169(3):985–90.

117. Studer UE, Burkhard FC, Schumacher M, et al. Twenty years experience with an ileal orthotopic low pressure bladder substitute–lessons to be learned. J Urol 2006;176(1):161–6.

118. Dahl D. Use of intestinal segments in urinary diversion. In: Wein AJ, Kavoussi LR, Partin AW, et al, editors. Campbell-walsh Urology, vol. 3, 11th edition. Philadelphia: Elsevier; 2016. p. 2281–316.

119. Collins JW, Patel H, Adding C, et al. Enhanced Recovery After Robot-assisted Radical Cystectomy: EAU Robotic Urology Section Scientific Working Group Consensus View. Eur Urol 2016;70(4):649–60.

120. Gustafsson UO, Scott MJ, Schwenk W, et al. Guidelines for perioperative care in elective colonic surgery: Enhanced Recovery After Surgery (ERAS(®)) Society recommendations. World J Surg 2013;37(2):259–84.

121. Xu W, Daneshmand S, Bazargani ST, et al. Postoperative Pain Management after Radical Cystectomy: Comparing Traditional versus Enhanced Recovery Protocol Pathway. J Urol 2015;194(5):1209–13.

122. Lee CT, Chang SS, Kamat AM, et al. Alvimopan accelerates gastrointestinal recovery after radical cystectomy: a multicenter randomized placebo-controlled trial. Eur Urol 2014;66(2):265–72.

123. Kouba EJ, Wallen EM, Pruthi RS. Gum chewing stimulates bowel motility in patients undergoing radical cystectomy with urinary diversion. Urology 2007;70(6): 1053–6.

124. Parekh DJ, Reis IM, Castle EP, et al. Robot-assisted radical cystectomy versus open radical cystectomy in patients with bladder cancer (RAZOR): an open-label, randomised, phase 3, non-inferiority trial. Lancet 2018;391(10139): 2525–36.

125. Venkatramani V, Reis IM, Castle EP, et al. Predictors of recurrence, and progression-free and overall survival following open versus robotic radical cystectomy: analysis from the RAZOR trial with a 3-year followup. J Urol 2020; 203(3):522–9.

126. Parekh DJ, Messer J, Fitzgerald J, et al. Perioperative outcomes and oncologic efficacy from a pilot prospective randomized clinical trial of open versus robotic assisted radical cystectomy. J Urol 2013;189(2):474–9.

127. Nix J, Smith A, Kurpad R, et al. Prospective randomized controlled trial of robotic versus open radical cystectomy for bladder cancer: perioperative and pathologic results. Eur Urol 2010;57(2):196–201.

128. Bochner BH, Sjoberg DD, Laudone VP, Memorial Sloan Kettering Cancer Center Bladder Cancer Surgical Trials Group. A randomized trial of robot-assisted laparoscopic radical cystectomy. N Engl J Med 2014;371(4):389–90.

129. Catto JWF, Khetrapal P, Ambler G, et al. Robot-assisted radical cystectomy with intracorporeal urinary diversion versus open radical cystectomy (iROC): protocol for a randomised controlled trial with internal feasibility study. BMJ Open 2018;8(8):e020500.

130. Solsona E, Climent MA, Iborra I, et al. Bladder preservation in selected patients with muscle-invasive bladder cancer by complete transurethral resection of the bladder plus systemic chemotherapy: long-term follow-up of a phase 2 nonrandomized comparative trial with radical cystectomy. Eur Urol 2009;55(4): 911–9.

131. Herr HW. Transurethral resection of muscle-invasive bladder cancer: 10-year outcome. J Clin Oncol 2001;19(1):89–93.

132. Siefker-Radtke A. Urachal adenocarcinoma: a clinician's guide for treatment. Semin Oncol 2012;39(5):619–24.

133. Golijanin D, Yossepowitch O, Beck SD, et al. Carcinoma in a bladder diverticulum: presentation and treatment outcome. J Urol 2003;170(5):1761–4.

134. Smith A, Matin S, Jarrett T. Urothelial tumors of the upper urinary tract and ureter. 11th ed.. In: Wein AJ, Kavoussi LR, Partin AW, et al, editors. Campbell-walsh Urology, 2 Philadelphia: Elsevier; 2016. p. 1365–402.

135. Rouprêt M, Babjuk M, Burger M, et al. European Association of Urology Guidelines on Upper Urinary Tract Urothelial Carcinoma: 2020 Update. Eur Urol 2020. https://doi.org/10.1016/j.eururo.2020.05.042.

136. Messer J, Shariat SF, Brien JC, et al. Urinary cytology has a poor performance for predicting invasive or high-grade upper-tract urothelial carcinoma. BJU Int 2011;108(5):701–5.

137. Lee KS, Zeikus E, DeWolf WC, et al. MR urography versus retrograde pyelography/ureteroscopy for the exclusion of upper urinary tract malignancy. Clin Radiol 2010;65(3):185–92.

138. Wang L-J, Wong Y-C, Chuang C-K, et al. Diagnostic accuracy of transitional cell carcinoma on multidetector computerized tomography urography in patients with gross hematuria. J Urol 2009;181(2):524–31 [discussion: 531].

139. Malm C, Grahn A, Jaremko G, et al. Diagnostic accuracy of upper tract urothelial carcinoma: how samples are collected matters. Scand J Urol 2017;51(2): 137–45.

140. Smith AK, Stephenson AJ, Lane BR, et al. Inadequacy of biopsy for diagnosis of upper tract urothelial carcinoma: implications for conservative management. Urology 2011;78(1):82–6.

141. Guo R-Q, Hong P, Xiong G-Y, et al. Impact of ureteroscopy before radical nephroureterectomy for upper tract urothelial carcinomas on oncological outcomes: a meta-analysis. BJU Int 2018;121(2):184–93.

142. Hendin BN, Streem SB, Levin HS, et al. Impact of diagnostic ureteroscopy on long-term survival in patients with upper tract transitional cell carcinoma. J Urol 1999;161(3):783–5.

143. Marchioni M, Primiceri G, Cindolo L, et al. Impact of diagnostic ureteroscopy on intravesical recurrence in patients undergoing radical nephroureterectomy for upper tract urothelial cancer: a systematic review and meta-analysis. BJU Int 2017;120(3):313–9.

144. Rouprêt M, Colin P, Yates DR. A new proposal to risk stratify urothelial carcinomas of the upper urinary tract (UTUCs) in a predefinitive treatment setting: low-risk versus high-risk UTUCs. Eur Urol 2014;66(2):181–3.

145. Seisen T, Colin P, Rouprêt M. Risk-adapted strategy for the kidney-sparing management of upper tract tumours. Nat Rev Urol 2015;12(3):155–66.

146. Seisen T, Peyronnet B, Dominguez-Escrig JL, et al. Oncologic outcomes of kidney-sparing surgery versus radical nephroureterectomy for upper tract urothelial carcinoma: a systematic review by the EAU Non-muscle Invasive Bladder Cancer Guidelines Panel. Eur Urol 2016;70(6):1052–68.

147. Chen GL, Bagley DH. Ureteroscopic management of upper tract transitional cell carcinoma in patients with normal contralateral kidneys. J Urol 2000;164(4): 1173–6.

148. Cutress ML, Stewart GD, Wells-Cole S, et al. Long-term endoscopic management of upper tract urothelial carcinoma: 20-year single-centre experience. BJU Int 2012;110(11):1608–17.

149. Cutress ML, Stewart GD, Zakikhani P, et al. Ureteroscopic and percutaneous management of upper tract urothelial carcinoma (UTUC): systematic review. BJU Int 2012;110(5):614–28.

150. Rouprêt M, Traxer O, Tligui M, et al. Upper urinary tract transitional cell carcinoma: recurrence rate after percutaneous endoscopic resection. Eur Urol 2007;51(3):709–13 [discussion: 714].

151. Colin P, Ouzzane A, Pignot G, et al. Comparison of oncological outcomes after segmental ureterectomy or radical nephroureterectomy in urothelial carcinomas of the upper urinary tract: results from a large French multicentre study. BJU Int 2012;110(8):1134–41.

152. Jeldres C, Lughezzani G, Sun M, et al. Segmental ureterectomy can safely be performed in patients with transitional cell carcinoma of the ureter. J Urol 2010;183(4):1324–9.

153. Foerster B, D'Andrea D, Abufaraj M, et al. Endocavitary treatment for upper tract urothelial carcinoma: A meta-analysis of the current literature. Urol Oncol 2019; 37(7):430–6.

154. Kleinmann N, Matin SF, Pierorazio PM, et al. Primary chemoablation of low-grade upper tract urothelial carcinoma using UGN-101, a mitomycin-containing reverse thermal gel (OLYMPUS): an open-label, single-arm, phase 3 trial. Lancet Oncol 2020;21(6):776–85.

155. Margulis V, Shariat SF, Matin SF, et al. Outcomes of radical nephroureterectomy: a series from the Upper Tract Urothelial Carcinoma Collaboration. Cancer 2009; 115(6):1224–33.

156. Peyronnet B, Seisen T, Dominguez-Escrig J-L, et al. Oncological Outcomes of Laparoscopic Nephroureterectomy Versus Open Radical Nephroureterectomy for Upper Tract Urothelial Carcinoma: An European Association of Urology Guidelines Systematic Review. Eur Urol Focus 2019;5(2):205–23.

157. Simone G, Papalia R, Guaglianone S, et al. Laparoscopic versus open nephroureterectomy: perioperative and oncologic outcomes from a randomised prospective study. Eur Urol 2009;56(3):520–6.

158. Aboumohamed AA, Krane LS, Hemal AK. Oncologic outcomes following robot-assisted laparoscopic nephroureterectomy with bladder cuff excision for upper tract urothelial carcinoma. J Urol 2015;194(6):1561–6.

159. Clements MB, Krupski TL, Culp SH. Robotic-assisted surgery for upper tract urothelial carcinoma: a comparative survival analysis. Ann Surg Oncol 2018;25(9): 2550–62.

160. Li W-M, Shen J-T, Li C-C, et al. Oncologic outcomes following three different approaches to the distal ureter and bladder cuff in nephroureterectomy for primary upper urinary tract urothelial carcinoma. Eur Urol 2010;57(6):963–9.

161. Xylinas E, Rink M, Cha EK, et al. Impact of distal ureter management on oncologic outcomes following radical nephroureterectomy for upper tract urothelial carcinoma. Eur Urol 2014;65(1):210–7.

162. Abercrombie GF, Eardley I, Payne SR, et al. Modified nephro-ureterectomy. Long-term follow-up with particular reference to subsequent bladder tumours. Br J Urol 1988;61(3):198–200.

163. McDONALD DF. Intussusception ureterectomy: a method of removal of the ureteral stump at time of nephrectomy without an additional incision. Surg Gynecol Obstet 1953;97(5):565–8.

164. Gill IS, Soble JJ, Miller SD, et al. A novel technique for management of the en bloc bladder cuff and distal ureter during laparoscopic nephroureterectomy. J Urol 1999;161(2):430–4.

165. Weight CJ, Gettman MT. The emerging role of lymphadenectomy in upper tract urothelial carcinoma. Urol Clin North Am 2011;38(4):429–37, vi.

166. Kondo T, Hara I, Takagi T, et al. Template-based lymphadenectomy in urothelial carcinoma of the renal pelvis: a prospective study. Int J Urol 2014;21(5):453–9.

167. Kondo T, Tanabe K. Role of lymphadenectomy in the management of urothelial carcinoma of the bladder and the upper urinary tract. Int J Urol 2012;19(8): 710–21.

168. Matin SF, Sfakianos JP, Espiritu PN, et al. Patterns of Lymphatic Metastases in Upper Tract Urothelial Carcinoma and Proposed Dissection Templates. J Urol 2015;194(6):1567–74.

169. Brausi MA, Gavioli M, De Luca G, et al. Retroperitoneal lymph node dissection (RPLD) in conjunction with nephroureterectomy in the treatment of infiltrative transitional cell carcinoma (TCC) of the upper urinary tract: impact on survival. Eur Urol 2007;52(5):1414–8.

170. Dominguez-Escrig JL, Peyronnet B, Seisen T, et al. Potential Benefit of Lymph Node Dissection During Radical Nephroureterectomy for Upper Tract Urothelial Carcinoma: A Systematic Review by the European Association of Urology Guidelines Panel on Non-muscle-invasive Bladder Cancer. Eur Urol Focus 2019;5(2):224–41.

171. Kondo T, Nakazawa H, Ito F, et al. Impact of the extent of regional lymphadenectomy on the survival of patients with urothelial carcinoma of the upper urinary tract. J Urol 2007;178(4 Pt 1):1212–7 [discussion: 1217].

172. Xylinas E, Kluth L, Passoni N, et al. Prediction of intravesical recurrence after radical nephroureterectomy: development of a clinical decision-making tool. Eur Urol 2014;65(3):650–8.

173. Fang D, Li X-S, Xiong G-Y, et al. Prophylactic intravesical chemotherapy to prevent bladder tumors after nephroureterectomy for primary upper urinary tract urothelial carcinomas: a systematic review and meta-analysis. Urol Int 2013;91(3): 291–6.

174. Ito A, Shintaku I, Satoh M, et al. Prospective randomized phase II trial of a single early intravesical instillation of pirarubicin (THP) in the prevention of bladder recurrence after nephroureterectomy for upper urinary tract urothelial carcinoma: the THP Monotherapy Study Group Trial. J Clin Oncol 2013;31(11): 1422–7.

175. O'Brien T, Ray E, Singh R, et al, British Association of Urological Surgeons Section of Oncology. Prevention of bladder tumours after nephroureterectomy for primary upper urinary tract urothelial carcinoma: a prospective, multicentre, randomised clinical trial of a single postoperative intravesical dose of mitomycin C (the ODMIT-C Trial). Eur Urol 2011;60(4):703–10.

Contemporary and Emerging Approaches to Bladder-Preserving Trimodality Therapy for Muscle-Invasive Bladder Cancer

David J. Konieczkowski, MD, PhD[a], Jason A. Efstathiou, MD, DPhil[b,1], Kent W. Mouw, MD, PhD[c,*,1]

KEYWORDS

- Muscle-invasive bladder cancer - Bladder preservation
- Combined modality therapy - Trimodality therapy - Radiation therapy
- Immunotherapy - Precision medicine - Biomarkers

KEY POINTS

- Bladder-preserving tri-modality therapy (TMT), consisting of trans-urethral resection of the bladder tumor followed by concurrent chemoradiotherapy, is a well-established standard of care for patients with muscle-invasive bladder cancer.
- Although a randomized trial comparing TMT to radical cystectomy has never been completed, TMT appears to offer comparable oncologic outcomes in selected patients while allowing patients to preserve their native bladder.
- Key to the excellent oncologic and functional outcomes now achieved with TMT is multi-disciplinary management and appropriate patient selection, which is currently based primarily on clinical and pathologic factors.
- Given preclinical evidence supporting the combination of immune checkpoint blockade (ICB) with RT, and the activity of ICB in advanced bladder cancer, studies incorporating ICB into bladder-preserving TMT are underway.
- Tumor molecular features may impact response to TMT (with or without ICB) and inform post-treatment surveillance, in the future enabling molecularly-informed precision approaches to treatment selection and patient monitoring.

[a] Department of Radiation Oncology, James Cancer Hospital, The Ohio State University, 460 West 10th Avenue, 2nd Floor, Columbus, OH 43210, USA; [b] Department of Radiation Oncology, Massachusetts General Hospital, Harvard Medical School, 55 Fruit Street, Cox 3, Boston, MA 02114, USA; [c] Department of Radiation Oncology, Dana-Farber Cancer Institute, Brigham & Women's Hospital, Harvard Medical School, 450 Brookline Avenue, HIM 328, Boston, MA 02215, USA
[1] Equal contribution.
* Corresponding author.
E-mail address: kent_mouw@dfci.harvard.edu

Hematol Oncol Clin N Am 35 (2021) 567–584
https://doi.org/10.1016/j.hoc.2021.02.006
0889-8588/21/© 2021 Elsevier Inc. All rights reserved.

BLADDER-PRESERVING TRIMODALITY THERAPY: A MODERN STANDARD OF CARE FOR MUSCLE-INVASIVE BLADDER CANCER

Radical cystectomy (RC) with or without perioperative chemotherapy has historically been the most common treatment of patients with localized, muscle-invasive bladder cancer (MIBC) in North America. Bladder-preserving trimodality therapy (TMT), which involves maximal safe transurethral resection of the bladder tumor (TURBT) followed by radiation therapy with concurrent chemotherapy, can provide oncologic outcomes similar to RC-based treatment in carefully selected patients while allowing these patients to preserve their native, functioning bladders. Initially pioneered at select high-volume centers in North America and Europe, TMT is now supported by the National Comprehensive Cancer Network (NCCN) (as a category 1 recommendation), European Society for Medical Oncology (ESMO), National Institute for Health and Care Excellence (NICE), and American Urological Association/American Society of Clinical Oncology/American Society for Radiation Oncology/Society of Urologic Oncology guidelines.[1–4]

Oncologic Outcomes of Bladder-Preserving Trimodality Therapy

Bladder-preserving TMT is supported by several large institutional case series as well as several prospective clinical trials (**Table 1**).

The largest single-institution retrospective study, from the Massachusetts General Hospital (MGH), reported on 475 patients with MIBC treated between 1986 and 2013 with TURBT followed by concurrent chemoradiation.[5] Patients with less than a complete response (CR) to TMT were managed with salvage cystectomy. With a median follow-up of 7.2 years among surviving patients, 5-year and 10-year disease-specific survival (DSS) was 66% and 59%, overall survival (OS) was 57% and 39%, and the 5-year risk of salvage cystectomy was 29%. On multivariate analysis, T2 disease and CR following TMT were associated with improved OS and DSS, whereas presence of tumor-associated carcinoma in situ (CIS) was associated with worse OS and DSS. Between the earliest (1986–1995) and latest (2005–2013) treatment eras, rates of clinical CR (cCR) improved from 66% to 88%, 5-year DSS improved from 60% to 84%, and the 5-year salvage RC rate decreased from 42% to 16%, highlighting the importance of improved patient selection and treatment delivery for achieving optimal outcomes.

Another large single-institution retrospective series has been reported from the University of Erlangen, where, between 1982 and 2002, 415 patients with high-risk T1 (n = 89) or MIBC (n = 326) were treated with TURBT followed by radiation therapy (RT) with (n = 289) or without (n = 126) chemotherapy.[6] Seventy-two percent of patients achieved a cCR to TMT, and, as in the MGH study, patients who did not were offered immediate salvage cystectomy. With a median follow-up of 60 months, 5-year and 10-year local control (LC) was not reported and 64%, DSS 56% and 42%, and OS 51% and 31%, respectively. On multivariate analysis, concurrent chemotherapy was associated with improved rates of cCR and OS. Two percent of patients (n = 3) required cystectomy for toxicity.

A pooled analysis of 486 patients from 6 completed Radiation Therapy Oncology Group (RTOG) studies of bladder-preserving TMT conducted between 1988 and 2007 has also been reported.[7] All patients received TURBT followed by concurrent chemoradiation, with substantial variation in chemoradiation regimens and/or use of additional (neoadjuvant or adjuvant) chemotherapy. Overall, 69% of patients achieved a cCR to TMT. With a median follow-up of 7.8 years among surviving patients, 5-year and 10-year OS was 57% and 36%, DSS 71% and 65%, and LF 43% and 48%.

Table 1
Selected studies supporting bladder-preserving trimodality therapy as a modern standard of care for muscle-invasive bladder cancer

Reference	Institution/Study	Years	Patients	Study Design	Median Follow-up	Outcomes	Notes
Giacalone et al,[5] 2017	MGH	1986–2013	475	Single-institution retrospective	7.2 y	DSS 5 y/10 y: 66%/59%; OS 5 y/10 y: 57%/39%; 5y salvage RC: 39%; Most recent era (2005–2013): cCR rate: 88%; 5-y DFS 84%; 5-y salvage RC: 16%	DSS event defined as any recurrence or death from disease
Rödel et al,[6] 2002	Erlangen	1982–2002	415	Single-institution retrospective	60 mo	LC 5 y/10 y: NR/64%; DSS 5 y/10 y: 56%/42%; OS 5 y/10 y: 51%/31%	30% (n = 126) without concurrent chemotherapy 21% (n = 89) with T1 (NMIBC) disease
Mak et al,[7] 2014	RTOG	1988–2007	486	Meta-analysis of 6 prospective studies	7.8 y	DSS 5 y/10 y: 71%/65%; OS 5 y/10 y: 57%/36%; LF 5 y/10 y: 43%/48%; cCR 69%	DSS event defined as death from disease
Hoskin et al,[28] 2010; Song et al,[29] 2019	BCON	2000–2006	333	Phase III RCT (concurrent CON vs none)	57 mo (RT alone) 60 mo (RT + CON)	3-y OS: 59% vs 46% (P = .04)	No concurrent chemotherapy. Benefit of CON limited to subgroup with hypoxic expression signatures[62]
James et al,[15] 2012	BC2001	2001–2008	360	Phase III RCT (concurrent chemotherapy vs none)	69.9 mo	Concurrent chemotherapy vs not: 2-y LRC 67% vs 54% (P = .03); 2-y salvage RC: 11.4% vs 16.8% (P = .07); 5-y OS: 48% vs 35% (P = .16)	2 × 2 factorial also randomizing between RT field design; no effect of RT field design on outcomes or toxicity[14,16]

Abbreviations: cCR, clinical complete response; CON, carbogen (inhaled 98% oxygen/2% carbon dioxide) and nicotinamide; DFS, disease-free survival; DSS, disease-specific survival; LC, local control; LRC, locoregional control; MGH, Massachusetts General Hospital; NR, not reported; NMIBC, non–muscle-invasive bladder cancer; RCT, randomized controlled trial; RT, radiation therapy.

These studies show that bladder-preserving TMT can provide disease outcomes in localized MIBC that are comparable with RC-based treatment. Whether these outcomes are truly noninferior to RC has historically been a matter of contention, because no prospective randomized trials of bladder-preserving TMT versus RC have been completed. The UK-based SPARE (Selective Bladder Preservation Against Radical Excision) trial was designed to test this comparison but closed early because of poor accrual, highlighting the challenges in patient preference, patient selection, differences in local practice patterns, and perceived lack of equipoise that are inherent in such a trial.[8] In the absence of randomized prospective data, numerous retrospective comparison studies have been performed. In a single-institution propensity score–matched analysis of 112 patients with MIBC managed with RC versus TMT, 5-year DSS was 73.2% with RC versus 76.6% with TMT ($P = .49$) at a median follow-up of 4.5 years.[9] Similarly, a recent meta-analysis examined 8 single-institution series enrolling 9554 patients, finding no differences in OS (hazard ratio [HR], 0.96, where HR<1 favors TMT; 95% confidence interval [CI], 0.72–1.29; $P = .778$), DSS (HR, 1.02; 95% CI, 0.73–1.49; $P = .905$), or progression-free survival (PFS) (HR, 0.85; 95% CI, 0.43–1.67; $P = .639$) between RC (with or without chemotherapy) and TMT.[10]

In summary, given the favorable long-term efficacy data from large single-institution retrospective and multi-institutional prospective studies of TMT, decades of experience with TMT across centers and countries, and oncologic outcomes comparable to cystectomy despite the lack of randomized comparative data, bladder-preserving TMT has now become an established standard of care for patients with localized MIBC.

Toxicity and Quality of Life Following Trimodality Therapy

In addition to providing oncologic outcomes that compare favorably with RC-based treatment, a key attraction of bladder-preserving TMT is the potential for the patients to retain their native bladders, which has important implications for patient quality of life (QoL). There is a robust body of literature describing QoL, patient-reported outcomes, and/or toxicity data following TMT.

One major study analyzed 285 patients treated between 1990 and 2002 on 4 prospective RTOG clinical trials.[11] At a median follow-up of 5.4 years, rates of investigator-assessed late grade 3 GU and gastrointestinal toxicity were 5.7% and 1.9%, respectively. In all but 1 patient, grade 3 toxicity had resolved at last follow-up, and there were no grade 4 to 5 toxicities. Another large study analyzed 226 patients treated with either TMT or RC between 1990 and 2011 at MGH and the University of North Carolina.[12] Although no baseline QoL data were available, patients were administered multiple validated QoL instruments in a post hoc fashion. At a median follow-up of 5.6 years, TMT patients had better overall QoL and functional scores, better bowel and sexual function, greater participation in informed decision making, and less concern about the negative effects of cancer than RC patients. Decision analytical modeling has also suggested that TMT offers a gain of expected quality-adjusted life years relative to RC.[13] More recently, data from the BC2001 study show that, although QoL measures declined significantly during and immediately after TMT, these metrics returned to baseline by 6 months posttreatment and remained stable thereafter.[14] Interestingly, there were no significant differences in QoL based on use of chemotherapy or on radiotherapy field design.

Thus, in summary, multiple studies have now shown that, although patients have an expected decrement in QoL during TMT caused by acute toxicity, long-term QoL/toxicity outcomes are excellent.

Treatment Paradigm for Bladder-Preserving Trimodality Therapy

The treatment paradigm for bladder-preserving TMT has been refined over decades of experience and its details are critical to achieving optimal outcomes.

Transurethral resection of the bladder tumor

Bladder-preserving TMT begins with a maximal safe TURBT with the goal of a visibly complete resection. In the previously described MGH and Erlangen series and the RTOG meta-analysis, a visibly complete TURBT was associated with improved outcomes.[5–7] In the MGH and RTOG studies, the relationship of complete TURBT with improved outcomes persisted even in a multivariate model incorporating primary tumor stage and other variables, suggesting that a visibly complete TURBT may provide therapeutic benefit rather than simply being correlated with less advanced disease; this hypothesis will be tested prospectively in the ongoing UK-based BladderPath trial (ISRCTN 35296862).

Radiation therapy

Following TURBT, patients undergo RT with concurrent chemotherapy (ie, concurrent chemoradiation). Although three-dimensional conformal radiation techniques are the historical standard, intensity modulated RT (IMRT) is now commonplace and can be useful in improving target coverage, reducing hotspots, and decreasing dose to adjacent organs at risk.

Conventional fractionation delivers a total dose of greater than 60 Gy (typically 64–65 Gy) in 1.8-Gy to 2.0-Gy daily fractions. Moderately hypofractionated regimens such as 55 Gy in 20 fractions seem to have similar disease control and toxicity outcomes to standard fractionation.[15] Most RTOG trials used an induction chemoradiation course to ~40 Gy followed by cystoscopic assessment. Patients with less than a cCR were recommended to undergo salvage cystectomy, whereas patients with cCR underwent a consolidation chemoradiation course to a total dose of greater than 60 Gy. This approach routed nonresponders to cystectomy before full-dose chemoradiation had been delivered, when surgical toxicity might be less, but had the radiobiological disadvantage of a treatment break allowing tumor cell repopulation. Therefore, many centers are now foregoing the interval cystoscopy and instead treating patients to the prescribed dose in a single course. Some RTOG trials have also used twice-daily RT, although this schedule can be logistically challenging.

The high-risk primary target volume (treated to the doses discussed earlier) can be defined either as the tumor bed (based on imaging and cystoscopy) plus a margin, or as the whole bladder plus a margin; no differences in disease control or toxicity were observed between these target volumes in the BC2001 study.[16] Although BC2001 did not include pelvic lymph nodes in the RT target volume, most completed RTOG trials have included treatment of a pelvic nodal field. If included, pelvic lymph nodes are typically treated to 40 to 45 Gy in 1.8-Gy to 2.0-Gy daily fractions.

Chemotherapy

The benefit of concurrent chemotherapy in TMT has been shown in 2 prospective randomized trials. The first, in Canada, randomized 99 patients between 1985 and 1989 to RT with or without concurrent weekly cisplatin.[17] At a median follow-up of 6.5 years, there was no difference in OS or PFS, but pelvic (ie, in-field) failure rates were reduced from 59% to 40% at 5 years (P = .038). The second, BC2001, randomized 360 patients in the United Kingdom between 2001 and 2008 to RT with or without concurrent fluorouracil (5-FU) and mitomycin C (MMC).[15] At a median follow-up of 69.9 months, concurrent chemotherapy significantly improved locoregional disease-free survival

(HR, 0.68, favoring concurrent chemotherapy; 95% CI, 0.48–0.96; P = .03), although not OS (HR, 0.82; 95% CI, 0.63–1.09; P = .16). Rates of acute or late grade 3 to 4 adverse events did not vary by treatment arm.

In practice, there is wide variability in the specific regimen used for concurrent chemotherapy. Cisplatin or a cisplatin-containing doublet is a commonly used regimen in North America. The combination of 5-FU and MMC is an established option based on the results from BC2001. Alternative approaches, particularly for patients who are ineligible for or refuse cisplatin-based concurrent chemotherapy, include single-agent gemcitabine or paclitaxel.[18–21]

There are no contemporary data showing a benefit to neoadjuvant or adjuvant chemotherapy as a part of bladder-preserving TMT. Two older studies evaluated the role of neoadjuvant chemotherapy (NAC). Although the BA06 30894 trial showed a benefit to 3 cycles of neoadjuvant cisplatin, methotrexate, and vinblastine (CMV) before RT (at median follow-up of 8 years; HR, 0.84 favoring CMV; 95% CI, 0.72–0.99; P = .037), this study did not use concurrent chemotherapy during RT.[22] In contrast, RTOG 8903 (which randomized patients to 2 cycles of neoadjuvant CMV vs no neoadjuvant therapy, followed in either case by concurrent chemoradiation) showed no benefit (in CR, DM, or OS) to NAC.[23,24] Adjuvant chemotherapy was used in RTOG 9706, RTOG 9906, and RTOG 0233; however, because all patients in these studies received adjuvant chemotherapy, it is difficult to make conclusions regarding its efficacy.[24–27] Given improvements in chemotherapy agents and dose/schedule of delivery, supportive care, patient selection, and other elements of TMT in the decades since these trials, the relevance of these data to current practice is uncertain. As such, neoadjuvant or adjuvant chemotherapy remains a reasonable consideration on an individualized basis, particularly for locally advanced disease (eg, T3b–T4 and/or N1 disease), but modern prospective data are needed to further clarify its role.

Modulation of tumor hypoxia is an alternative approach to achieve radiosensitization. In the Bladder Carbogen Nicotinamide (BCON) trial, 333 patients were randomized between 2000 and 2006 to receive RT alone or with carbogen (inhaled 98% oxygen plus 2% carbon dioxide, to mitigate diffusion-limited hypoxia by improving systemic oxygenation) and nicotinamide (delivered intravenously to mitigate perfusion-limited hypoxia by inducing local vasodilation) (CON). At a median follow-up of 57 months for RT alone and 60 months for RT + CON, 3-year OS was significantly improved with RT + CON (59% vs 46%, P = .04).[28] A recent abstract update indicates that this difference was maintained at 5-year and 10-year timepoints.[29] However, CON is not used routinely in North American practice and whether CON is beneficial in the setting of concurrent chemotherapy has not been assessed.

Immunotherapy. In light of the transformative impact of immune checkpoint blockade (ICB) in treatment of advanced bladder cancer, it is also the focus of numerous contemporary studies in localized disease. Immunotherapy is of particular interest for TMT given the complex interplay between the immune system and RT (**Fig. 1**). The immune system is a major determinant of RT response across disease sites; for example, it has been known for decades that immunodeficiency can attenuate the RT response.[30] RT has multifaceted effects on the antitumor immune response[31,32] and can have both immunostimulatory (eg, by increasing major histocompatibility complex class I expression, levels of chemokines and damage-associated molecular patterns, and tumor antigen cross-presentation) and immunosuppressive (eg, by directed toxicity to T cells within the RT field, programmed death-ligand 1 [PD-L1] upregulation, increasing regulatory T-cell [Treg] activity, and T-cell exhaustion) effects.

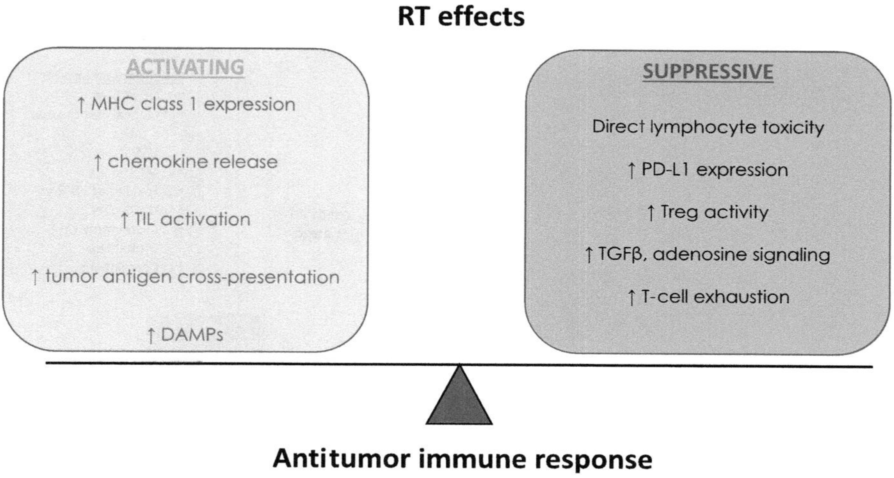

RT effects

ACTIVATING

↑ MHC class 1 expression

↑ chemokine release

↑ TIL activation

↑ tumor antigen cross-presentation

↑ DAMPs

SUPPRESSIVE

Direct lymphocyte toxicity

↑ PD-L1 expression

↑ Treg activity

↑ TGFβ, adenosine signaling

↑ T-cell exhaustion

Antitumor immune response

Fig. 1. Complex interplay between RT and the immune system. The interplay between RT and the host antitumor immune response is multifactorial and heterogeneous. RT can exert immune-activating effects via increased major histocompatibility complex class 1 expression, chemokine release, and other mechanisms. In contrast, RT also has immunosuppressive effects, including direct lymphocyte toxicity, increased regulatory T-cell (Treg) activity, and induction of T-cell exhaustion. ICB may provide an opportunity to tip this balance by attenuating RT-induced immunosuppression while preserving RT-induced immune activation, thus leading to a synergistic antitumor immune response.

These observations have led to principled preclinical and proof-of-concept clinical studies in multiple disease sites combining RT with immunotherapy in order to take advantage of RT's immunostimulatory properties while blunting its immunosuppressive effects. For example, anti–cytotoxic T lymphocyte–associated protein 4 (CTLA-4)–directed therapy might be used to suppress RT-induced Treg activation at the same time as RT enhances intratumoral interferon production and antitumor T-cell activation.[33,34] Similarly, anti–PD-L1 therapy might be used to counter RT-mediated PD-L1 upregulation at the same time as RT enhances programmed cell death protein 1 (PD-1)–mediated antigen cross-presentation.[33,35]

In bladder cancer, the mechanistic details of the interaction between RT and ICB remain to be fully elucidated.[4,36] However, multiple anti-PD1/PD-L1 agents have shown efficacy in bladder cancer and are US Food and Drug Administration approved for use in patients with advanced disease.[37–39] Based on these data from the advanced disease settings, as well as the established benefit of adjuvant ICB after chemoradiation in other disease sites, the randomized phase III SWOG/NRG 1806 trial (INTACT [Phase III Randomized Trial of Concurrent Chemoradiotherapy With or Without Atezolizumab in Localized Muscle Invasive Bladder Cancer], NCT03775265) is examining the role of concurrent and adjuvant atezolizumab in the setting of bladder-sparing TMT (**Fig. 2**A).[40,41] Similarly, the phase II ECOG-ACRIN/NRG EA8185 (INSPIRE [Phase II Study of Bladder-SparIng ChemoradiatioN With MEDI4736 (Durvalumab) in Clinical Stage III, Node PosItive BladdeR CancEr], NCT04216290) is investigating the role of concurrent durvalumab and chemoradiation in patients with node-positive bladder cancer. Both studies have extensive planned correlative studies, discussed further later, designed to identify the

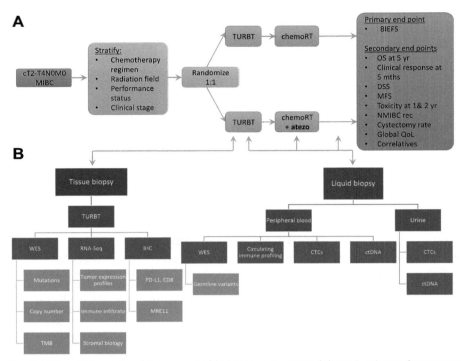

Fig. 2. ICB and biomarker-driven care in bladder-sparing TMT. (*A*) Study schema for SWOG/ NRG 1806, a randomized phase III trial of bladder-sparing TMT with or without concurrent and adjuvant atezolizumab (anti–PD-L1). The primary end point is bladder-intact event-free survival (BIEFS), a composite end point that includes muscle-invasive recurrence in the bladder, regional pelvic soft tissue or nodal recurrence, distant metastases, cystectomy, and death of any cause. (*B*) SWOG/NRG 1806 will provide many opportunities for multidimensional characterization of MIBC biology, tumor stromal/immune factors, and their interplay, both pretreatment via tissue biopsy (TURBT) and longitudinally via liquid biopsy (peripheral blood, urine). Given the multitude of biological factors that may influence tumor behavior and treatment response, unbiased and comprehensive profiling approaches paired with prospective clinical data generation are critical to understanding the molecular basis of clinical phenotypes. atezo, atezolizumab; chemoRT, chemoradiotherapy; CTCs, circulating tumor cells; ctDNA, circulating tumor DNA; QoL, quality of life; TMB, tumor mutational burden; WES, whole-exome sequencing.

molecular biomarkers of response to TMT with or without ICB (**Fig. 2**B). Although at least 1 case report of significant toxicity has emerged when combining ICB with markedly hypofractionated RT, given the overall favorable safety profile of RT in combination with ICB, there is reason for optimism regarding its safety with more conventionally fractionated RT.[42,43] If positive, these studies have the potential to fundamentally alter the treatment landscape of TMT.

Patient Selection for Trimodality Therapy: Clinical-Pathologic Variables

Long-term data from multiple published studies show that TMT is capable of achieving excellent disease control and QoL outcomes in localized MIBC. Critical to this success is thoughtful attention to patient selection. Several decades of experience has led to an understanding of the clinical-pathologic factors that can affect the success of TMT.

Broadly, the less tumor (both at diagnosis and at the start of chemoradiation), the more likely TMT is to succeed. Thus, as discussed earlier, the ability to achieve a visibly complete TURBT is associated with higher rates of CR, decreased rates of salvage cystectomy, and improved OS.[5–7] Likewise, although patients with clinical T2 to T4a disease have traditionally been eligible for bladder preservation trials, cT2 tumors have better outcomes than more advanced tumors, and cT2 to T3a tumors are considered to be the best candidates for TMT.[5,7] Unifocal tumors measuring less than 6 cm are also preferred. Similarly, tumor-associated hydronephrosis, which can reflect either initial bulky disease or disease impinging on the ureteral orifice, where visibly complete TURBT may be challenging, is associated with inferior outcomes.[5,7] However, unilateral hydronephrosis is not an absolute contraindication to TMT. Most studies of TMT have restricted enrollment to urothelial histology; however, tumors with a component of urothelial variant histology (eg, mixed variant urothelial histology with squamous cell carcinoma differentiation) may respond comparably well to TMT, although this is less clear for pure nonurothelial histologies.[44,45] Evidence supporting the use of TMT for non-MIBC (ie, T1 disease) is limited, and, for MIBC, presence of tumor-associated CIS is associated with inferior outcomes.[5,6] In addition, because the key differentiator of bladder-conserving TMT versus RC is the opportunity to retain the patient's native bladder, adequate baseline bladder function is essential. In other words, patients must have a bladder worth sparing.

OPPORTUNITIES TO INCORPORATE MOLECULAR PROFILING
Selection of Patients for Trimodality Therapy

Although the clinical-pathologic factors discussed earlier have been critical to identifying suitable candidates for bladder-preserving TMT, the emerging understanding of the molecular and genomic landscape of bladder cancer may provide additional opportunities to refine patient and treatment selection (**Fig. 3**). Molecular markers that

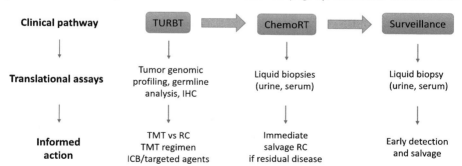

Fig. 3. Opportunities to integrate molecular profiling for bladder-sparing TMT. Bladder-sparing TMT involves maximal safe TURBT followed by concurrent chemoradiation and posttreatment surveillance cystoscopies and imaging. Opportunities for molecular profiling exist at each step in this paradigm. Pretreatment tumor and germline profiling could inform selection of TMT versus RC or selection of specific TMT regimen (such as chemotherapy agent, radiation dose/field, and use of concurrent ICB or other targeted agents). Disease monitoring during and immediately following chemoRT via minimally invasive urine or serum analyses could enable sensitive identification of local disease persistence and appropriate early salvage cystectomy. Posttreatment monitoring could enable early detection of relapse and initiation of salvage therapy.

are causal to or even simply associated with differential response to TMT versus RC could help guide patients to the most appropriate treatment paradigm. Likewise, such markers associated with differential response to an individual element of TMT (eg, radiation or a specific systemic therapy agent) could improve selection of the specific TMT regimen from the spectrum of clinically acceptable options. Markers associated with worse prognosis regardless of treatment assignment may identify patients who would benefit from studies of treatment intensification.

Critical to such efforts is knowledge of the underlying molecular and genomic landscape of bladder cancer, which has been mapped in significant detail.[46] Key features include recurrent mutations in established oncogenes and tumor suppressors such as *TP53*, *PIK3CA*, and *RB1*; a high tumor mutational burden (TMB), largely driven by APOBEC-induced mutagenesis with contributions from other DNA damage repair genes, including *ERCC2*; and frequent copy-number variants.[47] Regarding gene expression, a recent consensus classification scheme has described 6 transcriptional classes, broadly reflecting a distinction between basal and luminal phenotypes, which may reflect both distinct oncogenic mechanisms and differential contributions of tumor microenvironment and interaction with the immune compartment.[48] The potential role of ICB as a component of TMT may provide further opportunities for biologically principled clinical decision making. Together, this wealth of genomic and transcriptional information has provided several emerging possibilities for genomically guided treatment selection, monitoring of response, and posttreatment surveillance.

DNA damage repair alterations

Alterations in several DNA damage repair (DDR) genes have been proposed as predictive markers of response to TMT. The most studied to date is MRE11, a component of the MRN (Mre11/Rad50/Nbs1) complex critical to the cellular response to DNA double-strand breaks. Increased MRE11 protein expression by immunohistochemistry (IHC) has been associated in some studies with improved DSS after RT but not RC, and a low nuclear/cytoplasmic MRE11 ratio is associated with increased disease-specific mortality.[49–51] The association between increased expression of a DNA repair protein and worse response to DNA-damaging therapy is counterintuitive but may reflect a futile attempt of an otherwise repair-deficient cell to upregulate DNA repair in the face of genomic insult. However, attempts to validate a relationship between MRE11 protein expression and treatment outcomes in the BCON and BC2001 trials were hindered by technical challenges related to IHC, and ultimately the association could not be validated in these datasets.[52] MRE11 expression was also not associated with outcomes in an additional TMT cohort.[53] Thus, despite the extensive interest in MRE11 as a possible biomarker of TMT response, more work is required.

An additional DDR gene potentially associated with TMT response is *ERCC2*. Mutations in *ERCC2*, a core member of the nucleotide excision repair pathway critical for repairing cisplatin-induced DNA adducts, are detected in MIBC at a frequency of approximately 9% based on The Cancer Genome Atlas data.[46] Such mutations were first associated with improved response to cisplatin-based chemotherapy in the neoadjuvant and metastatic settings and have also been associated with improved outcomes following TMT.[53–56] The same TMT study also identified a trend toward improved outcomes following TMT among patients with other DDR pathway alterations, similar to prior findings in the neoadjuvant setting.[57] Thus, *ERCC2* mutations and other DDR pathway alterations represent an increasingly promising, mechanistically plausible predictive biomarker of response to cisplatin-based chemotherapy in the neoadjuvant and TMT settings. At present, several trials are evaluating the possibility of omitting RC in patients who experience a cCR to cisplatin-based NAC; whether such patients could be managed instead with cisplatin-containing TMT represents a promising question for future studies.[58]

Although no DDR pathway gene has yet been associated with response to RT specifically in MIBC, a recent study has identified inactivating *ATM* mutations as predictive of RT response in patients with advanced cancers.[59] This finding serves as a proof of principle that specific gene mutations are associated with clinical RT response, and could prove important in the rational selection of patients for RT-based therapy, including TMT.

In addition to modulating repair of RT-induced or chemotherapy-induced DNA damage, DDR pathway alterations may also influence response to ICB in bladder cancer. The precise mechanism of this relationship is uncertain but may involve increased TMB/neoantigen burden or enhanced innate immune pathway activation via cGAS/STING.[60] In the metastatic setting, mutations in DDR genes have been associated with increased likelihood of response to ICB.[61] In the neoadjuvant setting, a similar relationship has been described, with potential additional effects of TMB.[62] The recent findings that up to 14% of patients with bladder cancer harbor deleterious germline DDR pathway mutations also raises the possibility that not only somatic but also germline variants may contribute to tumor response to ICB or DNA-damaging agents.[63] Although there is not yet an established role for ICB in bladder-preserving TMT, the ongoing SWOG/NRG 1806 INTACT and ECOG-ACRIN/NRG INSPIRE clinical trials may define a role for ICB in bladder-preserving TMT.

Gene expression classes

Although identification of somatic mutations and copy-number alterations provides tumor-specific information, assessment of messenger RNA expression patterns offers an opportunity to assess not only tumor but also stromal and immune biology. This approach may thus provide complementary opportunities to identify modulators of response to TMT in tumor and host compartments.

Distinct transcriptional subtypes of MIBC have been associated with differential clinical outcomes. For example, luminal tumors had superior outcomes and claudin-low tumors had inferior outcomes regardless of receipt of NAC before RC, whereas basal-type tumors had the most significant improvement in outcomes with NAC.[64] These findings provide proof of principle that RNA expression patterns may be not only prognostic but also predictive for response to chemotherapy and raise the possibility that similar such correlates of TMT response may exist. In support of this possibility, a single-institution study from MGH found that, among 136 patients with MIBC treated with TMT and 223 with NAC-RC, signatures of T-cell activation and interferon-gamma signaling were associated with improved outcomes following TMT but not following NAC-RC.[65] In addition, higher stromal infiltration was associated with worse outcomes following NAC-RC but not TMT. The observation that an immune-activated subset of patients has improved outcomes with TMT suggests that these patients may derive even greater benefit from the addition of ICB, as is being tested in SWOG/NRG 1806.

Gene expression patterns may also modulate the response to hypoxia-modifying therapies. A recent correlative analysis of the BCON trial showed that the benefit to hypoxia-modification treatment was restricted to patients whose tumors had high hypoxic gene expression signatures.[66]

Expression signatures have also recently been shown to be correlated to response to ICB. In the PURE-01 study, which examined neoadjuvant pembrolizumab before RC, expression of an immune activation signature was associated with higher rates of pathologic CR at the time of RC; no such association was observed in patients treated with NAC.[62,67] However, the association of immune expression signature with CR to pembrolizumab may be most prominent in patients whose tumors display an increased TMB.[68] This finding illustrates the potential challenges to a reductionist approach to biomarkers of ICB response; determinants of ICB response are almost certainly multifactorial.[69] One method to potentially mitigate this challenge is to build comprehensive translational correlatives into the design of future studies. For example, patients enrolled on the SWOG/NRG 1806 trial will have not only TURBT samples collected for transcriptome, whole-exome sequencing, and IHC analyses but also peripheral blood collected for germline DNA analysis and circulating immune cell subsets. This integrative molecular profiling approach has the potential to be highly informative in determining which sets of biomarkers are most associated with response to TMT with or without concurrent ICB.

Monitoring Response During and After Treatment

Before treatment, tissue-based biomarkers as outlined earlier have the potential to identify which patients are most likely to respond to a given treatment. After treatment, evaluation of response and surveillance for relapse represent additional opportunities for novel molecular approaches. At present, cystoscopy is the mainstay of monitoring local response after TMT. A posttreatment cystoscopy is used to identify patients with less than a CR, for whom salvage cystectomy is typically offered, and regular surveillance cystoscopies aim to promptly identify bladder recurrences. However, this approach is limited in its sensitivity to detect residual disease or early recurrence; for example, in series of patients who manifested a cCR to NAC from cystoscopy with biopsy, and who subsequently declined RC, in-bladder recurrence rates of 30% to 50% have been documented, suggesting the presence of at least microscopic residual disease that was not detected by conventional methods.[70,71]

Molecularly informed markers could be useful in multiple contexts following TMT. They may enable more sensitive detection of residual disease after TMT, prompting consideration of further therapy. They may also enable earlier detection of disease recurrence, enabling earlier salvage therapy. In principle, bladder cancer is a uniquely favorable context for noninvasive molecular monitoring because the bladder routinely sheds cells into urine, which is readily collectible. This principle not only is the basis of traditional urine cytology but also enables molecular analyses. Springer and colleagues[72] have shown that a custom sequencing panel can identify bladder cancer genomic alterations in patients with MIBC. Localized MIBC can also contribute to the circulating tumor cell (CTC) and circulating cell-free DNA pool, and the presence of CTCs is associated with unfavorable outcomes following RC.[73,74] A recent abstract also suggests that expression profiling of pretreatment CTCs can identify patients at high risk of recurrence after TMT.[75] In addition, such liquid biopsy approaches can be used to monitor for recurrence; for example, in patients with locally advanced MIBC treated with NAC-RC, ultradeep plasma sequencing was able to detect recurrences a median of 96 days earlier than radiographic imaging.[76] Liquid biopsies may be informative regarding not only the existence but also the mechanism of resistance and relapse. Taken together, these studies suggest that urine and/or plasma liquid biopsy approaches have the potential to provide increased sensitivity to detect residual or recurrent disease and may also provide novel insights by revealing mechanisms of treatment resistance.

SUMMARY

Based on robust clinical evidence, bladder-preserving TMT is now an accepted paradigm for the treatment of MIBC and can provide favorable oncologic and QoL outcomes in carefully selected patients. Key elements of TMT are a maximal safe TURBT, RT with concurrent chemotherapy, and close posttreatment monitoring. The documented success with TMT in large modern series is due in large part to thoughtful patient selection. Although current decision making between RC and TMT is largely driven by clinical factors and patient/physician preference, there are emerging opportunities for molecular and genomic insights to influence clinical care in this disease. In particular, mutations and/or expression patterns may help determine which patients are likely to fare better with TMT versus RC, may help select specific TMT regimens (including choice among accepted chemotherapy options and/or potential integration of ICB), may more sensitively detect residual disease following TMT, and may facilitate early detection and mechanistic understanding of recurrence after treatment. There is strong preclinical and clinical rationale supporting the addition of ICB to TMT, and several trials are ongoing to assess its clinical impact in this setting. The results of these trials have the potential to alter the treatment paradigm for TMT, and planned correlative studies may provide novel mechanistic insight into the determinants of ICB response. Although the true application of molecular insights to routine clinical practice is in its infancy, the TMT paradigm provides an opportunity to study molecularly informed precision approaches that may ultimately improve both disease outcomes and patient QoL for patients with localized MIBC.

CLINICS CARE POINTS

- Bladder-conserving TMT is now a well-established standard of care for patients with MIBC and is best delivered by a multidisciplinary team including urologic oncology, medical oncology, and radiation oncology.

- Although never compared with RC in a randomized study, TMT seems to offer comparable oncologic outcomes in carefully selected patients while allowing patients to preserve their native bladders.

- Ideal candidates for bladder-conserving TMT include patients with (1) unifocal tumors less than 6 cm; (2) cT2 to T3a tumors; (3) urothelial histology (although a component of variant histology may also be acceptable); (4) no or limited tumor-associated CIS; (5) no or unilateral tumor-associated hydronephrosis; and (6) good baseline bladder function. Patients who do not meet all criteria may still be candidates for TMT on an individualized basis.

- The key elements of TMT are (1) a maximal safe TURBT; (2) radiotherapy (conventionally fractionated to 60–66 Gy in daily fractions of 1.8–2.0 Gy, or moderately hypofractionated [eg, 55 Gy in 20 fractions], encompassing either the whole bladder or the bladder tumor bed plus a margin, and with treatment of pelvic nodes to 40–45 Gy considered on an individualized basis); (3) concurrent chemotherapy (with options including cisplatin, a cisplatin-containing doublet, 5-FU–MMC, single-agent gemcitabine, single-agent paclitaxel), or hypoxia-modifying agents (CON); and (4) posttreatment surveillance imaging and cystoscopies with urine cytology and, as indicated, biopsy.

- There is a preclinical rationale for combination of RT and ICB in bladder cancer and clinical evidence for ICB activity in advanced disease; ongoing trials are investigating the role of ICB as a component of TMT.

In the future, molecular features such as tumor mutations or gene expression patterns may be useful in guiding patient selection and informing treatment approaches for TMT. Similarly, novel methods for tumor detection through urine or circulating biomarkers (such as circulating tumor DNA or CTCs) may inform response evaluation and guide posttreatment surveillance.

DISCLOSURE

D.J. Konieczkowski: none. J.A. Efstathiou: consulting (Blue Earth Diagnostics, Boston Scientific, AstraZeneca), Advisory Board (Roivant); honoraria (UpToDate). K.W. Mouw: research funding (Pfizer); consulting (EMD Serono/Pfizer); honoraria (UpToDate, OncLive).

REFERENCES

1. Bellmunt J, Orsola A, Wiegel T, et al. Bladder cancer: ESMO Clinical Practice Guidelines for diagnosis, treatment and follow-up. Ann Oncol 2011; 22(suppl_6):vi45–9.
2. Flaig TW, Spiess PE, Agarwal N, et al. Bladder Cancer, Version 3.2020, NCCN clinical practice guidelines in oncology. J Natl Compr Canc Netw 2020;18(3): 329–54.
3. Chang SS, Bochner BH, Chou R, et al. Treatment of Non-Metastatic Muscle-Invasive Bladder Cancer: AUA/ASCO/ASTRO/SUO Guideline. J Urol 2017;198(3): 552–9.
4. Solanki AA, Bossi A, Efstathiou JA, et al. Combining Immunotherapy with Radiotherapy for the Treatment of Genitourinary Malignancies. Eur Urol Oncol 2018; 2(1):79–87.
5. Giacalone NJ, Shipley WU, Clayman RH, et al. Long-term outcomes after bladder-preserving tri-modality therapy for patients with muscle-invasive bladder cancer: an updated analysis of the Massachusetts General Hospital experience. Eur Urol 2017;71(6):952–60.
6. Rödel C, Grabenbauer GG, Kühn R, et al. Combined-modality treatment and selective organ preservation in invasive bladder cancer: long-term results. J Clin Oncol 2002;20(14):3061–71.
7. Mak RH, Hunt D, Shipley WU, et al. Long-term outcomes in patients with muscle-invasive bladder cancer after selective bladder-preserving combined-modality therapy: A Pooled Analysis of Radiation Therapy Oncology Group Protocols 8802, 8903, 9506, 9706, 9906, and 0233. J Clin Oncol 2014. https://doi.org/10.1200/jco.2014.57.5548.
8. Huddart RA, Hall E, Lewis R, et al. Life and death of spare (selective bladder preservation against radical excision): reflections on why the spare trial closed. BJU Int 2010;106(6):753–5.
9. Kulkarni GS, Hermanns T, Wei Y, et al. Propensity Score Analysis of Radical Cystectomy Versus Bladder-Sparing Trimodal Therapy in the Setting of a Multidisciplinary Bladder Cancer Clinic. J Clin Oncol 2017;35(20). JCO.2016.69.232.
10. Vashistha V, Wang H, Mazzone A, et al. Radical cystectomy compared to combined modality treatment for muscle-invasive bladder cancer: a systematic review and meta-analysis. Int J Radiat Oncol Biol Phys 2017;97(5):1002–20.
11. Efstathiou JA, Bae K, Shipley WU, et al. Late Pelvic Toxicity After Bladder-Sparing Therapy in Patients With Invasive Bladder Cancer: RTOG 89-03, 95-06, 97-06, 99-06. J Clin Oncol 2009;27(25):4055–61.
12. Mak KS, Smith AB, Eidelman A, et al. Quality of Life in Long-term Survivors of Muscle-Invasive Bladder Cancer. Int J Radiat Oncol Biol Phys 2016;96(5): 1028–36.
13. Royce TJ, Feldman AS, Mossanen M, et al. Comparative Effectiveness of Bladder-preserving Tri-modality Therapy Versus Radical Cystectomy for Muscle-invasive Bladder Cancer. Clin Genitourin Canc 2018;17(1):23–31.e3.

14. Huddart RA, Hall E, Lewis R, et al. Patient-reported Quality of Life Outcomes in Patients Treated for Muscle-invasive Bladder Cancer with Radiotherapy ± Chemotherapy in the BC2001 Phase III Randomised Controlled Trial. Eur Urol 2019;77(2):260–8.
15. James ND, Hussain SA, Hall E, et al. Radiotherapy with or without Chemotherapy in Muscle-Invasive Bladder Cancer. N Engl J Med 2012;366(16):1477–88.
16. Huddart RA, Hall E, Hussain SA, et al. Randomized Noninferiority Trial of Reduced High-Dose Volume Versus Standard Volume Radiation Therapy for Muscle-Invasive Bladder Cancer: Results of the BC2001 Trial (CRUK/01/004). Int J Radiat Oncol Biol Phys 2013;87(2):261–9.
17. Coppin CM, Gospodarowicz MK, James K, et al. Improved local control of invasive bladder cancer by concurrent cisplatin and preoperative or definitive radiation. The National Cancer Institute of Canada Clinical Trials Group. J Clin Oncol 1996;14(11):2901–7.
18. Kent E, Sandler H, Montie J, et al. Combined-Modality Therapy With Gemcitabine and Radiotherapy As a Bladder Preservation Strategy: Results of a Phase I Trial. J Clin Oncol 2004;22(13):2540–5.
19. Choudhury A, Swindell R, Logue JP, et al. Phase II Study of Conformal Hypofractionated Radiotherapy With Concurrent Gemcitabine in Muscle-Invasive Bladder Cancer. J Clin Oncol 2011;29(6):733–8.
20. Coen JJ, Zhang P, Saylor PJ, et al. Bladder Preservation With Twice-a-Day Radiation Plus Fluorouracil/Cisplatin or Once Daily Radiation Plus Gemcitabine for Muscle-Invasive Bladder Cancer: NRG/RTOG 0712—A Randomized Phase II Trial. J Clin Oncol 2019;37(1):44–51.
21. Michaelson MD, Hu C, Pham HT, et al. A Phase 1/2 Trial of a Combination of Paclitaxel and Trastuzumab With Daily Irradiation or Paclitaxel Alone With Daily Irradiation After Transurethral Surgery for Noncystectomy Candidates With Muscle-Invasive Bladder Cancer (Trial NRG Oncology RTOG 0524). Int J Radiat Oncol Biol Phys 2017;97(5):995–1001.
22. Trialists IC of, Group) MRCABCWP (now the NCRIBCCS, Group EO for R and T of CG-UTC, et al. International Phase III Trial Assessing Neoadjuvant Cisplatin, Methotrexate, and Vinblastine Chemotherapy for Muscle-Invasive Bladder Cancer: Long-Term Results of the BA06 30894 Trial. J Clin Oncol 2011;29(16):2171–7.
23. Tester W, Caplan R, Heaney J, et al. Neoadjuvant combined modality program with selective organ preservation for invasive bladder cancer: results of Radiation Therapy Oncology Group phase II trial 8802. J Clin Oncol 1996;14(1):119–26.
24. Shipley WU, Winter KA, Kaufman DS, et al. Phase III trial of neoadjuvant chemotherapy in patients with invasive bladder cancer treated with selective bladder preservation by combined radiation therapy and chemotherapy: initial results of Radiation Therapy Oncology Group 89-03. J Clin Oncol 1998;16(11):3576–83.
25. Kaufman DS, Winter KA, Shipley WU, et al. Phase I-II RTOG Study (99-06) of patients with muscle-invasive bladder cancer undergoing transurethral surgery, paclitaxel, cisplatin, and twice-daily radiotherapy followed by selective bladder preservation or radical cystectomy and adjuvant chemotherapy. Urology 2009;73(4):833–7.
26. Mitin T, Hunt D, WU Shipley, et al. Transurethral surgery and twice-daily radiation plus paclitaxel-cisplatin or fluorouracil-cisplatin with selective bladder preservation and adjuvant chemotherapy for patients with muscle invasive bladder cancer (RTOG 0233): a randomised multicentre phase 2 trial. Lancet Oncol 2013;14(9):863–72.

27. Mitin T, George A, Zietman AL, et al. Long-Term Outcomes Among Patients Who Achieve Complete or Near-Complete Responses After the Induction Phase of Bladder-Preserving Combined-Modality Therapy for Muscle-Invasive Bladder Cancer: A Pooled Analysis of NRG Oncology/RTOG 9906 and 0233. Int J Radiat Oncol Biol Phys 2016;94(1):67–74.

28. Hoskin PJ, Rojas AM, Bentzen SM, et al. Radiotherapy With Concurrent Carbogen and Nicotinamide in Bladder Carcinoma. J Clin Oncol 2010;28(33):4912–8.

29. Song YP, Mistry H, Choudhury A, et al. Long-term outcomes of hypoxia modification in bladder preservation: Update from BCON trial. J Clin Oncol 2019; 37(7_suppl):356.

30. Stone HB, Peters LJ, Milas L. Effect of host immune capability on radiocurability and subsequent transplantability of a murine fibrosarcoma. J Natl Cancer 1979; 63(5):1229–35.

31. Sharabi AB, Lim M, DeWeese TL, et al. Radiation and checkpoint blockade immunotherapy: radiosensitisation and potential mechanisms of synergy. Lancet Oncol 2015;16(13):e498–509.

32. Kordbacheh T, Honeychurch J, Blackhall F, et al. Radiotherapy and anti-PD-1/PD-L1 combinations in lung cancer: building better translational research platforms. Ann Oncol 2018;29(2):301–10.

33. Victor CT-S, Rech AJ, Maity A, et al. Radiation and dual checkpoint blockade activate non-redundant immune mechanisms in cancer. Nature 2015;520(7547): 373–7.

34. Formenti SC, Rudqvist N-P, Golden E, et al. Radiotherapy induces responses of lung cancer to CTLA-4 blockade. Nat Med 2018;24(12):1845–51.

35. Sharabi AB, Nirschl CJ, Kochel CM, et al. Stereotactic radiation therapy augments antigen-specific PD-1–mediated antitumor immune responses via cross-presentation of tumor antigen. Cancer Immunol Res 2015;3(4):345–55.

36. Buchwald ZS, Efstathiou JA. Immunotherapy and radiation – a new combined treatment approach for bladder cancer? Bladder Cancer 2015;1(1):15–27.

37. Rosenberg JE, Hoffman-Censits J, Powles T, et al. Atezolizumab in patients with locally advanced and metastatic urothelial carcinoma who have progressed following treatment with platinum-based chemotherapy: a single-arm, multicentre, phase 2 trial. Lancet 2016;387(10031):1909–20.

38. Powles T, Durán I, van der Heijden MS, et al. Atezolizumab versus chemotherapy in patients with platinum-treated locally advanced or metastatic urothelial carcinoma (IMvigor211): a multicentre, open-label, phase 3 randomised controlled trial. Lancet 2018;391(10122):748–57.

39. Galsky MD, Arija JÁA, Bamias A, et al. Atezolizumab with or without chemotherapy in metastatic urothelial cancer (IMvigor130): a multicentre, randomised, placebo-controlled phase 3 trial. Lancet 2020;395(10236):1547–57.

40. Antonia SJ, Villegas A, Daniel D, et al. Overall Survival with Durvalumab after Chemoradiotherapy in Stage III NSCLC. N Engl J Med 2018;379(24):2342–50.

41. Gray JE, Villegas A, Daniel D, et al. Brief report: Three-year overall survival with durvalumab after chemoradiotherapy in Stage III NSCLC - Update from PACIFIC. J Thorac Oncol 2019;15(2):288–93.

42. Tree AC, Jones K, Hafeez S, et al. Dose-limiting urinary toxicity with Pembrolizumab combined with weekly hypofractionated radiotherapy in bladder cancer. Int J Radiat Oncol Biol Phys 2018;101(5):1168–71.

43. Hwang WL, Pike LRG, Royce TJ, et al. Safety of combining radiotherapy with immune-checkpoint inhibition. Nat Rev Clin Oncol 2018;15(8):477–94.

44. Krasnow RE, Drumm M, Roberts HJ, et al. Clinical outcomes of patients with histologic variants of urothelial cancer treated with trimodality bladder-sparing therapy. Eur Urol 2017;72(1):54–60.

45. Arslan B, Bozkurt IH, Yonguc T, et al. Clinical features and outcomes of nontransitional cell carcinomas of the urinary bladder: Analysis of 125 cases. Urol Ann 2015;7(2):177–82.

46. Robertson AG, Kim J, Al-Ahmadie H, et al. Comprehensive molecular characterization of muscle-invasive bladder cancer. Cell 2017;171(3):540–56.e25.

47. Kim J, Mouw KW, Polak P, et al. Somatic ERCC2 mutations are associated with a distinct genomic signature in urothelial tumors. Nat Genet 2016;48(6):600–6.

48. Kamoun A, Reyniès A de, Allory Y, et al. A consensus molecular classification of muscle-invasive bladder cancer. Eur Urol 2019;77(4):420–33.

49. Choudhury A, Nelson LD, Teo MTW, et al. MRE11 Expression Is Predictive of Cause-Specific Survival following Radical Radiotherapy for Muscle-Invasive Bladder Cancer. Cancer Res 2010;70(18):7017–26.

50. Laurberg JR, Brems-Eskildsen AS, Nordentoft I, et al. Expression of TIP60 (tat-interactive protein) and MRE11 (meiotic recombination 11 homolog) predict treatment-specific outcome of localised invasive bladder cancer. Bju Int 2012; 110(11c):E1228–36.

51. Magliocco A, Moughan J, Simko J, et al. The Impact of MRE11 in Nuclear to Cytoplasmic Ratio on Outcomes in Muscle Invasive Bladder Cancer: an Analysis of NRG/RTOG 8802, 8903, 9506, 9706, 9906, and 0233. Int J Radiat Oncol Biol Phys 2017;99(2):S117–8.

52. Walker AK, Karaszi K, Valentine H, et al. MRE11 as a predictive biomarker of outcome following radiotherapy in bladder cancer. Int J Radiat Oncol Biol Phys 2019;104(4):809–18.

53. Desai NB, Scott SN, Zabor EC, et al. Genomic characterization of response to chemoradiation in urothelial bladder cancer. Cancer 2016;122(23):3715–23.

54. Allen EMV, Mouw KW, Kim P, et al. Somatic ERCC2 mutations correlate with cisplatin sensitivity in muscle-invasive urothelial carcinoma. Cancer Discov 2014;4(10):1140–53.

55. Liu D, Plimack ER, Hoffman-Censits J, et al. Clinical Validation of Chemotherapy Response Biomarker ERCC2 in Muscle-Invasive Urothelial Bladder Carcinoma. JAMA Oncol 2016;2(8):1094–6.

56. Teo MY, Bambury RM, Zabor EC, et al. DNA Damage Response and Repair Gene Alterations Are Associated with Improved Survival in Patients with Platinum-Treated Advanced Urothelial Carcinoma. Clin Cancer Res 2017;23(14):3610–8.

57. Plimack ER, Dunbrack RL, Brennan TA, et al. Defects in DNA repair genes predict response to neoadjuvant cisplatin-based chemotherapy in muscle-invasive bladder cancer. Eur Urol 2015;68(6):959–67.

58. Grivas P. DNA damage response gene alterations in urothelial cancer: ready for practice? Clin Cancer Res 2018;25(3). clincanres.2512.2018.

59. Pitter KL, Casey DL, Lu YC, et al. Pathogenic ATM Mutations in Cancer and a Genetic Basis for Radiotherapeutic Efficacy. J Natl Cancer 2020. https://doi.org/10.1093/jnci/djaa095.

60. Mouw KW, Goldberg MS, Konstantinopoulos PA, et al. DNA Damage and Repair Biomarkers of Immunotherapy Response. Cancer Discov 2017;7(7):675–93.

61. Teo MY, Seier K, Ostrovnaya I, et al. Alterations in DNA Damage Response and Repair Genes as Potential Marker of Clinical Benefit From PD-1/PD-L1 Blockade in Advanced Urothelial Cancers. J Clin Oncol 2018;36(17):1685–94.

62. Necchi A, Anichini A, Raggi D, et al. Pembrolizumab as Neoadjuvant Therapy Before Radical Cystectomy in Patients With Muscle-Invasive Urothelial Bladder Carcinoma (PURE-01): An Open-Label, Single-Arm, Phase II Study. J Clin Oncol 2018;36(34). JCO.18.01148.

63. Carlo MI, Ravichandran V, Srinavasan P, et al. Cancer susceptibility mutations in patients with urothelial malignancies. J Clin Oncol 2020;38(5):406–14.

64. Seiler R, Ashab HAD, Erho N, et al. Impact of molecular subtypes in muscle-invasive bladder cancer on predicting response and survival after neoadjuvant chemotherapy. Eur Urol 2017;72(4):544–54.

65. Efstathiou JA, Mouw KW, Gibb EA, et al. Impact of immune and stromal infiltration on outcomes following bladder-sparing trimodality therapy for muscle-invasive bladder cancer. Eur Urol 2019;76(1):59–68.

66. Yang L, Taylor J, Eustace A, et al. A gene signature for selecting benefit from hypoxia modification of radiotherapy for high-risk bladder cancer patients. Clin Cancer Res 2017;23(16):4761–8.

67. Necchi A, Raggi D, Gallina A, et al. Impact of molecular subtyping and immune infiltration on pathological response and outcome following neoadjuvant pembrolizumab in muscle-invasive bladder cancer. Eur Urol 2020;77(6):701–10.

68. Bandini M, Ross JS, Raggi D, et al. Predicting the pathologic complete response after neoadjuvant pembrolizumab in muscle-invasive bladder cancer. Jnci J Natl Cancer Inst 2020. https://doi.org/10.1093/jnci/djaa076.

69. Konieczkowski DJ, Johannessen CM, Garraway LA. A convergence-based framework for cancer drug resistance. Cancer Cell 2018;33(5):801–15.

70. Solsona E, Climent MA, Iborra I, et al. Bladder preservation in selected patients with muscle-invasive bladder cancer by complete transurethral resection of the bladder plus systemic chemotherapy: long-term follow-up of a Phase 2 Nonrandomized Comparative Trial with Radical Cystectomy. Eur Urol 2009;55(4):911–21.

71. Herr HW. Outcome of patients who refuse cystectomy after receiving neoadjuvant chemotherapy for muscle-invasive bladder cancer. Eur Urol 2008;54(1):126–32.

72. Springer SU, Chen C-H, Pena MDCR, et al. Non-invasive detection of urothelial cancer through the analysis of driver gene mutations and aneuploidy. eLife 2018;7:e32143.

73. Zhang Z, Fan W, Deng Q, et al. The prognostic and diagnostic value of circulating tumor cells in bladder cancer and upper tract urothelial carcinoma: a meta-analysis of 30 published studies. Oncotarget 2015;5(0):59527–38.

74. Rink M, Chun FK, Dahlem R, et al. Prognostic Role and HER2 Expression of Circulating Tumor Cells in Peripheral Blood of Patients Prior to Radical Cystectomy: A Prospective Study. Eur Urol 2012;61(4):810–7.

75. Hwang W, Pleskow H, Czapla JAA, et al. Integrated Gene Expression Score in Circulating Tumor Cells to Predict Treatment Response in Muscle-Invasive Bladder Cancer. Int J Radiat Oncol Biol Phys 2019;105(1):E663.

76. Christensen E, Birkenkamp-Demtröder K, Sethi H, et al. Early detection of metastatic relapse and monitoring of therapeutic efficacy by ultra-deep sequencing of plasma cell-free DNA in patients with urothelial bladder carcinoma. J Clin Oncol 2019;37(18). JCO.18.02052.

Emerging Targeted Therapy for Bladder Cancer

Constance Thibault, MD[a], Yohann Loriot, MD, PhD[b],*

KEYWORDS

- Urothelial carcinoma • Targeted therapies • FGFR inhibitors • PARP inhibitors
- Conjugated antibodies • Antiangiogenic

KEY POINTS

- Around 15% of metastatic urothelial carcinoma harbor *FGFR* alterations that can be targeted with fibroblast growth factor receptor inhibitors.
- PARP inhibitors failed to show efficacy as a single agent in unselected urothelial carcinoma but are currently evaluated as maintenance after platinum chemotherapy, in combination with checkpoint inhibitors and in selected patients with DNA damage repair deficiency.
- Several antibody-drug conjugates are currently evaluated in unselected metastatic urothelial carcinoma with promising results on the preliminary studies.

INTRODUCTION

Until recently, bladder cancer was one of several rare tumors in which no targeted therapies had shown efficacy. However, since the publication of the results of The Cancer Genome Atlas project conducted on 131 cases of muscle-invasive bladder cancer (MIBC), several teams have incrementally mapped out the alterations of the landscape in signaling pathways, such as p53/Rb and RTK/RAS/MAP-Kinase. Among genetic alterations on RTK, several can be targeted by systemic treatments, such as vascular endothelial growth factor (VEGF), epidermal growth factor receptors 1 and 2 (EGFR and HER2/*neu*), and fibroblast growth factor receptor (FGFR). In this review, the authors summarize the therapeutic treatments that are currently evaluated in clinical trials (**Table 1**).

[a] Medical Oncology Department, European Georges Pompidou Hospital, APHP.5, 20 rue Leblanc, Paris 75015, France; [b] Département de médicine oncologique, Gustave Roussy, Université Paris-Saclay, Gustave Roussy 114 rue Edouard Vaillant, 94805 Villejuif, France
* Corresponding author.
E-mail address: yohann.loriot@gustaveroussy.fr

Hematol Oncol Clin N Am 35 (2021) 585–596
https://doi.org/10.1016/j.hoc.2021.02.011
0889-8588/21/© 2021 Elsevier Inc. All rights reserved.

Table 1
Clinical trials with targeted therapies in urothelial carcinoma

Class	Drug	Study	Design	Population	Results	Adverse Events
FGFR inhibitors	Erdafitinib	Phase II (BLC2001) NCT02365597	Single arm	mUC with FGFR mut/trans previously treated N = 99	ORR: 40% PFS: 5.5 mo OS: 13.8 mo	Hyperphosphatemia stomatitis Diarrhea Onycholysis Retinal detachment
		Phase III (THOR) NCT	Randomized vs pembrolizumab or Chemotherapy (taxane or vinflunine)	mUC with FGFR mut/trans (post gem platinum ± pembrolizumab)	Ongoing	Ongoing
	Rogaratinib	Phase I extension cohort	Single arm	mUC with mRNA FGFR1-3 overexpression or FGFR3 mutations N = 99	ORR 24% DCR 73%	Not reported
		Phase II/III (FORT-1) NCT03410693	Randomized vs taxane or vinflunine	mUC with mRNA FGFR1-3 overexpression	Not reported	Not reported
	Pemigatinib	Phase II (FIGHT 201) NCT02872714	Single arm	mUC with FGFR3 mutations/fusions (cohort A) (n = 64) or others FGFR3 alterations (cohort B) (n = 36)	ORR 25% (cohort A) ORR 3% (cohort B)	Diarrhea Alopecia Constipation Dry mouth
		Phase II (FIGHT-205) NCT04003610	Randomized pemigatinib alone vs pemigatinib + pembrolizumab vs chemotherapy	mUC with FGFR3 mutation or rearrangement	Ongoing	Ongoing
	Vofatamab	Phase Ib/II (FIERCE-21) NCT02401542	Randomized alone or with docetaxel	mUC with FGFR3 genomic alteration N = 42	ORR 24% (with docetaxel) ORR 5% (without docetaxel)	Anorexia Diarrhea Pyrexia Asthenia Anemia
		Phase Ib/II (FIERCE-22) NCT03123055	Single arm with pembrolizumab	mUC N = 35	ORR 30%	

Class	Drug	Phase/NCT	Design	Population	Results	Toxicity/Status
PARP inhibitors	Rucaparib	Phase II (ATLAS) NCT03397394	Single arm	mUC previously treated (n = 97)	ORR 28% PFS 1.8 mo	Asthenia Nausea Anemia
	Olaparib	Phase I NCT03375307	Single arm	mUC previously treated with DDR alterations	Ongoing	Ongoing
		Phase I (BISCAY)	Single arm with durvalumab	mUC previously treated with DDR alterations	ORR: 36%	Not reported
		Phase II (BAYOU) NCT03459846	Randomized Durvalumab + olaparib/placebo	mUC as first-line treatment in cisplatin-ineligible patients	Ongoing	Ongoing
		Phase II (NEODURVARIB) NCT03534492	Single arm Neoadjuvant treatment	Localized bladder cancer	Ongoing	Ongoing
	Niraparib	Phase II (MORPHEUS) NCT03869190	Single arm in combination with atezolizumab	mUC previously treated	Ongoing	Ongoing
	Talazoparib	Phase II (TALASUR)	Single arm Avelumab + talazoparib	mUC as maintenance after chemo	Ongoing	Ongoing
Antibody-drug conjugate	Enfortumab vedotin (EV)	Phase I (EV-103)	Single arm EV + pembrolizumab	mUC previously cisplatin ineligible	ORR 71%	Fatigue Neuropathy Alopecia Rash Decreased appetite dysgeusia
		Phase II (EV-201)	Single arm	mUC previously treated with chemo and IO N = 125	ORR 44% DOR: 7.6 mo	

(continued on next page)

Table 1
(continued)

Class	Drug	Study	Design	Population	Results	Adverse Events
		Phase III (EV-301) NCT03474107	Randomized EV vs chemo (taxane or vinflunine)	mUC previously treated with chemo and IO	Ongoing	Ongoing
	Sacituzumab govitecan	Phase II (TROPHY-U-01) NCT03547973	Single arm (multiple cohort)	mUC previously treated with chemo and IO n = 113	ORR: 27% DOR: 5.9 mo	Neutropenia Diarrhea Nausea Fatigue Alopecia
		Phase III (TROPiCS-04) NCT04527991	Randomized vs physician's choice	mUC previously treated with chemo and IO	Ongoing	
	RC 48-ADC	Phase II NCT03507166	Single arm	mUC previously treated with chemo HER2 positive (IHC 2+/3+) N = 43	ORR 51%	Hypoesthesia Alopecia Neutropenia Fatigue ALT/AST increase
Antiangiogenic	Bevacizumab	Phase III (CALGB90601) NCT00942331	Randomized Cis gem + bevacizumab/placebo	mUC as first-line treatment n = 506	OS 14.5 vs 14.3 mo	Not reported
	Ramucirumab	Phase III (RANGE) NCT02426125	Randomized Docetaxel + ramucirumab/placebo	mUC previously treated with chemo n = 530	PFS 4.07 vs 2.76 mo	Hypertension Neutropenia Febrile neutropenia
	Lenvatinib	Phase III (LEAP-011) NCT 03898180	Randomized pembrolizumab + lenvatinib/placebo	mUC as first-line treatment	Ongoing	Ongoing
	Cabozantinib	Phase I/II (COSMI-021) NCT03170960	Single arm In combination with atezolizumab	mUC as first-line treatment and after platinum failure	Ongoing	Ongoing

Abbreviations: Chemo, chemotherapy; cis, cisplatin; DDR, DNA damage responsive; DOR, duration of response; gem, gemcitabine; GI, gastrointestinal; IO, immune-oncology; trans, translocation.

FIBROBLAST GROWTH FACTOR RECEPTOR INHIBITORS

FGFR is a family of transmembrane receptors composed of extracellular ligand-binding domains, a transmembrane domain, and an intracellular tyrosine-kinase domain. FGFRs play roles both during embryonic development in organogenesis and in the adult organism by regulating tissue homeostasis (cell proliferation, survival to growth arrest, migration, and differentiation).[1] They are encoded by 4 genes (FGFR1, FGFR2, FGFR3, FGFR4), making 7 receptors. FGFR signaling can be activated in tumor cells through mutations/amplifications/fusions in encoding regions, through the alterations of epigenetic regulators, or through upregulation of ligands.[2] In urothelial carcinoma (UC), the most frequent altered genes are FGFR1 and FGFR3. Amplification is the most frequent alteration on FGFR1, whereas mutation is the most frequent alteration on FGFR3. Their incidence in UC depends on the stage of UC (muscle invasive vs no muscle invasive) and on the location of the tumors (bladder vs upper tract). FGFR1 amplification is found in 7% of UC, and FGFR3 mutations have been reported in 70% of non–muscle-invasive bladder cancer NMIBC, 15% of MIBC, 30% in upper tract UC, and fusions in 6% of UC (the most common being FGFR3-TACC3).[2,3] Two therapeutic classes are currently being tested in patients with FGFR alterations UC: tyrosine kinase inhibitor and antibody.

Among tyrosine kinase inhibitors, erdafitinib (JNJ-42756493) is the most advanced drug. This oral FGFR1-4 inhibitor had demonstrated clinical activity in a phase II trial BLC2001 (NCT02365597) that included 99 patients with metastatic urothelial carcinoma (mUC) with FGFR alteration (either mutations or fusions).[4] The dose was 8 mg/d in a continuous regimen with uptitration to 9 mg based on phosphate level assessed during the first 3 weeks. Almost all patients had previously received chemotherapy (88%); 43% have been treated with at least 2 previous courses of treatment, and 79% had visceral metastases. The objective response rate (ORR; primary endpoint of the study) was 40%. The median progression-free survival (PFS) and overall survival (OS) were 5.5 and 13.8 months, respectively. Half of the patients (46%) had a grade 3 or higher adverse event. The most frequent were hyperphosphatemia, stomatitis, diarrhea, hand-foot syndrome, fatigue, and onycholysis. Detachment of the retinal pigment epithelium is a classic side effect that has been reported in 27% of patients.[5] The main reason for treatment discontinuation was disease progression, and 16% of patients stopped because of toxicity. Based on those results, the Food and Drug Administration (FDA) granted accelerated approval to erdafitinib for mUC with FGFR2 or 3 genetic alterations that has progressed after platinum-based chemotherapy. A phase III study (THOR, NCT03390504) is currently enrolling patients to compare erdafitinib versus chemotherapy (vinflunine or docetaxel) and anti– programmed cell death-1 (PD-1) agent (pembrolizumab) in mUC with selected FGFR gene alterations previously treated with platinum-based chemotherapy. Another trial (phase Ib/II, NORSE, NCT02699606) is now investigating the combination of erdafitinib with cetrelimab (PD-1 inhibitor) in patients with mUC who are ineligible for cisplatin-based chemotherapy. Three doses of erdafitinib are evaluated in the phase Ib: 6 mg, 8 mg, and 8 mg with uptitration to 9 mg. The results of the 22 patients enrolled in the phase 1b have been presented at the European Society for Medical Oncology (ESMO) meetings 2020: 3 patients (14%) had a serious treatment-related adverse event (grade 2 events of central serous retinopathy). The ORR was 52% (n = 11/21), and the disease control rate (DCR) was 100%. The combination erdafitinib (8 mg/d) + cetrelimab is now being explored in the ongoing randomized phase II portion of this study as first-line treatment for patients ineligible for cisplatin.[6] Given the frequency of FGFR3 gene alterations in NMIBC, erdafitinib is currently assessed in a randomized phase II trial in patients with recurrent NMIBC Bacillus Calmette–Guérin-unresponsive who refuse or are not eligible for cystectomy (THOR-2, NCT04172675). Patients are randomized between erdafitinib (experimental arm) and investigator choice (gemcitabine or mitomycin C).

Rogaratinib (BAY 1163877) is pan-FGFR. Unlike other FGFR TKI, its efficacy correlated not only with mutations/fusion of FGFR but also with the messenger RNA (mRNA) FGFR1-3 expression. A phase I study (NCT01976741) has therefore been conducted in patients with solid tumors overexpressing FGFR1-3.[7] In the expansion cohort of UC, 219 patients were screened for mRNA FGFR1-3 expression, and 99 patients (45%) were considered FGFR-positive (mRNA FGFR1-3 overexpression or FGFR3 activating mutations). Patients were treated with rogaratinib 800 mg twice daily. Fifty-one patients were evaluable for response. The ORR was 24%, and the DCR was 73% with a favorable toxicity profile. A randomized phase II/III study (FORT-1, ClinicalTrials.gov identifier: NCT03410693) was conducted in patients with mUC with high expression of FGFR1 and mRNA expression previously treated with platinum-based chemotherapy. After enrollment of 175 patients, there was no difference between rogaratinib and chemotherapy groups with regards to ORR and DCR, and the study accrual stopped early.[8] A phase Ib/II (FORT-2, NCT03473756) is also evaluating rogaratinib in combination with atezolizumab as first-line treatment in cisplatin-ineligible patients with mUC FGFR mRNA overexpression. Among the 27 patients enrolled in the phase Ib, the most common treatment-emergent adverse events (TEAEs) were diarrhea (63%), hyperphosphatemia (44%), and urinary tract infection (37%), leading to interruption or reduction in 67% and 37% of the patients, respectively. The maximum tolerated dose was 600 mg twice a day. The ORR was 39% (13% of complete response, 26% of partial response), and 26% of the patients had a stable disease. The combination rogaratinib (600 mg twice a day) + atezolizumab is now being evaluated in the second part of the trial.[9]

Pemigatinib (INCB054828) is also a TKI but it inhibits only FGFR 1, 2, and 3. A phase II clinical trial FIGHT-201 (ClinicalTrials.gov identifier: NCT02872714) has investigated the antitumor activity of the drug in metastatic or unresectable UC with FGFR alterations that failed after 1 therapy or as first-line treatment if platinum ineligible.[10] Patients receive oral INCB054828 13.5 mg once daily on a 21-day cycle (2 weeks on, 1 week off). Depending on the FGFR alterations, 64 patients were enrolled in cohort A (FGFR3 mutations/fusions) and 36 patients were enrolled in cohort B (other FGFR alterations). In cohort A, 64 patients were eligible for evaluation, and the ORR was 25% (95% confidence interval [CI], 14%–40%). In cohort B, only 1 patient with FGF10 amplification had an unconfirmed partial response. Common TEAEs in all patients were diarrhea (40%), alopecia (32%), fatigue (29%), constipation (28%), and dry mouth (28%). Grade 3 TEAEs in greater than 5% of patients were urinary tract infections (7%) and fatigue (6%). Another phase II trial (FIGHT-205) is currently enrolling cisplatin-ineligible patients with mUC FGFR alterations (FGFR3 mutation or rearrangement) to compare efficacy and safety of pemigatinib alone versus pemigatinib + pembrolizumab versus chemotherapy as first-line treatment study (ClinicalTrials.gov identifier: NCT04003610). Pemigatinib is also evaluated in NMIBC in a phase II trial (NCT03914794) for recurrent tumors after transurethral resection.

Infigrantinib is an oral selective pan-FGFR antagonist that has been evaluated in 67 patients with an mUC harboring FGFR3 alteration at a dose of 125 mg/d on a 3 weeks' on, 1 week off schedule. The ORR was 25%, and the DCR was 39% with an acceptable safety profile.[11] A phase III trial is ongoing evaluating the efficacy of infigrantinib as adjuvant treatment in MIBC and Upper Tract Urothelial Cancer with FGFR3 alterations (PROOF-302, ClinicalTrials.gov identifier: NCT04197986).

Other FGFR-TKI are currently evaluated in clinical trials with pending results: debio 1347, dovitinib. Of note, derazantinib (ARQ087) is another orally administered pan-FGFR inhibitor with multikinase activity. In biochemical studies, it showed potent activity against both wild-type and variants of the FGFR kinases (FGFR1-3), and to a lesser extent against FGFR4 with a favorable safety profile (only 5% of grade 1 hyperphosphatemia and no ocular toxicity).[10] A phase Ib/II study (NCT04045613) is now ongoing to evaluate the efficacy of this drug alone or in combination with atezolizumab with advanced UC harboring FGFR alterations as first-line treatment if cisplatin ineligible or if progressed after either first-line treatment or prior FGFR inhibitors.

Vofatamab (B-701) is a fully human antibody against FGFR3 that blocks activation of the wild-type and genetically activated receptor. FIERCE-21 and FIERCE-22 are 2 dose escalation and expansion phase Ib/II studies (NCT02401542 and NCT03123055) that evaluated vofatamab alone or in combination with docetaxel (FIERCE-21) or with pembrolizumab (FIERCE-22) in patients with mUC previously treated with at least 1 prior line of chemotherapy.[12–14] Only patients with FGFR mutation/fusions were enrolled in FIERCE-21. The dose selected was 25 mg/kg every 3 weeks. The toxicity profile was favorable: anorexia, diarrhea, pyrexia, asthenia, anemia, but no ocular or hyperphosphatemia. In FIERCE-21, 42 patients were included (21 in vofatamab alone arm and 21 in vofatamab + docetaxel arm). Five patients had a partial response in the combination arm, and only 1 patient had a partial response in the vofatamab alone arm. In FIERCE-22, 35 patients were treated, among which 6 with FGFR wild-type tumors had responses. To date, no phase III trial is ongoing.

PARP INHIBITORS

The characterization of the genomic landscape of MIBC reported that defects in DNA repair genes have been observed in one-third of tumors (such as *CHK1/2*, *RAD51*, *BRCA1/2*, *ATM*, *ATR*, *MDC1*, and *FANCF*), suggesting that PARP inhibitors might have activity in patients with MIBC.[15,16] Some of DNA repair genes (ATM and FANCC) have been associated with response to neoadjuvant cisplatin-based chemotherapy and a better prognosis.[17] The rationale for the use of PARP inhibitors in UC was therefore high. However, ATLAS is a phase II trial (NCT03397394) that evaluated efficacy of rucaparib in mUC previously treated with at least 1 first-line treatment.[18] The study has been stopped after first interim analysis for futility. Of note, patients were enrolled in the study regardless of DNA repairs genes status. Olaparib, another PARP inhibitor, is evaluated in a phase II trial conducted in mUC patients with DDR genes alterations (NCT03375307).

Previous studies suggested that DDR gene alterations might be predictive markers of immune checkpoints inhibitors (ICI).[19] Moreover, the use of PARP inhibitors increases DNA damage, and therefore, the tumor mutational load that is known to be also a biomarker of ICI efficacy.[20] Therefore, the combination of ICI with a PARP inhibitor is currently evaluated in UC. The combination of olaparib with durvalumab (anti–PD-L1) has been evaluated in the basket trial BISCAY in which the treatment was decided based on molecular analysis to maximize outcomes.[21] All patients treated with olaparib + pembrolizumab therefore had DNA damage repair genes alterations tumors. The ORR was 35.7%. Two other phase II trials with the same combination are now ongoing: one in mUC as first-line treatment in cisplatin-ineligible patients (BAYOU, NCT03459846) and 1 phase II in localized bladder cancer as neoadjuvant treatment (NEODURVARIB, NCT03534492). Another association of PARP inhibitor and ICI (niraparib + atezolizumab) is also evaluated as second-line treatment in an umbrella study with multiple arms of treatment in patients with mUC previously treated with platinum-based chemotherapy (MORPHEUS, NCT03869190).

Another approach is to use PARP inhibitor as maintenance treatment after platinum-based chemotherapy as in ovarian cancer. Niraparib is currently being evaluated in this indication in a phase II randomized trial (NCT03945084).

ANTIBODY-DRUG CONJUGATES

Antibody-drug conjugate (ADC) belongs to a new pharmaceutical class based on an antibody targeting a specific tumor antigen linked with a cytotoxic agent. After internalization of the ADC, the cytotoxic agent is released inducing cell death by DNA damage or targeting microtubule to inhibit mitosis.

Enfortumab vedotin (EV) is an ADC targeting Nectin-4 that is overexpressed in several cancers, including UC. The cytotoxic agent linked to the antibody is monomethyl auristatin E (MMAE), a known microtubule-disrupting agent. EV has been evaluated in a phase I trial (EV-101) that determined a dose of 1.25 mg/kg on days 1, 8, and 15 every 4 weeks.[22] In the phase II trial (EV-201), 125 patients previously treated with platinum chemotherapy and anti-PD-1/L1 therapy were treated for an mUC. The ORR was 44% (95% CI, 31.5%–53.2%), including 12% of complete response, with a median duration of response of 7.6 months (0.95–11.30).[23] The most common treatment-related adverse events were fatigue (50%), peripheral neuropathy (50%), alopecia (49%), rash (48%), decreased appetite (44%), and dysgeusia (40%). Based on those results, FDA granted accelerated approval to EV for patients with locally advanced or metastatic urothelial cancer who have previously received a PD-1/L1 inhibitor and a platinum-containing chemotherapy. The results of the phase III trial (EV-301, NCT03474107) comparing EV with chemotherapy in the same population of patients are pending, but a press release revealed in September 2020 that the trial stopped early because of positive results of the primary endpoint (OS) at planned interim analysis. EV is also currently evaluated at an earlier stage and in combination with pembrolizumab, based on very promising results of the combination with an ORR reported of 73.3% in the phase I trial (EV-103).[24]

Sacituzumab govitecan (SG) is another ADC that targets Trop-2, another tumor antigen overexpressed by almost 90% of tumor urothelial cells, linked with the active metabolic agent of irinotecan: SN-38. SG has been evaluated in a 3-cohort phase II trial (TROPHY-U-01) at a dose of 10 mg/kg on days 1 and 8 every 21 days. In cohort 1 and 2, patients included received SG after platinum chemotherapy and anti–PD-1/L-1 inhibitor, or after anti–PD-1/L-1 inhibitor, respectively, whereas in cohort 3, patients received SG + pembrolizumab as second-line treatment after platinum chemotherapy. The results of the 113 patients enrolled in the cohort 1 have been presented at an ESMO meeting in 2020, with an ORR of 27% (95% CI: 19–37) and a median duration of response of 5.9 months (95% CI: 4.70–8.60).[25] The main treatment-related adverse events were neutropenia (46%), diarrhea (65%), nausea (58%), fatigue (50%), and alopecia (47%). A phase III trial (TROPiCS-04, NCT04527991) is currently enrolling patients with mUC after platinum chemotherapy and anti–PD-1/L-1 inhibitors failure to compare efficacy of SG versus treatment of physician's choice.

Other ADC targeting HER-2 are currently evaluated in UC overexpressing HER-2 (approximately 30% of mUC).[26] RC 48-ADC is an ADC anti-HER2 combined with MMAE evaluated in a phase II study in HER2-positive (immunohistochemistry [IHC] 2+ or 3+) mUC previously treated with at least 1 chemotherapy regimen.[27] A total of 43 patients were treated, and the ORR was 51% with an acceptable safety profile. DS-8201a (trastuzumab deruxtecan) is also an ADC that combined trastuzumab with a topoisomerase I inhibitor (DX-8951 derivative) that is tested in a phase I cohort in patients with breast or urothelial cancer (NCT03523572).

ANTIANGIOGENIC THERAPIES

Angiogenesis is known to play a key role in migration, proliferation, and metastasis in several cancers. Tumor VEGF expression is associated with a poor prognosis in mUC, and preclinical models have shown a promising activity of antiangiogenic drug, such as VGFR TKI or antibody. Several phase II trials have evaluated the efficacy of bevacizumab in combination with platinum gemcitabine in the first-line setting in mUC.[28,29] However, the phase III study (CALGB 90601) conducted failed to show a benefit, adding bevacizumab to cisplatin gemcitabine in the first-line treatment in mUC, with a median OS of 14.5 months with bevacizumab versus 14.3 months with placebo (hazard ratio [HR] 0.87; 95% CI: 0.72–1.06).[30] Ramucirumab is another VEGF antibody that has been tested in a phase III trial (RANGE) in combination with docetaxel after chemotherapy failure in mUC.[31] A total of 530 patients have been randomized between docetaxel 75 mg/m^2 + ramucirumab 10 mg/kg or placebo. The study was positive with a PFS significantly prolonged in patients allocated ramucirumab plus docetaxel versus placebo plus docetaxel (median, 4.07 months [95% CI: 2.96–4.47] vs 2.76 months [2.60–2.96]; HR, 0.757; 95% CI: 0.607–0.943; P = .0118). However, no benefit on OS was observed, and the ramucirumab has not been approved by either the FDA or the European Medicines Agency. However, several studies are currently conducted to evaluate the efficacy of antiangiogenic therapy (either antibody or TKI) in combination with checkpoint inhibitors. The combination of cabozantinib + atezolizumab has been evaluated in a multitumor phase I study with promising results in cohort 2 that included 30 patients with mUC previously treated with platinum chemotherapy (COSMIC-021, NCT03170960). The ORR was 27%, and the PFS was 5.4 months. Grade 3/4 treatment-related adverse events occurred in 57% of patients. The most common adverse events were fatigue (37%), diarrhea (27%), decreased appetite (23%), increased transaminases (23%), and mucosal inflammation (20%).[32] In addition, the combination of sitravatinib, a VEGF receptor TKI that also targets the TAM kinases (Tyro, Axl, Mer) to enhance the immune microenvironment, appeared promising in combination with nivolumab.[33] A phase III trial evaluating pembrolizumab + lenvatinib is currently enrolling patients with mUC cisplatin-ineligible PD-L1+ (CPS [Combined Positive Score] >10) or ineligible for platinum chemotherapy regardless of PD-L1 status (LEAP-011, NCT03898180).

OTHER PROMISING TARGETED THERAPIES

PI3K/AKT/mTOR might be also a promising pathway to target in UC. Everolimus failed to show a clinical benefit in a phase II trial.[34] However, some patients harbored a spectacular response, raising the question whether a combination of treatment or a molecular selection might help to increase the efficacy of PI3K/AKT/mTOR inhibitors in UC. BISCAY is a randomized phase I trial based on biomarker selection to maximize response to systemic treatment. Vistusertib is a TORC1/2 inhibitor that was administered in combination with durvalumab in patients with an RICTOR amplification or TSC1/2 mutations. A total of 29 patients were treated with this combination. The main adverse events were fatigue (44.8%), diarrhea (37.9%), constipation (34.5%), abdominal pain (34.5%), nausea (31%), urinary tract infection (31%), and decreased appetite (31%).[21] The ORR was 24.1% (14.0%–37.2%) and a PFS rate at 6 months of 35% (24%–47%). However, those efficacy results were quite similar to those observed with durvalumab alone. Another phase Ib/II randomized umbrella study (MORPHEUS mUC, NCT03869190) is exploring several treatments in combination with atezolizumab in mUC that have progressed during or following a platinum-containing regimen. Multiple drugs are tested with atezolizumab: EV, SG, niraparib (PARP inhibitor), Hu5F9-G4 (anti-CD47), tiragolumab (anti-TIGIT), tocilizumab (anti-IL6), RO7122290 (4-1BB agonist simultaneously targeting fibroblast activation protein). The primary study endpoint is investigator-assessed ORR, and the study is currently ongoing.

DISCUSSION

In the last decade, 4 types of targeted therapies have been evaluated in UC with promising results: FGFR inhibitors, ADC, PARP inhibitors, and antiangiogenics. FDA has already approved several new targeted therapies based on phase II trials even before the results of the phase III trial, such as erdafitinib or EV in mUC. Even if the results of the phase III trials are pending, there is a high probably that several targeted therapies will be approved soon. Several of those new drugs are evaluated as a single treatment and in the metastatic stage, and the next steps will be to evaluate them at an earlier stage and in combination with other drugs, such as checkpoints inhibitors.

CLINICS CARE POINTS

- Many targeted targeted therapies are currently investigated across different stages of urothelial cancers.
- The pan FGFR inhibitor erdafitinib is the only one approved TKI in US for patients with metastatic urothelial cancers and selected FGFR2/3 gene alterations.
- Anti-nectin 4 antibody drug conjugate, enfortumab Vedotin is approved in US for patients with metastatic urothelial cancers who had received prior treatment with a PD-1/PD-L1 inhibitor and platinum-based chemotherapy.

DISCLOSURE

Conflict-of-interest disclosure: C. Thibault: Sanofi, Astellas, Janssen, Pfizer, Ipsen, BMS, AstraZeneca; Y. Loriot reports personal fees from Immunomedics; personal fees and nonfinancial support from Roche, AstraZeneca, BMS, Pfizer, Astellas, and Seattle Genetics; and grant support, personal fees, and nonfinancial support from MSD and Janssen.

REFERENCE

1. Haugsten EM, Wiedlocha A, Olsnes S, et al. Roles of fibroblast growth factor receptors in carcinogenesis. Mol Cancer Res 2010;8(11):1439–52.
2. Helsten T, Elkin S, Arthur E, et al. The FGFR landscape in cancer: analysis of 4,853 tumors by next-generation sequencing. Clin Cancer Res 2016;22(1):259–67.
3. Sfakianos JP, Cha EK, Iyer G, et al. Genomic characterization of upper tract urothelial carcinoma. Eur Urol 2015;68(6):970–7.
4. Loriot Y, Necchi A, Park SH, et al. Erdafitinib in locally advanced or metastatic urothelial carcinoma. N Engl J Med 2019;381(4):338–48.
5. Siefker-Radtke AO, Necchi A, Park SH, et al. Erdafitinib in locally advanced or metastatic urothelial carcinoma (mUC): long-term outcomes in BLC2001. J Clin Oncol 2020;38(15_suppl):5015.

6. Siefker-Radtke AO, Loriot Y, Siena S, et al. 752P Updated data from the NORSE trial of erdafitinib (ERDA) plus cetrelimab (CET) in patients (pts) with metastatic or locally advanced urothelial carcinoma (mUC) and specific fibroblast growth factor receptor (FGFR) alterations. Ann Oncol 2020;31:S584–5.
7. Joerger M. Rogaratinib in patients with advanced urothelial carcinomas pre-screened for tumor FGFR mRNA expression and effects of mutations in the FGFR signaling pathway.. Available at: https://ascopubs.org/doi/10.1200/JCO.2018.36.15_suppl.4513. Accessed October 16, 2020.
8. Quinn DI, Petrylak DP, Bellmunt J, et al. FORT-1: Phase II/III study of rogaratinib versus chemotherapy (CT) in patients (pts) with locally advanced or metastatic urothelial carcinoma (UC) selected based on *FGFR1/3* mRNA expression. J Clin Oncol 2020;38(6_suppl):489.
9. Rosenberg JE, Gajate P, Morales-Barrera R, et al. Safety and preliminary efficacy of rogaratinib in combination with atezolizumab in a phase Ib/II study (FORT-2) of first-line treatment in cisplatin-ineligible patients (pts) with locally advanced or metastatic urothelial cancer (UC) and FGFR mRNA overexpression. J Clin Oncol 2020;38(15_suppl):5014.
10. Papadopoulos KP, El-Rayes BF, Tolcher AW, et al. A phase 1 study of ARQ 087, an oral pan-FGFR inhibitor in patients with advanced solid tumours. Br J Cancer 2017;117(11):1592–9.
11. Pal SK, Rosenberg JE, Hoffman-Censits JH, et al. Efficacy of BGJ398, a fibroblast growth factor receptor 1-3 inhibitor, in patients with previously treated advanced urothelial carcinoma with FGFR3 alterations. Cancer Discov 2018;8(7):812–21.
12. Bellmunt J, Picus J, Kohli M, et al. FIERCE-21: phase 1b/2 study of docetaxel + b-701, a selective inhibitor of FGFR3, in relapsed or refractory (R/R) metastatic urothelial carcinoma (mUCC). J Clin Oncol 2018;36(15_suppl):4534.
13. Necchi A, Castellano DE, Mellado B, et al. Fierce-21: phase II study of vofatamab (B-701), a selective inhibitor of FGFR3, as salvage therapy in metastatic urothelial carcinoma (mUC). J Clin Oncol 2019;37(7_suppl):409.
14. Siefker-Radtke AO, Currie G, Abella E, et al. FIERCE-22: clinical activity of vofatamab (V) a FGFR3 selective inhibitor in combination with pembrolizumab (P) in WT metastatic urothelial carcinoma, preliminary analysis. J Clin Oncol 2019;37(15_suppl):4511.
15. Cancer Genome Atlas Research Network. Comprehensive molecular characterization of urothelial bladder carcinoma. Nature 2014;507(7492):315–22.
16. Robertson AG, Kim J, Al-Ahmadie H, et al. Comprehensive molecular characterization of muscle-invasive bladder cancer. Cell 2017;171(3):540–56.e25.
17. Plimack ER, Dunbrack RL, Brennan TA, et al. Defects in DNA repair genes predict response to neoadjuvant cisplatin-based chemotherapy in muscle-invasive bladder cancer. Eur Urol 2015;68(6):959–67.
18. Grivas P, Loriot Y, Feyerabend S, et al. Rucaparib for recurrent, locally advanced, or metastatic urothelial carcinoma (mUC): results from ATLAS, a phase II open-label trial. J Clin Oncol 2020;38(6_suppl):440.
19. Teo MY, Seier K, Ostrovnaya I, et al. Alterations in DNA damage response and repair genes as potential marker of clinical benefit from PD-1/PD-L1 blockade in advanced urothelial cancers. J Clin Oncol 2018;36(17):1685–94.
20. Brown JS, Sundar R, Lopez J. Combining DNA damaging therapeutics with immunotherapy: more haste, less speed. Br J Cancer 2018;118(3):312–24.
21. Powles T, Balar A, Gravis G, et al. An adaptive, biomarker directed platform study in metastatic urothelial cancer (BISCAY) with durvalumab in combination with targeted therapies. Ann Oncol 2019;30:v356–7.

22. Rosenberg J, Sridhar SS, Zhang J, et al. EV-101: a phase I study of single-agent enfortumab vedotin in patients with nectin-4-positive solid tumors, including metastatic urothelial carcinoma. J Clin Oncol 2020;38(10):1041–9.

23. Petrylak DP, Balar AV, O'Donnell PH, et al. EV-201: Results of enfortumab vedotin monotherapy for locally advanced or metastatic urothelial cancer previously treated with platinum and immune checkpoint inhibitors. J Clin Oncol 2019; 37(18_suppl):4505.

24. Rosenberg JE, Flaig TW, Friedlander TW, et al. Study EV-103: Preliminary durability results of enfortumab Vedotin plus pembrolizumab for locally advanced or metastatic urothelial carcinoma. J Clin Oncol 2020;38: 6_suppl:441-441.

25. Loriot Y, Balar AV, Petrylak DP, et al. TROPHY-U-01 cohort 1 final results: A phase II study of sacituzumab govitecan (SG) in metastatic urothelial cancer (mUC) that has progressed after platinum (PLT) and checkpoint inhibitors (CPI). Ann Oncol 2020; 31(suppl_4):S1142-S215. TROPHY-U-01 cohort 1 final results: a phase 2 study of sacituzumab govitecan (SG) in metastatic urothelial cancer that has progressed after platinum and checkpoint inhibitors. In: ; 2020.

26. Thibault C, Khodari W, Lequoy M, et al. HER2 status for prognosis and prediction of treatment efficacy in adenocarcinomas: a review. Crit Rev Oncol Hematol 2013;88(1):123–33.

27. Sheng X, Zhou A-P, Yao X, et al. A phase II study of RC48-ADC in HER2-positive patients with locally advanced or metastatic urothelial carcinoma. J Clin Oncol 2019;37(15_suppl):4509.

28. Hahn NM, Stadler WM, Zon RT, et al. Phase II trial of cisplatin, gemcitabine, and bevacizumab as first-line therapy for metastatic urothelial carcinoma: Hoosier Oncology Group GU 04-75. J Clin Oncol 2011;29(12):1525–30.

29. Balar AV, Apolo AB, Ostrovnaya I, et al. Phase II study of gemcitabine, carboplatin, and bevacizumab in patients with advanced unresectable or metastatic urothelial cancer. J Clin Oncol 2013;31(6):724–30.

30. Rosenberg JE, Ballman KV, Halabi S, et al. CALGB 90601 (Alliance): randomized, double-blind, placebo-controlled phase III trial comparing gemcitabine and cisplatin with bevacizumab or placebo in patients with metastatic urothelial carcinoma. J Clin Oncol 2019;37(15_suppl):4503.

31. Petrylak DP, de Wit R, Chi KN, et al. Ramucirumab plus docetaxel versus placebo plus docetaxel in patients with locally advanced or metastatic urothelial carcinoma after platinum-based therapy (RANGE): a randomised, double-blind, phase 3 trial. Lancet 2017;390(10109):2266–77.

32. Pal SK, Agarwal N, Loriot Y, et al. Cabozantinib in combination with atezolizumab in urothelial carcinoma previously treated with platinum-containing chemotherapy: results from cohort 2 of the COSMIC-021 study. J Clin Oncol 2020; 38(15_suppl):5013.

33. Msaouel P, Thall PF, Yuan Y, et al. A phase I/II trial of sitravatinib (sitra) combined with nivolumab (nivo) in patients (pts) with advanced clear cell renal cell cancer (aCCRCC) that progressed on prior VEGF-targeted therapy. J Clin Oncol 2020; 38(6_suppl):612.

34. Milowsky MI, Iyer G, Regazzi AM, et al. Phase II study of everolimus in metastatic urothelial cancer. BJU Int 2013;112(4):462–70.

Real World Outcomes of Patients with Bladder Cancer
Effectiveness Versus Efficacy of Modern Treatment Paradigms

John L. Pfail, BS[a], Alexander C. Small, MD[a],
Shiviram Cumarasamy, MD[a], Matthew D. Galsky, MD[b],*

KEYWORDS

- Bladder cancer • Nonmuscle invasive bladder cancer
- Muscle invasive bladder cancer • Metastatic bladder cancer • Intravesical therapy
- Radical cystectomy • Neoadjuvant chemotherapy • Immunotherapy

KEY POINTS

- Bladder cancer remains a common and insidious disease in the United States. There have been several advances in the understanding of the biology of bladder cancer, novel diagnostic tools, improvements in multidisciplinary care pathways, and new therapeutics for advanced disease over the past few decades.
- Clinical trials have demonstrated efficacy for new treatments in each disease state, but additional work is needed to advance the effectiveness of bladder cancer care.
- Real world data provide critical information regarding patterns of care, adverse events, and outcomes helping to bridge the efficacy versus effectiveness gap.

INTRODUCTION

Bladder cancer remains a common and insidious disease in the United States, with more than 81,400 new cases and 17,980 deaths in 2020.[1] Its disproportionate effect on the elderly, proclivity for recurrence, and aggressive nature make the management of bladder cancer particularly difficult. Moreover, each state of urothelial carcinoma of the bladder, non–muscle invasive (NMIBC), muscle invasive (MIBC), and advanced disease, presents its own unique challenges. Despite advances in the understanding of the biology of bladder cancer, novel diagnostic tools, improvements in multidisciplinary care pathways, and new therapeutics for advanced disease, little progress has been made in improving survival in the past 30 years.[2]

[a] Department of Urology, Icahn School of Medicine at Mount Sinai, 1425 Madison Avenue, New York, NY 10029, USA; [b] Division of Oncology, Department of Medicine, Icahn School of Medicine at Mount Sinai, 1425 Madison Avenue, New York, NY 10029, USA
* Corresponding author. One Gustave Levy Place, Box 1079, New York, NY 10029.
E-mail address: matthew.galsky@mssm.edu

Hematol Oncol Clin N Am 35 (2021) 597–612
https://doi.org/10.1016/j.hoc.2021.01.005
0889-8588/21/© 2021 Elsevier Inc. All rights reserved.

hemonc.theclinics.com

The American Cancer Society estimates that the 5-year survival for patients with localized bladder cancer is approximately 69% and falls to 35% in those with locally advanced disease. However, survival rates in clinical trials appear much better, with patients' 10-year survival approaching 79% after radical cystectomy (RC), 85% after neoadjuvant chemotherapy (NAC) plus RC, and 69% after chemotherapy plus radiation.[3] Although clinical trials and basic science research have led to many advancements in the treatment of bladder cancer, the potential disconnect between the performance of treatment approaches in the clinical trial setting versus the "real world" warrants careful consideration.

Efficacy is defined as the performance of an intervention under ideal, controlled conditions with a highly selected population, for example, in a randomized controlled trial (RCT). On the other hand, *effectiveness* is the performance of the same intervention in uncontrolled, real world practice with a heterogeneous population.[4] Efficacy studies have strictly enforced protocols administered by highly experienced providers, whereas effectiveness studies like population or case series represent flexible application of interventions by providers in clinical practice.

RCTs are the gold standard of evidence-based medicine. In bladder cancer, there is often a disconnect between efficacy in RCTs and effectiveness in real world studies.[5] Numerous factors may influence this divide, including patient age, comorbidities, organ function, fitness for treatment, and clinician experience. Furthermore, genetic heterogeneity in bladder cancer is now known to contribute to progression, relapse, and poor outcomes, and real world patient cohorts may be much more heterogeneous than previously understood.[6] Finally, bladder cancer significantly impacts physical, mental, and social quality of life (QoL),[7] yet few RCTs report QoL outcomes.[8] Real world outcomes are often described in case series, population studies, and meta-analyses. Bias in these studies must be taken into consideration: institutional case series are fraught with selection bias and referral bias, and population studies are prone to classification bias and may ignore unmeasured confounding factors. Nonetheless, these real world experiences should be viewed as complementary to RCTs and can help inform clinical decision making.

This review explores real world outcomes of patients with NMIBC, MIBC, and advanced bladder cancer with particular focus on case series, population studies, and meta-analyses to better understand the effectiveness of modern treatment paradigms.

NON–MUSCLE INVASIVE BLADDER CANCER

Most new cases (70%–80%) of bladder cancer in the United States are non–muscle invasive. Although a subset of these patients will progress to more advanced disease, most have a long course requiring frequent surveillance, invasive procedures, and multiple treatments of intravesical therapies. One series of 726 patients with NMIBC showed 55% recurrence at a median of 5.6 years of follow-up and recurrence-free survival (RFS) time of 4.2 years.[9] Risk stratification is particularly important in patients with NMIBC because it is a heterogeneous category of tumors with widely varying recurrence and progression rates.

Risk Stratification and Transurethral Resection of Bladder Tumor

Various risk stratification systems have been published including from the European Organization for Research and Treatment of Cancer,[10] the Club Urologico Español de Tratamiento Oncologo,[11] and the American Urologic Association (AUA). Risk groups provide a framework to inform patients and providers on surveillance plans, intravesical therapies, and surgical options. The latest 2016 AUA guidelines recommend classifying patients as low, intermediate, or high risk based on tumor stage (Ta, T1, or Tis), tumor size, number of tumors, recurrence time, high versus low grade histology, variant histology, lymphovascular invasion, and bacillus Calmette-Guérin (BCG) failure.[12] A single-institutional study performed retrospectively with 398 patients with NMIBC showed acceptable validity of this system.[13] Five-year progression-free survival (PFS) rate and 5-year RFS rate was 95%/43% for low risk, 74%/33% for intermediate risk, and 54%/23% for high risk. On multivariate analysis compared with low risk, classification as intermediate risk showed almost a 10-fold increase in progression (hazard ratio [HR] 9.7, 95% confidence interval [CI] 2.23–42.0, P<.01) and high-risk showed a 36-fold increase in progression (HR 36, 95% CI 8.16–159, P<.001). Proper assessment of risk strata is essential in the initial workup of patients with NMIBC.

Transurethral resection of bladder tumor (TURBT) is critical for proper diagnosis, risk stratification, and often definitive treatment of bladder cancer. Initial high-quality TURBT involves complete resection of tumors and resection deep enough to adequately sample the muscularis propria.[14] In reality, primary resection can often leave residual tumor and/or inadequately sample muscularis propria. Guidelines strongly recommend repeat TURBT for intermediate-risk and high-risk patients.[12] A classic 1999 study from Memorial Sloan Kettering Cancer Center (MSKCC) showed that 75% of 96 patients with NMIBC who underwent repeat TURBT had residual noninvasive tumors, and 29% were upstaged to invasive tumors.[15] Repeat TURBT changed management in one-third of patients. A contemporary meta-analysis of 31 studies including 8409 patients with intermediate-risk and high-risk NMIBC, residual tumor at repeat TURBT was identified 17% to 67% of Ta patients and in 20% to 71% T1 patients, and upstaging occurred in 0% to 8% of Ta patients and 0% to 32% of T1 patients.[16] Recurrence risk was also significantly lower in the repeat-TURBT group for Ta patients (16% vs 58%). Repeat resection becomes particularly important before high-risk patients go on to receive intravesical treatment with chemotherapy or immunotherapy. A retrospective review of 1021 patients at MSKCC receiving BCG therapy showed that 56% had viable tumors at repeat TURBT.[17] Furthermore, the patients who refused repeat TURBT showed worse 5-year recurrence (odds ratio [OR] 2.1, 95% CI 1.3–3.3, P = .01) and shorter time to recurrence (median 22 vs 36 months, P<.001). New technology including fluorescence endoscopy with blue light and hexaminolevulinic acid (Cysview, Photocure, Inc., Princeton, NJ) and new urinary biomarkers may improve the early detection and treatment of small tumors.

Intravesical Therapy

Intravesical treatment with chemotherapy like mitomycin, epirubicin, and gemcitabine and/or with BCG immunotherapy remains a pillar of NMIBC treatment. In patients with low-risk and intermediate-risk cancer, a single postoperative instillation of chemotherapy has been repeatedly shown to reduce recurrence risk.[18] A 2018 RCT of 2243 patients who received immediate versus delayed intravesical instillation of mitomycin-C for NMIBC showed a 27% relative recurrence risk reduction for those who received immediate treatment after TURBT (3-year recurrence 27% vs 36% for no chemotherapy, P<.001).[19] In a real world cohort of 363 patients with NMIBC at Kyoto University, not receiving immediate postoperative instillation of chemotherapy was independently associated with increased recurrence risk in low-risk and intermediate-risk patients (2-year recurrence, HR 2.33; 95% CI 1.14–4.88, P = .02).[20] There were no significant differences in local or systemic toxicity rates in those who received postoperative chemotherapy. Despite strong evidence, a survey of American urologists by the Bladder Cancer Advocacy Network showed that only 63% reported routinely using perioperative intravesical chemotherapy, with an even lower rate among private practitioners (54%) versus academic urologists (80%).[21] Another survey of 489 European urologists showed that although 87% stated that they followed clinical practice guidelines, only 60% routinely administered intravesical chemotherapy within 24 hours after TURBT.[22] And similarly, in the United Kingdom, an audit of a tertiary care center showed that only 40% of eligible patients received intravesical chemotherapy following TURBT.[23] Certainly reasons for forgoing intravesical treatment occur, such as deep resection with concern for chemotherapy extravasation, bleeding, or appearance of muscle invasive disease, but in practice, logistical barriers and provider preference often translate into missed opportunities for improving patient outcomes.

Intravesical BCG induction and maintenance therapy is recommended for high-risk NMIBC and is an option for intermediate-risk NMIBC, but its real world implementation has been limited, especially due to global drug shortages. Multiple clinical trials and meta-analyses have shown the benefits of BCG treatment in reducing recurrence and progression risk.[24] Contemporary surveys suggest much higher rates of provider preference for utilization of BCG, up to 99%.[21] BCG derives its anticancer effects by inducing local and systemic inflammatory and immune responses. However, this same inflammatory effect can cause undesired toxicities, including urinary frequency, cystitis, fever, and hematuria in approximately 85% of patients. Regardless of the BCG strain, patients who cannot tolerate treatment often reduce the BCG dose, modify the administration schedule, or take antibiotics or antituberculostatic agents.[25] In fact, side effects can be so severe that many patients cannot complete BCG therapy. In a pivotal trial of maintenance BCG therapy, only 16% of the study population was able to complete all scheduled treatments due to side effects.[26] Adequate BCG therapy, BCG intolerance, and BCG failure have been heterogeneously defined in the literature, making comparing data from historical studies difficult. In a real world cohort from the Surveillance, Epidemiology, and End Results (SEER) database of 4776 patients with NMIBC diagnosed with high-grade disease between 1992 and 2002 and followed until 2007, Lenis and colleagues[27] showed that only 7.1% received full-induction BCG, 7.5% received treatment beyond induction, and fewer than 1% received both on schedule.

Among those eligible for BCG treatment, worldwide shortages have limited its implementation. BCG has a lengthy and costly manufacturing process and few companies produce the drug, prompting escalating costs and limited availability.[28] A French institutional series showed that disruptions to BCG supplies during a 10-year period (2005–2015) resulted in 18% of their patients completing fewer than 6 installations during BCG induction and another 53% of patients skipping their maintenance instillations.[29] Dose and protocol modifications and second-line intravesical chemotherapies have been increasingly used due to BCG scarcity.[30] A 2016 RCT of half-dose BCG compared with full-dose BCG showed no significant difference between the groups (complete response 79% low dose vs 85% full dose, $P = .119$). Induction and maintenance intravesical chemotherapy with mitomycin-C, doxorubicin, epirubicin, and thiotepa have also been associated with a decreased risk of NMIBC recurrence, but no difference in risk of progression.[31] Of note, a cost analysis showed +99% to +146% spikes in costs of mitomycin, valrubicin, and thiotepa after the 2012 and 2014 BCG shortages.[32] New combination regimens have also shown promising outcomes. In heavily pretreated NMIBC patient cohorts, intravesical combinations of gemcitabine/docetaxel and cabazitaxel/gemcitabine/cisplatin have shown potential efficacy.[33,34] Effectiveness in real world practice remains to be seen.

Surveillance and Quality of Life

NMIBC carries a unique set of diagnostic, surgical, and therapeutic challenges. Its proclivity to reoccur and progress mandates lifelong surveillance, making bladder cancer the most costly type of cancer per patient in the United States. One model calculated 5-year cumulative costs at $52,125 for low-risk, $146,250 for intermediate-risk, and $366,143 for high-risk NMIBC, with higher costs driven by progression to MIBC.[35] Beyond financial impact, patients must endure a burden on their psychological health and QoL. A study of health-related QoL among 398 patients with NMIBC in North Carolina showed significant impact on sexual function, fatigue, insomnia, and financial difficulties.[36] Negative effects persisted even after 6+ years of follow-up. Patients who experience financial impacts related to bladder cancer are more likely to delay care and experience worse physical and mental QoL. When we reflect on real world outcomes of NMIBC treatment, it is imperative to consider the QoL impact of this disease and integrate these outcomes into future prospective trials.

MUSCLE INVASIVE BLADDER CANCER

MIBC (cT2-T4N0M0) is a highly aggressive disease state in which real world outcomes often fail to match data from clinical trials. Even with advances in diagnostic techniques and availability of new biomarkers, the proportion of patients initially diagnosed with MIBC has remained stable over time at roughly 20%.[37,38] In addition, progression to MIBC occurs in 20% to 50% of patients with NMIBC, and once a patient develops progression, their prognosis is generally unfavorable.[10] A retrospective study comparing the prognosis of primary and progressive MIBC showed that the 3-year cancer-specific survival was 67% in the primary MIBC group and 37% in the progressive group.[39] If MIBC is left untreated, approximately 38% of patients will develop metastasis with resultant 5-year overall survival as low as 5%.[40] Notwithstanding local control, approximately 50% of patients with MIBC will go on to develop metastatic disease.

Treatment with Curative Intent

The gold standard for treatment with curative intent of MIBC is RC with pelvic lymphadenectomy and neoadjuvant chemotherapy (NAC) for eligible patients, or alternatively combination bladder-sparing trimodal therapy with TURBT, concurrent chemotherapy, and external beam radiation therapy.[41] Regardless of strong evidence, many patients do not receive treatment with curative intent (TCI). Gray and colleagues[42] used the National Cancer Database (NCDB) to analyze treatment patterns in patients with MIBC between 2004 and 2008 and showed that overall only 52.5% of the cohort received potentially curative therapy for MIBC: 28.7% of patients received RC alone, 1.9% received NAC plus RC, 10.7% received RC plus adjuvant chemotherapy, 3.7% of patients underwent partial cystectomy, and 7.6% underwent radiation therapy. Likewise, Gore and colleagues[43] identified 3205 patients with stage II disease from 1992 to 2002 in the SEER database and found that only 21% underwent RC, whereas 51% of patients were treated with surveillance. RC resulted in a 42% 5-year overall survival (OS) rate, whereas surveillance carried a dismal 15% 5-year OS rate. Over the next 10 years from 2002 to 2011 in SEER, the utilization rate dropped even further to 18.9% of patients with MIBC undergoing RC.[44] A similar trend can also be seen outside of the United States. A recent analysis of the Swedish National Bladder Cancer Database from 1997 to 2014 showed that 55% of men and 62% of women with nonmetastatic MIBC did not receive TCI.[45] A subanalysis looking at the 1352 patients with T2 or T3 disease treated without curative intent showed a median OS of 12 months for T2 and 9 months for those with T3 disease. Furthermore, there was no improvement in overall or cancer-specific mortality rates over time.

This begs the question: why do so few patients with MIBC receive TCI? Patient factors, tumor characteristics, provider motivators, and economic incentives all contribute to the low rates of treatment with RC.[42,43] Williams and colleagues[46] conducted a systematic review analyzing the utilization of RC for MIBC. This review included 14 studies and concluded that age, race, marital status, socioeconomic factors, cancer severity, comorbidity burden, surgeon volume, and facility type and location significantly determined RC receipt. In addition, there has been disagreement among urologists, radiation oncologists, and oncologists in selecting optimal patients and optimal treatment regimens for TCI.[47] Regarding patient selection, OS and cancer-specific survival worsen significantly with age older than 70 years for both RC and radiotherapy regimens in patients with nonmetastatic MIBC.[48] Another major concern is the relatively high complication rates associated with this procedure, which may cause many surgeons to shy away from offering RC. Although there are more than 12,000 practicing urologists in the United States, case logs indicate that just over 2000 urologists perform this operation.[49] The 90-day major and minor complication rates following RC have been reported to be 24% and 54%, and furthermore the 90-day emergency room visit, readmission, and mortality rates were 37.9%, 29.6%, and 4.0%, respectively.[50] The most common complications are infectious or gastrointestinal, which can result in prolonged hospitalizations. Finally, socioeconomic and racial disparities contribute to access to care, surgical outcomes, and long-term survival.[44,51]

Neoadjuvant Chemotherapy

Similarly, evidence from RCTs supports the use of NAC, but real world utilization remains low.[52,53] A meta-analysis conducted by Yin and colleagues[54] analyzed 3285 individuals included in 15 RCTs to study the effectiveness of neoadjuvant single-agent platinum or combination therapy. Overall, there was a significant benefit associated with NAC plus local treatment compared with local treatment alone, with a 13% improvement in overall survival (HR 0.87, 95% CI 0.79–0.96, $P = .004$). Guidelines now strongly recommend cisplatin-based NAC to eligible patients before RC as standard of care.[41] Even though data from prospective RCTs have shown the benefits associated with cisplatin-based NAC, retrospective cohort studies have not shown the same associations. Hanna and colleagues[55] queried the NCDB for patients with nonmetastatic MIBC treated from 2004 to 2012 and found that receipt of NAC was not associated with a survival benefit in 1619 patients of 8732 who underwent RC (19%) (HR 0.97; $P = .591$). They also found that although pT0 rates were higher in patients who received NAC, the overall rates of pT0 (13%) were much lower than was seen in the pivotal SWOG-8710 trial (38%).[56] In addition, Zargar and colleagues[57] conducted a retrospective study of pT0 rates at 19 centers for patients receiving NAC (methotrexate, vinblastine, doxorubicin, cisplatin [MVAC] or gemcitabine-cisplatin [GC]) and also found lower response rates (24.5% or MVAC or 23.9% for GC) than those reported in the SWOG-8710 trial (38%).

NAC has persistently underwhelming uptake in clinical practice. Pfail and colleagues[58] queried the NCDB from 2004 to 2015 for all patients with cT2-4aN0M0 disease who had undergone RC and found a modest increase in the usage of multiagent NAC before RC: from 8% in 2004 to 38% in 2015. In this study, the usage of adjuvant chemotherapy stayed relatively constant at 10%. Using the NCDB from 2006 to 2014, Duplisea and colleagues[59] concluded that several patient factors were associated with lower use of NAC, such as older age, higher comorbidity score, lower cT stage, lower hospital RC volume, treatment at a nonacademic facility, lower patient income, and receipt of partial cystectomy. In addition to these US studies, Booth and colleagues[60] conducted a population-based study using the Ontario Cancer Registry to identify all patients with bladder cancer treated with cystectomy from 1994 to 2013. In 5582 patients with MIBC, utilization of NAC increased from 4% in 1994 to 2008 to 19% in 2009 to 2013. Meanwhile, the usage of adjuvant chemotherapy during 2009 to 2013 was a constant 20%.

Even though NAC usage rates have been rising, there remains a significant disconnect between the evidence-based gold standard and the treatment of real world patients. This disconnect may be caused by the fact that a significant proportion of patients in practice are considered to be "cisplatin-ineligible." Historically, adequate renal function (creatinine clearance $\geq$60 mL/min) has been required for enrollment trials exploring perioperative chemotherapy in urothelial carcinoma. However, it has long been recognized that a large proportion of patients with bladder cancer have impaired renal function, thereby excluding them from cisplatin-based treatments.[61] Decline in renal function may be attributable to many factors, such as medical comorbidities, age-related decline in glomerular filtrationrate, and ureteral obstruction. Carboplatin may be substituted for cisplatin, however, non–cisplatin-based regimens such as gemcitabine plus carboplatin have consistently underperformed GC and are generally not recommended for NAC.[62] Split-dose cisplatin with gemcitabine may be a good alternative,[63] and multiple clinical trials of neoadjuvant chemoimmunotherapy are ongoing.[64]

In addition to cisplatin ineligibility, another commonly cited concern from surveyed urologists regarding NAC administration is the potential for delay to definitive treatment with RC.[65] Prior studies analyzing RC for MIBC have shown that a delay from diagnosis to surgery greater than 12 weeks resulted in higher pathologic tumor stage, worse PFS after 5 years, and higher mortality.[66,67] Using the SEER database from 2004 to 2012, Chu and colleagues[68] identified 1509 patients with MIBC who underwent RC and showed that delays in time to RC increased overall mortality, regardless of the use of NAC (HR without NAC 1.34; 95% CI 1.03–1.76; HR after NAC 1.63; 95% CI, 1.06–2.52). Interestingly, in 2012 Alva and colleagues[69] used a single-institution cohort of 153 patients with MIBC from 1990 to 2007 who received NAC before RC and found that RC within 10 weeks of NAC completion did not compromise patient survival. In this study, procedural scheduling was the most common cause of RC after 10 weeks, and this occurred disproportionately in patients receiving NAC at an outside institution. Given these findings, mechanisms to improve the time from NAC to RC are critical to optimize survival.

High-level evidence and guidelines are often not translated into widespread clinical practice. For MIBC, underutilization of RC and NAC remain major challenges. The Ontario data suggested several possible barriers to utilization of NAC and adjuvant chemotherapy including the simple fact that most patients who underwent cystectomy for MIBC were not referred to a medical oncologist.[70] This finding emphasizes the association between upstream decision making by surgeons and utilization of perioperative chemotherapy in MIBC. There are now dozens of ongoing clinical trials for new neoadjuvant, adjuvant and bladder-sparing immunotherapy drugs that may revolutionize the care of MIBC.[71] Despite these issues, potentially curative therapy should still be considered for many patients with MIBC who are presently only receiving surveillance. With hopes of increasing uptake and adherence to guidelines, urologists and medical oncologists should create a team-based approach to maximize patient consideration for NAC. Collaboration should be encouraged between centers of excellence and community practices.

ADVANCED BLADDER CANCER

Although early diagnosis and multimodal therapy can potentially result in cure for those harboring NMIBC or MIBC, metastatic disease is generally incurable for the 10% to 15% of patients who present in this state.[72] The prognosis for these patients is extremely poor with a median survival of 3 to 6 months without treatment, and up to 12 to 15 months with treatment.[73,74] The preferred choice of initial treatment for fit patients with metastatic urothelial cancer (mUC) is cisplatin-based combination chemotherapy, specifically GC or MVAC.[75] Carboplatin-based regimens have been previously used for those who are deemed cisplatin ineligible, and in the past few years, immunotherapies have rapidly redefined this space.

Cisplatin-Based Chemotherapy

The efficacy of cisplatin-based combination chemotherapy for treatment of mUC was first reported in the 1990s by Loehrer and colleagues,[76] who showed a significant survival benefit associated with the use of MVAC compared with cisplatin alone (median OS: 12.5 vs 8.2 months, respectively, $P = .0002$). Toxicities associated with MVAC such as myelosuppression, neutropenia, sepsis, mucositis, nausea, and vomiting, and a mortality rate up to 3% to 4% have been major concerns and have guided treatment toward more tolerable combinations like GC. Based on a phase III trial, treatment with GC demonstrated a similar survival benefit (median OS 13.8 months) and objective response rate (49%) as well as a better safety profile than treatment with MVAC.[73,74] Once again, despite the high-level evidence supporting cisplatin-based chemotherapy, the effectiveness, toxicity, and uptake of these treatments in real world practice is widely variable.

Population studies of advanced bladder cancer are limited, but several recent analyses lend insight into patterns of treatment selection, practical barriers to care, and real world effectiveness of therapy. Using the SEER database, Galsky and colleagues[77] reported that only 42% of the 1703 patients identified with mUC between 2004 to 2011 were treated with first-line chemotherapy. GC was the most common treatment regimen (43%) followed by cisplatin-based regimens (27%). First-line–treated patients had a shorter median OS (8.5 months) than those previously reported in clinical trials. Patients who received first-line cisplatin-based chemotherapy tended to be younger, have fewer comorbidities, and have metastatic disease limited to lymph nodes compared with their non–cisplatin-treated counterparts. Fisher and colleagues[78] aimed to answer the same questions, but retrospectively reviewed the medical records of adults diagnosed with stage IV bladder cancer between 2008 and 2015 at community oncology practices in the United States. Overall, 56% of patients received first-line platinum-based chemotherapy with the most common regimens being gemcitabine/carboplatin (23.6%) and GC (17%). The median OS was 9.4 months from stage IV bladder cancer diagnosis and 8.4 months from start of first-line therapy. Finally, Flannery and colleagues[79] used the SEER database to analyze treatment cost and utilization among patients with mBC. Less than half of mBC patients received first-line cisplatin combination therapy, and for those patients receiving second-line compared with only first-line treatment, there was a significant decrease in the 1-year (32.8% vs 56.5%), 2-year (14.9% vs 25.6%), and 3-year (7.7% vs 15.5%) survival rates. Furthermore, there were drastic differences in costs associated between the first-line (mean: $36,793, SD: $28,753) and second-line (mean: $26,732, SD: $21,143) treatments. Identifying proper candidates for platinum-based chemotherapy, risk stratification and high costs all likely contribute to disconnects in efficacy found in the real world.

Like cisplatin-based NAC before cystectomy, up to 50% of patients with advanced bladder cancer are deemed ineligible for cisplatin chemotherapy due to age or comorbidities.[80] Cisplatin ineligibility for mBC has been more specifically defined as having any of the following: Eastern Cooperative Oncology Group (ECOG) performance status ≥2, creatinine clearance less than 60 mL/min, grade ≥2 hearing loss, grade ≥2 peripheral neuropathy, or New York Heart Association class III heart failure.[81] Galsky and colleagues[82] surveyed 301 US oncologists in 2017 on preferences related to cisplatin-ineligible patients with mBC. They found that the most commonly identified clinical factors for cisplatin ineligibility were renal dysfunction (78%) and poor performance status (77%), followed by neuropathy (47%), solitary kidney (43%), hearing loss (43%), advanced age (43%), and cardiovascular dysfunction (41%). Patients were typically deemed ineligible for cisplatin at diagnosis (58%) or on initiation of first-line metastatic therapy (61%).

Immunotherapy

Although cisplatin-based chemotherapy remains the preferred first-line treatment for patients with advanced bladder cancer, it is clear that many patients are unable to undergo treatment. Recent advancements in understanding of bladder cancer tumor biology have led to the development of several immune checkpoint inhibitors (ICI) that confer a meaningful response in advanced bladder cancer. In the IMvigor210 phase 2 study of the PD-L1 inhibitor atezolizumab, Rosenberg and colleagues[83] showed that a subset of patients with cisplatin-refractory disease achieved a durable objective response rate of 15%, compared with a historical control cohort of 10%. In patients who expressed high levels of PD-L1, response rates rose to 27%. Furthermore, atezolizumab had a favorable side-effect profile with only 15% of patients experiencing grade 3 or 4 adverse events. This led to Food and Drug Administration (FDA) approval of atezolizumab for treatment of advanced UC in cisplatin-refractory patients in May 2016. In a follow-up study to IMvigor210, Balar and colleagues[84] demonstrated that similar durable responses with a favorable safety profile can be achieved in previously untreated patients who are cisplatin-ineligible. Between February and May 2017, 4 additional ICIs (nivolumab, pembrolizumab, durvalumab, and avelumab) were approved in the use of advanced bladder cancer. Notably, atezolizumab and pembrolizumab both were considered first-line therapy for cisplatin-ineligible patients, regardless of PD-L1 level expression. Approval for these agents underwent an accelerated process on the basis of phase 2 clinical trials. As such, many clinicians rapidly began to use immunotherapy when treating advanced bladder cancer. The survey by Galsky and colleagues[82] of US oncologists indicated that 75% of respondents preferred ICIs as first-line non-cisplatin treatment for advanced bladder cancer, followed by just 19% who preferred carboplatin-based chemotherapy.

As FDA approvals led to increased clinician use of immunotherapy, continued research with phase 3 trials and surveillance monitoring demonstrated that the rapid embrace of ICI use in advanced bladder cancer may have been premature. IMvigor130 and KEYNOTE-361 were both phase 3 trials investigating the use of combination immunotherapy and chemotherapy versus chemotherapy alone versus PD-1/PD-L1 blockade alone.[85] Notably, before these trials completed accrual, the data and safety monitoring committees of both trials performed unplanned analyses after identifying that patients with low PD-L1 expressing tumors randomized to immune checkpoint blockade alone were dying at a faster rate compared with those randomized to chemotherapy. As such, on August 16, 2018, the FDA restricted use of ICIs as first-line treatment for cisplatin-ineligible patients to those with tumors expressing high levels of PD-L1 expression. A study of treatment utilization rates before and after this FDA restriction showed how real world practice can adjust rapidly to such data, demonstrating a reversal of prior trends of rising ICI utilization with a precipitous 37% drop in ICI use, 35% rise in and 12% increase in PD-L1 testing.[86]

Suffice to say, immunotherapy is still in its infancy, and its use, although promising, should be hedged with caution as clinicians continue to accrue data that indicate exactly which patients will benefit from such treatments in real world settings. A retrospective cohort study conducted by Khaki and colleagues[87] comprised 519 patients treated with ICIs at 18 institutions across the globe. In patients treated with first-line ICI therapy, a favorable ECOG performance status 0 to 1 was associated with much better outcomes compared with those with ECOG performance status greater than 1 (median OS 15.2 vs 7.2 months, HR 0.62, $P = .01$). Interestingly, objective response rates were similar in both groups. Of the 55% of patients in the cohort who died, ICIs were initiated in the last 30 and 90 days of life in 10% and 32%, respectively, yet ICI initiation in the last 30 days of life was associated with a nearly threefold increase in hospital death. These findings suggest that the more favorable tolerability profile of ICI compared with conventional systemic therapy, and the potential for durable responses in a small subset of patients has lowered the bar for "trying" such treatments in patients with borderline functional status. However, the high costs associated with ICIs and the low likelihood of benefit in such populations still warrants more thoughtful utilization of ICIs in this setting. A cost-effectiveness analysis of pembrolizumab as second-line therapy for advanced urothelial carcinoma demonstrated an incremental cost of 69,852 Euros, but the drug still met cost-effectiveness criteria at willingness to pay threshold of 100,000 Euro/quality-adjusted-life-year.[88] Together, these real world data underscore the need to approach implementation of ICIs judiciously as more data become available.

Table 1		
Real world barriers to improving bladder cancer care		
Disease State	High-Level Evidence	Real World
Non–muscle-invasive bladder cancer	High-quality TURBT and accurate staging	Inadequate resection and under staging
	Single postoperative instillation of chemotherapy	Underutilization due to provider preference and logistical issues
	Intravesical BCG induction and maintenance therapy	Patient intolerance; worldwide drug shortages
	Lifelong surveillance	Financial burden; quality of life impact
Muscle-invasive bladder cancer	Treatment with curative intent (RC + NAC or trimodal therapy)	Patient factors, tumor characteristics, provider motivators, geography and economic incentives influence treatment decisions
	Neoadjuvant platinum-based chemotherapy	Cisplatin ineligibility; delay of cystectomy may reduce oncology referrals
Advanced bladder cancer	Platinum-based chemotherapy	Cisplatin ineligibility; low uptake
	Immunotherapy	Data immature; expensive drugs

Abbreviations: BCG, bacillus Calmette-Guérin; NAC, neoadjuvant chemotherapy; RC, radical cystectomy; TURBT, transurethral resection of bladder tumor.

SUMMARY

Real world data can supplement results from clinical trials to inform clinicians about practice patterns, barriers to care, and adverse effects. NMIBC, MIBC, and advanced bladder cancer each have unique challenges, but together as new data from prospective studies evolve, adjustments in care pathways will be critical. Ultimately a multidisciplinary approach to bladder cancer care, informed by rigorous evidence-based guidelines and acknowledging real world barriers (**Table 1**) will continue to improve patient outcomes.

CLINICS CARE POINTS

- Even though there exists high level evidence for the efficacy of treatment for bladder cancer there is a disconnect between clinical trials and real world outcomes.
- For the treatment of non-muscle invasive bladder cancer, there is an inadequate initial resection and therefore leading to understaging. Additionally, there is an underutilization of postoperative chemotherapy due to provider preference, patient intolerance, drug shortages, and other logistical issues.
- For the treatment of both muscle-invasive bladder cancer and advanced bladder cancer, there is low uptake of platinum-based chemotherapy due to high rates of cisplatin ineligibility.

DISCLOSURES

None.

REFERENCES

1. Siegel RL, Miller KD, Jemal A. Cancer statistics, 2020. CA Cancer J Clin 2020; 70:7–30.
2. de Vere White R, Lara PN Jr, Black PC, et al. Framing pragmatic strategies to reduce mortality from bladder cancer: an endorsement from the society of urologic oncology. J Clin Oncol 2020;38:1760–2.
3. Fahmy O, Khairul-Asri MG, Schubert T, et al. A systematic review and meta-analysis on the oncological long-term outcomes after trimodality therapy and radical cystectomy with or without neoadjuvant chemotherapy for muscle-invasive bladder cancer. Urol Oncol 2018;36:43–53.
4. Singal AG, Higgins PD, Waljee AK. A primer on effectiveness and efficacy trials. Clin Transl Gastroenterol 2014;5:e45.
5. Robinson AG, Izard JP, Booth CM. The role of population-based observational research in bladder cancer. Bladder Cancer 2015;1:123–31.
6. Meeks JJ, Al-Ahmadie H, Faltas BM, et al. Genomic heterogeneity in bladder cancer: challenges and possible solutions to improve outcomes. Nat Rev Urol 2020;17:259–70.
7. Smith AB, Jaeger B, Pinheiro LC, et al. Impact of bladder cancer on health-related quality of life. BJU Int 2018;121:549–57.
8. Feuerstein MA, Jacobs M, Piciocchi A, et al. Quality of life and symptom assessment in randomized clinical trials of bladder cancer: a systematic review. Urol Oncol 2015;33:331.e17-23.
9. Wyszynski A, Tanyos SA, Rees JR, et al. Body mass and smoking are modifiable risk factors for recurrent bladder cancer. Cancer 2014;120:408–14.

10. Sylvester RJ, van der Meijden APM, Oosterlinck W, et al. Predicting recurrence and progression in individual patients with stage Ta T1 bladder cancer using EORTC risk tables: a combined analysis of 2596 patients from seven EORTC trials. Eur Urol 2006;49:466–77.

11. Fernandez-Gomez J, Madero R, Solsona E, et al. Predicting nonmuscle invasive bladder cancer recurrence and progression in patients treated with bacillus Calmette-Guerin: the CUETO scoring model. J Urol 2009;182:2195–203.

12. Chang SS, Boorjian SA, Chou R, et al. Diagnosis and treatment of non-muscle invasive bladder cancer: AUA/SUO guideline. J Urol 2016;196:1021–9.

13. Ritch CR, Velasquez MC, Kwon D, et al. Use and validation of the AUA/SUO risk grouping for nonmuscle invasive bladder cancer in a contemporary cohort. J Urol 2020;203:505–11.

14. Akand M, Muilwijk T, Raskin Y, et al. Quality control indicators for transurethral resection of non-muscle-invasive bladder cancer. Clin Genitourin Cancer 2019; 17:e784–92.

15. Herr HW. The value of a second transurethral resection in evaluating patients with bladder tumors. J Urol 1999;162:74–6.

16. Cumberbatch MGK, Foerster B, Catto JWF, et al. Repeat transurethral resection in non-muscle-invasive bladder cancer: a systematic review. Eur Urol 2018;73: 925–33.

17. Sfakianos JP, Kim PH, Hakimi AA, et al. The effect of restaging transurethral resection on recurrence and progression rates in patients with nonmuscle invasive bladder cancer treated with intravesical bacillus Calmette-Guerin. J Urol 2014;191:341–5.

18. Perlis N, Zlotta AR, Beyene J, et al. Immediate post-transurethral resection of bladder tumor intravesical chemotherapy prevents non-muscle-invasive bladder cancer recurrences: an updated meta-analysis on 2548 patients and quality-of-evidence review. Eur Urol 2013;64:421–30.

19. Bosschieter J, Nieuwenhuijzen JA, van Ginkel T, et al. Value of an immediate intravesical instillation of Mitomycin C in patients with non-muscle-invasive bladder cancer: a prospective multicentre randomised study in 2243 patients. Eur Urol 2018;73:226–32.

20. Murakami K, Hamada A, Teramoto Y, et al. Efficacy of immediate postoperative instillation of chemotherapy for primary non-muscle-invasive bladder cancer in real-world clinical practice. Clin Genitourin Cancer 2019;17:e1003–10.

21. Nielsen ME, Smith AB, Pruthi RS, et al. Reported use of intravesical therapy for non-muscle-invasive bladder cancer (NMIBC): results from the Bladder Cancer Advocacy Network (BCAN) survey. BJU Int 2012;110:967–72.

22. Hendricksen K, Aziz A, Bes P, et al. Discrepancy between European Association of Urology guidelines and daily practice in the management of non-muscle-invasive bladder cancer: results of a European Survey. Eur Urol Focus 2019;5: 681–8.

23. Sountoulides P, Mutomba WF, Bouras E, et al. How well do we manage non-muscle invasive bladder tumors? A UK audit of real-life practices. Urologia 2020;87:142–8.

24. Sylvester RJ, van der MA, Lamm DL. Intravesical bacillus Calmette-Guerin reduces the risk of progression in patients with superficial bladder cancer: a meta-analysis of the published results of randomized clinical trials. J Urol 2002; 168:1964–70.

25. Krajewski W, Matuszewski M, Poletajew S, et al. Are there differences in toxicity and efficacy between various bacillus calmette-guerin strains in bladder cancer patients? Analysis of 844 patients. Urol Int 2018;101:277–84.
26. Lamm DL, Blumenstein BA, Crissman JD, et al. Maintenance bacillus Calmette-Guerin immunotherapy for recurrent TA, T1 and carcinoma in situ transitional cell carcinoma of the bladder: a randomized Southwest Oncology Group Study. J Urol 2000;163:1124–9.
27. Lenis AT, Donin NM, Litwin MS, et al. Association between number of endoscopic resections and utilization of Bacillus Calmette-Guerin therapy for patients with high-grade, non-muscle-invasive bladder cancer. Clin Genitourin Cancer 2017; 15:e25–31.
28. Golla V, Lenis AT, Faiena I, et al. Intravesical therapy for non-muscle invasive bladder cancer-current and future options in the age of Bacillus Calmette-Guerin shortage. Rev Urol 2019;21:145–53.
29. Alhogbani MM, Picard JA, Fassi-Fehri MH, et al. Prognostic impact of Bacillus Calmette-Guerin interruption at the time of induction and consolidation. Urol Ann 2017;9:315–20.
30. Fankhauser CD, Teoh JY, Mostafid H. Treatment options and results of adjuvant treatment in nonmuscle-invasive bladder cancer (NMIBC) during the Bacillus Calmette-Guerin shortage. Curr Opin Urol 2020;30:365–9.
31. Chou R, Selph S, Buckley DI, et al. Intravesical therapy for the treatment of non-muscle invasive bladder cancer: a systematic review and meta-analysis. J Urol 2017;197:1189–99.
32. Bandari J, Maganty A, MacLeod LC, et al. Manufacturing and the market: rationalizing the shortage of Bacillus Calmette-Guerin. Eur Urol Focus 2018;4:481–4.
33. Daniels MJ, Barry E, Milbar N, et al. An evaluation of monthly maintenance therapy among patients receiving intravesical combination gemcitabine/docetaxel for nonmuscle-invasive bladder cancer. Urol Oncol 2020;38:40.e17-24.
34. DeCastro GJ, Sui W, Pak JS, et al. A phase I trial of intravesical cabazitaxel, gemcitabine and cisplatin for the treatment of nonmuscle invasive bacillus calmette-guerin unresponsive or recurrent/relapsing urothelial carcinoma of the bladder. J Urol 2020;204:247–53.
35. Mossanen M, Wang Y, Szymaniak J, et al. Evaluating the cost of surveillance for non-muscle-invasive bladder cancer: an analysis based on risk categories. World J Urol 2019;37:2059–65.
36. Jung A, Nielsen ME, Crandell JL, et al. Health-related quality of life among non-muscle-invasive bladder cancer survivors: a population-based study. BJU Int 2020;125:38–48.
37. Charlton ME, Adamo MP, Sun L, et al. Bladder cancer collaborative stage variables and their data quality, usage, and clinical implications: a review of SEER data, 2004-2010. Cancer 2014;120(Suppl 23):3815–25.
38. Smith AB, Deal AM, Woods ME, et al. Muscle-invasive bladder cancer: evaluating treatment and survival in the National Cancer Data Base. BJU Int 2014;114:719–26.
39. Schrier BP, Hollander MP, van Rhijn BW, et al. Prognosis of muscle-invasive bladder cancer: difference between primary and progressive tumours and implications for therapy. Eur Urol 2004;45:292–6.
40. Martini A, Sfakianos JP, Renström-Koskela L, et al. The natural history of untreated muscle-invasive bladder cancer. BJU Int 2020;125:270–5.
41. Chang SS, Bochner BH, Chou R, et al. Treatment of non-metastatic muscle-invasive bladder cancer: AUA/ASCO/ASTRO/SUO guideline. J Urol 2017;198:552–9.

42. Gray PJ, et al. Use of potentially curative therapies for muscle-invasive bladder cancer in the United States: results from the National Cancer Data Base. Eur Urol 2013;63:823–9.
43. Gore JL, Litwin MS, Lai J, et al. Use of radical cystectomy for patients with invasive bladder cancer. J Natl Cancer Inst 2010;102:802–11.
44. Williams SB, Huo J, Chamie K, et al. Underutilization of radical cystectomy among patients diagnosed with clinical stage T2 muscle-invasive bladder cancer. Eur Urol Focus 2017;3:258–64.
45. Westergren DO, Gardmark T, Lindhagen L, et al. A nationwide, population based analysis of patients with organ confined, muscle invasive bladder cancer not receiving curative intent therapy in Sweden from 1997 to 2014. J Urol 2019; 202:905–12.
46. Williams SB, Hudgins HK, Ray-Zack MD, et al. Systematic review of factors associated with the utilization of radical cystectomy for bladder cancer. Eur Urol Oncol 2019;2:119–25.
47. Ploussard G, Daneshmand S, Efstathiou JA, et al. Critical analysis of bladder sparing with trimodal therapy in muscle-invasive bladder cancer: a systematic review. Eur Urol 2014;66:120–37.
48. Fonteyne V, Ost P, Bellmunt J, et al. Curative treatment for muscle invasive bladder cancer in elderly patients: a systematic review. Eur Urol 2018;73:40–50.
49. Flum A, Oberlin D, Bachrach L, et al. Characteristics of certifying urologists performing cystectomies in the United States. J Urol 2014;191:E536–7.
50. Djaladat H, Katebian B, Bazargani ST, et al. 90-Day complication rate in patients undergoing radical cystectomy with enhanced recovery protocol: a prospective cohort study. World J Urol 2017;35:907–11.
51. Golombos DM, O'Malley P, Lewicki P, et al. The impact of socioeconomic status on perioperative complications and oncologic outcomes in patients undergoing radical cystectomy. World J Urol 2017;35:1063–71.
52. International Collaboration of Trialists; Medical Research Council Advanced Bladder Cancer Working Party (now the National Cancer Research Institute Bladder Cancer Clinical Studies Group); European Organisation for Research and Treatment of Cancer Genito-Urinary Tract Cancer Group, et al. International phase III trial assessing neoadjuvant cisplatin, methotrexate, and vinblastine chemotherapy for muscle-invasive bladder cancer: long-term results of the BA06 30894 trial. J Clin Oncol 2011;29:2171–7.
53. Kitamura H, Tsukamoto T, Shibata T, et al. Randomised phase III study of neoadjuvant chemotherapy with methotrexate, doxorubicin, vinblastine and cisplatin followed by radical cystectomy compared with radical cystectomy alone for muscle-invasive bladder cancer: Japan Clinical Oncology Group Study JCOG0209. Ann Oncol 2014;25:1192–8.
54. Yin M, Joshi M, Meijer RP, et al. Neoadjuvant chemotherapy for muscle-invasive bladder cancer: a systematic review and two-step meta-analysis. Oncologist 2016;21:708–15.
55. Hanna N, Trinh Q-D, Seisen T, et al. Effectiveness of neoadjuvant chemotherapy for muscle-invasive bladder cancer in the current real world setting in the USA. Eur Urol Oncol 2018;1:83–90.
56. Grossman HB, Natale RB, Tangen CM, et al. Neoadjuvant chemotherapy plus cystectomy compared with cystectomy alone for locally advanced bladder cancer. N Engl J Med 2003;349:859–66.
57. Zargar H, Espiritu PN, Fairey AS, et al. Multicenter assessment of neoadjuvant chemotherapy for muscle-invasive bladder cancer. Eur Urol 2015;67:241–9.

58. Pfail JL, Audenet F, Martini A, et al. Survival of patients with muscle-invasive urothelial cancer of the bladder with residual disease at the time of cystectomy following neoadjuvant chemotherapy: an analysis of the national cancer database. J Urol 2020;203:E839.

59. Duplisea JJ, Mason RJ, Reichard CA, et al. Trends and disparities in the use of neoadjuvant chemotherapy for muscle-invasive urothelial carcinoma. Can Urol Assoc J 2019;13:24–8.

60. Booth CM, Karim S, Brennan K, et al. Perioperative chemotherapy for bladder cancer in the general population: are practice patterns finally changing? Urol Oncol 2018;36:89 e13–e20.

61. Dash A, Galsky MD, Vickers AJ, et al. Impact of renal impairment on eligibility for adjuvant cisplatin-based chemotherapy in patients with urothelial carcinoma of the bladder. Cancer 2006;107:506–13.

62. Koie T, Ohyama C, Hashimoto Y, et al. Efficacies and safety of neoadjuvant gemcitabine plus carboplatin followed by immediate cystectomy in patients with muscle-invasive bladder cancer, including those unfit for cisplatin: a prospective single-arm study. Int J Clin Oncol 2013;18:724–30.

63. Osterman CK, Babu DS, Geynisman DM, et al. Efficacy of split schedule versus conventional schedule neoadjuvant cisplatin-based chemotherapy for muscle-invasive bladder cancer. Oncologist 2019;24:688–90.

64. Einstein DJ, Sonpavde G. Treatment approaches for cisplatin-ineligible patients with invasive bladder cancer. Curr Treat Options Oncol 2019;20:12.

65. Cowan N, Chen YY, La Rochelle J, et al. Neoadjuvant chemotherapy use in bladder cancer: a survey of current practice and opinions. J Urol 2013;189:E587–8.

66. Gore JL, Lai J, Setodji CM, et al. Mortality increases when radical cystectomy is delayed more than 12 weeks results from a surveillance, epidemiology, and end results-medicare analysis. Cancer 2009;115:988–96.

67. Sanchez-Ortiz RF, Huang WC, Mick R, et al. An interval longer than 12 weeks between the diagnosis of muscle invasion and cystectomy is associated with worse outcome in bladder carcinoma. J Urol 2003;169:110–5.

68. Chu AT, Holt SK, Wright JL, et al. Delays in radical cystectomy for muscle-invasive bladder cancer. Cancer 2019;125:2011–7.

69. Alva AS, Tallman CT, He C, et al. Efficient delivery of radical cystectomy after neoadjuvant chemotherapy for muscle-invasive bladder cancer. Cancer 2012;118:44–53.

70. Booth CM, Siemens DR, Peng YP, et al. Patterns of referral for perioperative chemotherapy among patients with muscle-invasive bladder cancer: a population-based study. Urol Oncol 2014;32:1200–8.

71. Patel VG, Oh WK, Galsky MD. Treatment of muscle-invasive and advanced bladder cancer in 2020. CA Cancer J Clin 2020;70(5):404–23.

72. Kamat AM, Hegarty PK, Gee JR, et al. ICUD-EAU international consultation on bladder cancer 2012: screening, diagnosis, and molecular markers. Eur Urol 2013;63:4–15.

73. von der Maase H, Hansen SW, Roberts JT, et al. Gemcitabine and cisplatin versus methotrexate, vinblastine, doxorubicin, and cisplatin in advanced or metastatic bladder cancer: results of a large, randomized, multinational, multicenter, phase III study. J Clin Oncol 2000;18:3068–77.

74. von der Maase H, Sengelov L, Roberts JT, et al. Long-term survival results of a randomized trial comparing gemcitabine plus cisplatin, with methotrexate,

vinblastine, doxorubicin, plus cisplatin in patients with bladder cancer. J Clin Oncol 2005;23:4602–8.

75. Stenzl A, Cowan NC, De Santis M, et al. Treatment of muscle-invasive and metastatic bladder cancer: update of the EAU guidelines. Eur Urol 2011;59:1009–18.
76. Loehrer PJ Sr, Einhorn LH, Elson PJ, et al. A randomized comparison of cisplatin alone or in combination with methotrexate, vinblastine, and doxorubicin in patients with metastatic urothelial carcinoma: a cooperative group study. J Clin Oncol 1992;10:1066–73.
77. Galsky MD, Pal SK, Lin S-W, et al. Real-world effectiveness of chemotherapy in elderly patients with metastatic bladder cancer in the United States. Bladder Cancer 2018;4:227–38.
78. Fisher MD, Shenolikar R, Miller PJ, et al. Treatment patterns and outcomes in stage IV bladder cancer in a community oncology setting: 2008-2015. Clin Genitourin Cancer 2018;16:e1171–9.
79. Flannery K, Cao X, He J, et al. Real world treatment costs and resource utilization among patients with metastatic bladder cancer. Ann Oncol 2017;28.
80. Galsky MD, Hahn NM, Rosenberg JE, et al. Defining "cisplatin ineligible" patients with metastatic bladder cancer. J Clin Oncol 2011;29. https://doi.org/10.1200/jco.2011.29.7_suppl.238.
81. Galsky MD, Hahn NM, Rosenberg J, et al. A consensus definition of patients with metastatic urothelial carcinoma who are unfit for cisplatin-based chemotherapy. Lancet Oncol 2011;12:211–4.
82. Galsky MD, Ma E, Shah-Manek B, et al. Cisplatin ineligibility for patients with metastatic urothelial carcinoma: a survey of clinical practice perspectives among US oncologists. Bladder Cancer 2019;5:281–8.
83. Rosenberg JE, Hoffman-Censits J, Powles T, et al. Atezolizumab in patients with locally advanced and metastatic urothelial carcinoma who have progressed following treatment with platinum-based chemotherapy: a single-arm, multicentre, phase 2 trial. Lancet 2016;387:1909–20.
84. Balar AV, Galsky MD, Rosenberg JE, et al. Atezolizumab as first-line treatment in cisplatin-ineligible patients with locally advanced and metastatic urothelial carcinoma: a single-arm, multicentre, phase 2 trial. Lancet 2017;389:67–76.
85. Galsky MD, Arija JÁA, Bamias A, et al. Atezolizumab with or without chemotherapy in metastatic urothelial cancer (IMvigor130): a multicentre, randomised, placebo-controlled phase 3 trial. Lancet 2020;395:1547–57.
86. Parikh RB, et al. Association between FDA label restriction and immunotherapy and chemotherapy use in bladder cancer. JAMA 2019;322:1209–11.
87. Khaki AR, Li A, Diamantopoulos LN, et al. Impact of performance status on treatment outcomes: a real-world study of advanced urothelial cancer treated with immune checkpoint inhibitors. Cancer 2020;126:1208–16.
88. Srivastava T, Prabhu VS, Li H, et al. Cost-effectiveness of pembrolizumab as second-line therapy for the treatment of locally advanced or metastatic urothelial carcinoma in Sweden. Eur Urol Oncol 2018. https://doi.org/10.1016/j.euo.2018.09.012.

Preclinical Models for Bladder Cancer Research

Shaoming Zhu, MD[a,b], Zheng Zhu, PhD[c], Ai-Hong Ma, MD, PhD[d],
Guru P. Sonpavde, MD[e], Fan Cheng, MD[a,*], Chong-xian Pan, MD, PhD, MS[c,f,*]

KEYWORDS

- Bladder cancer • Organoid • Conditionally reprogrammed cell culture
- Genetically engineered mouse model • Patient-derived xenograft
- Humanized mouse

KEY POINTS

- Cell lines and their derived in vivo models are readily available and easy to manipulate, but may behave differently from human bladder cancer in the clinic.
- Carcinogen-induced models recapitulate the natural oncogenesis of human cancer.
- Genetically engineered mouse models have more uniform and defined genetic alterations, but lack tumor heterogeneity.
- Patient-derived models of cancer (organoids, conditionally reprogrammed cell cultures, and xenografts) retain most of the genetic alterations of their parent cancers and have high concordance of drug response.
- Humanized mice have human immune systems and can be implanted with human cancers for research in immunotherapy.

Bladder cancer (BC) is the most common tumor in the urinary system, ranking 11th among all human malignancies worldwide. It is more common in men than in women, with a ratio of 3:1 to 5:1.[1] In 2017, approximately 430,000 new cases were diagnosed with BC (330,000 men and 99,000 women) worldwide, with 51,000 deaths in the European Union and 18,000 deaths in North America.[2] The risk factors include smoking, occupational chemical exposure, male gender, and socioeconomic status.[2–4]

S. Zhu and Z. Zhu contributed equally to this work.
[a] Department of Urology, Renmin Hospital of Wuhan University, 99 Zhangzhidong Road, Wuchang District, Hubei Province, 430060, China; [b] Division of Hematology and Oncology, Department of Internal Medicine, School of Medicine, University of California Davis, Sacramento, USA; [c] Department of Medicine, Brigham and Women's Hospital, Harvard Medical School, 75 Francis Street, Boston, MA 02115, USA; [d] Department of Biochemistry and Molecular Medicine, University of California Davis, 2700 Stockton BLVD, Sacramento, CA 95817, USA; [e] Dana-Farber Cancer Institute, Harvard University, 450 Brookline Ave, Boston, MA 02215, USA; [f] VA Boston Healthcare System, West Roxbury, MA, USA
* Corresponding authors. Harvard Medical School, Building 3, Research administration, 1400 VFW Parkway, West Roxbury, MA 02132, USA.
E-mail addresses: urology1969@163.com (F.C.); chongxian_pan@hms.harvard.edu (C.-x.P.)

Hematol Oncol Clin N Am 35 (2021) 613–632
https://doi.org/10.1016/j.hoc.2021.02.007
0889-8588/21/Published by Elsevier Inc.
hemonc.theclinics.com

Depending on whether cancer cells invade into the muscle layer of the bladder wall, BC is divided into non–muscle-invasive BC (NMIBC) and advanced BC, which includes locally advanced and metastatic cancer. NMIBC includes Ta, T1, and cancer in situ, and accounts for approximately 75% of newly diagnosed BC cases.[2] The standard of care for NMIBC is transurethral resection followed by intravesical therapy for high-risk patients. With this treatment, more than 70% of patients develop cancer recurrence and one-third of patients have cancer progression to advanced stages.[5] For advanced BC, the standard of care for locally advanced muscle-invasive BC (MIBC) is neoadjuvant chemotherapy followed by radical cystectomy, and approximately 55% of patients with MIBC survive at 5 years. The standard treatment of metastatic BC is systemic therapy and the median survival is less than 2 years.[6]

There has been no significant improvement in BC treatment until recently with the approval of immunotherapy for both advanced and NMIBC, as well as 1 targeted therapy with a fibroblast growth factor receptor inhibitor, erdafitinib, and 1 antibody-drug conjugate, enfortumab vedotin, for advanced BC. The development of therapeutic interventions is still disappointing, and advanced BC is generally incurable. For example, recurrent genomic alterations have been identified in BC.[7] However, so far, only erdafitinib has been approved and it yields a modest incremental benefit and no cures. Immunotherapy using programmed cell death protein 1 (PD-1)/programmed cell death ligand 1 (PD-L1) inhibitors has shown promising activity, but the response rate is only around 20% in advanced BC.[8] This article reviews various in vitro and in vivo models that can be used to advance BC research and care for both NMIBC and advanced BC.

IN VITRO TWO-DIMENSIONAL MODELS
Cancer Cell Lines

Compared with animal models, cancer cell lines are faster, cheaper, easier to manipulate, more widely available, and have been extensively used in BC research. They are the most used models for cancer research.

BC is classified as low or high grade based on differentiation. Accordingly, human BC cell lines can also be classified into low-grade cancer cell lines, such as RT4 and RT112, and high-grade ones, such as T24, J82, 5637, UM-UC1, UM-UC3, HB-CLS-2, TCCSUP, and EJ-1.[9] Furthermore, the genetic characteristics and drug sensitivity information of cell lines can be found at some of the commonly used databases, such as Catalog of Somatic Mutations In Cancer (COSMIC),[10] Cancer Cell Line Encyclopedia (CCLE),[11] and the Genomics of Drug Sensitivity in Cancer.[12] Based on gene expression profiling, BC cell lines can recapitulate the expression profiles of different molecular subtypes of human BC.[13]

Besides human BC, cell lines from dog, rat, and mouse BC have also been developed.[13–15] The advantage of rat and mouse BC cell lines is that they can be implanted into immunocompetent syngeneic hosts to allow studies in immunotherapy. When human and canine cell lines are implanted in vivo, immunodeficient animals are usually used that do not permit studies in immunotherapy.

There are several major drawbacks associated with cell lines. First, cell lines and human BCs may have different genetic and epigenetic alterations. Cancer cell lines have been cultured in vitro for a long time, leading to the acquisition and accumulation of additional genetic and epigenetic aberrations that can be dramatically different from the original cancers. Even after a few generations, there was a great irreversible genetic divergence between a primary tumor and a cell line derived from that tumor.[16] Hence it is not surprising that prediction models based on cell lines frequently fail to predict drug efficacy in the clinic.[17] Second, cell lines use synthetic artificial culture medium. Different culture environment, nutrition availability, and different endocrine/paracrine/autocrine growth factor support during cell culture apply selection pressure to cells, skew cancer cell composition, and cause genetic and epigenetic alterations of the survived cancer cells. Furthermore, long-term culture in vitro enables tumor cells adapted to the culture environment, selects the fittest cells, and loses the heterogeneity seen in primary tumor tissues. Third, lack of three-dimensional (3D) structure and supporting environment can alter cell behavior. In vivo cancer cells grow in a 3D environment and communicate with other components, such as epithelial cells, stromal cells, immune cells, and matrix. The communication plays important roles in tumorigenesis and progression. Fourth, for in vivo studies, human and dog BC cell lines can only be implanted into mice or rats that are immunocompromised and, hence, are not suitable for research in immunotherapy.

Conditionally Reprogrammed Cell Culture

Conditionally reprogrammed cell (CRC) culture has recently emerged as a promising primary culture of both normal and cancer cells.[18] To establish CRC, after specimens are reviewed by pathology, they are digested with enzymes to generate single-cell suspension and cocultured with irradiated 3T3-J2 mouse fibroblasts (these serve as feeder cells) in a medium containing a Rho-associated kinase inhibitor Y-27632. Under this culture condition, cells rapidly convert to a stemlike state, are highly proliferative, but retain the original karyotype.[19] After its development, this method has been used to establish CRC cultures of many normal epithelial tissues, including skin, prostate, lung, breast, kidney, salivary gland, and liver cells, and cells across many species, such as mouse, rat, dog, ferret, horse, and cow. CRC can be established for all cancer types that have been tested so far.

CRC has been extensively studied in BC. CRC can be easily established using urine specimens, with an overall success rate of 83.3% (50 out of 60), including 85.4% for high-grade BC (41 out of 48) and 75.0% (9 out of 12) for low-grade BC.[20] This finding suggests that patient-derived CRC models can be established in most patients without requiring biopsy. CRC retains the genetic alterations and shares similar drug sensitivities to their corresponding in vivo parental cancer models.[21]

There are several advantages associated with CRC. First, CRC cells can be propagated in long-term culture but retain cell lineage commitment with the capacity to fully differentiate into the original tissue types they are derived from.[18] Second, CRC is highly efficient in establishing cultures. Epithelial colonies are readily observed at 2 days and proliferate rapidly. Third, CRC maintains the heterogeneity of cells present in a biopsy. The drawbacks of CRC are similar to those of cell lines except that CRCs are directly derived from cancer tissues, retain genetic alterations and high concordance of drug sensitivity as the in vivo counterparts, and can differentiate into the original tissues that CRC was developed from.

IN VITRO THREE-DIMENSIONAL MODELS
Organoid

An organoid is a miniaturized and simplified version of an organ produced in vitro from differentiated cells, embryonic stem cells, or induced pluripotent stem cells that self-organize in a 3D structure and can self-renew and replicate. Compared with traditional two-dimensional (2D) cell line culture models, organoids better retain the intrinsic characteristics of tumor and its microenvironment, including cell-cell interaction, cell-stroma interaction, tissue polarity, and nutrition gradients. With the development of culture matrix, a variety of organoid culture models are increasingly applied to BC research, such as BC stem cells and coculture system. However, there is still a lack of unified quantitative standards in correlating primary BCs and cultured organoids. Genomic and transcriptomic sequencing have been widely used in analyzing the consistency between organoids and primary BCs, whereas sensitivity to treatments has been used to correlate and predict the response of primary BCs to the same treatments.

The most common sources of organoids include cell lines (murine and human BC cell lines), patient-derived organoids, and cancer tissue–originated spheroid (CTOS).[22] To grow BC organoids, cell suspensions from cell lines or cancer specimens are implanted into a medium containing growth factors and cell matrix to grow into 3D structures (**Fig. 1**).[23] Cells of different tissue and cancer types have different success rates. For BC, papillary BC is more likely to survive and has a success rate up to 80%, whereas nonpapillary BC has a success rate of less than 30%.[24,25] It is particularly important to optimize the medium and matrix.[26] After organoids are established, they are characterized phenotypically, such as immunohistochemistry (IHC), flow cytometry, western blot, and proteomics, and genomically, such as exome sequencing, transcriptome sequencing, and methylation profile. Mullecci and colleagues[26] optimized the culture conditions and established a variety of organoid models, including murine bladder basal cell organoids, murine ureter and suprabasal bladder organoids, and human urothelial organoids. By comparing various biomarkers in mouse BC tissues and in organoids, such as basal (keratin 5, Ck5), intermediate (p63), and suprabasal/umbrella (keratin 20, Ck20, and UpkIII), organoids were able to retain the main features of mouse BC; by comparing different biomarkers of BC subtypes, such as basal (KRT5 and KRT6), luminal (KRT20, UPK1A, and UPK3A), and potential tumor-initiating cells (cluster of differentiation [CD] 44), human BC organoids were found to retain these features of the human BC subtypes. Okuyama and colleagues[23] analyzed E-cadherin, Ki67, uroplakin III (differentiation marker), and

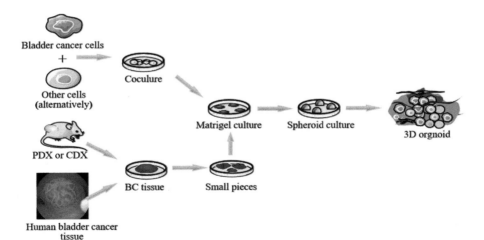

Fig. 1. Organoid models. Organoids can be developed from clinical cancer specimens, cell lines, or other models. After the initial pathology review and process (mincing and/or digestion), cells or tissues are seeded into culture dishes with supporting materials, such as Matrigel, which then grow in 3D structures and form spheroids. Organoids retain some of the 3D cancer structure and tumor microenvironment and recapitulate some of the cancer behaviors in vivo. CDX, cancer-derived xenograft; PDX, patient-derived xenograft.

p63 (basal cell marker) of BC CTOSs and found that CTOSs retained the differentiation status of the primary tumors.

The tumorigenesis and progression of BC always involve the interaction between BC cells and the tumor microenvironment (TME). TME contains cellular components, such as tumor cells, normal epithelial cells, immune cells, and stromal fibroblasts, and noncellular components, such as cytokines, fibers, and collagen. Although the traditional coculture technology can increase the communication among cells, tumor cells are very active in communicating with other components in TME in a 3D space. Therefore, the 3D culture can better simulate TME and provides better communication for the interaction between BC and TME.[27] For example, macrophages can be divided into tumor-suppressive (M1), tumor-supportive (M2), and regulatory macrophages (Mreg).[28,29] Cancer-associated fibroblasts (CAFs) affect the microenvironment by secreting a series of cytokines, which play important roles in tumorigenesis, progression, and resistance. Miyake and colleagues[30] found that cocultured CAFs and tumor-associated macrophages promoted cell adhesion and interaction between these cells and BC cells by secreting the chemokine CXCL1 in 3D models; compared with 2D cultures, tumor cells in a 3D culture showed higher cell survival rate and cell proliferation rate.

So far, extensive studies in organoids have been performed in BC. Lee and colleagues[31] established a BC organoid biobank by 3D culturing of primary and recurrent BC tissues from operation and biopsy in vitro. These organoids highly retained the human BC mutational spectrum, tumor evolution, phenotypic stability, plasticity, and some other characteristics. Xenograft models and organoids had similar resistance and mutational profiles. Mullenders and colleagues[26] collected tissues from 53 patients with BC and established an organoid biobank. Furthermore, they established primary murine basal cell organoids and found that organoids had high fidelity of primary cancer tissues through analysis of cellular surface molecules and functional validation. Different organoids differed in sensitivity to the same chemotherapy drugs, indicating the heterogeneity of BC organoids.

Goulet and colleagues[32] extracted the urothelial cells, fibroblasts, and endothelial cells from bladder biopsy tissues and spread the fibroblasts on sheets to form 3D vesical stroma. Then noninvasive or invasive BC cells were seeded and cultured as compact spheroids. Invasive BC cells crossed the basement membrane and invaded the stromal compartment, whereas noninvasive BC cells were confined to the urothelium. Thus the 3D culture model can possibly be used to study cancer behavior and drug effects.

Compared with the 2D cultures, organoids provide a 3D structure that partially retains the interaction of cancer cells with their TME. However, some of the drawbacks are obvious. First, even though vasculature can be established and maintained, organoids lack blood circulation and cells obtain nutrients mainly through concentration gradient and diffusion. Second, the culture medium supplemented with growth factors differs with that of the in vivo native TME and can change cancer cell behavior. Third, even though immune cells can be embedded, organoids lack the dynamic interaction of immune components in organoids with the immune system in the whole body.

Three-dimensional Printing

3D bioprinting deposits layers of bioinks, such as cells, extracellular matrix, and supporting materials, in accordance with the specifications that are predesigned and stored in a digital model to generate a spatially defined viable 3D construct. In contrast with other 3D models that take advantage of the intrinsic properties of biological materials, as seen in organoids, or that use extrinsic physical properties to aggregate biomaterials, as seen in hanging drops, ultralow attachment plates, and microchambers, 3D printing precisely deposits building materials, biological or synthetic, in spatially predefined manners.

Compared with other in vitro 2D and 3D models, there are several advantages of 3D printing. First, extracellular matrix properties are controllable. With predesigned models, cellular composition and density, matrix stiffness, and the concentration and gradients of bioactive molecules can all be controlled and adjusted to study cellular behavior in the microenvironment. Extracellular mechanics plays important roles in cancer cell behaviors. Polyethylene glycol–based photocross-linked scaffold with tunable stiffness has been used to study cancer cell migration,[33] whereas precisely controlled spatiotemporal gradients of bioactive molecules mimic the physiochemical microenvironment of cancer cells and allow the study of cancer cell behavior in desired manners.[34]

Second, high-throughput fabrication of replicable cancer models. Although other cancer models usually rely on the natural growth/expansion of cancer models and generate heterogenicity among individual models with the same origin, identical cancer models can be rapidly fabricated with 3D bioprinting, which allows rapid drug screening and biological studies with high precision.

Third, perfusable vasculature can be fabricated. All 3 bioprinting modalities, extrusion, droplet, and laser based, have been explored to fabricate vasculature in cancer models.[35] Both scaffold-based and scaffold-free bioprinting have been used to integrate vasculature in the models.[36] With the scaffold-based approach, cells are bioprinted in an exogenous biomaterial (ie, hydrogel or decellularized matrix components) resembling the target tissue structure, whereas cell assembly and fusion/remodeling are the driving mechanisms of vasculature formation in the cancer models.[37] Furthermore, to study cancer cell behavior, including cancer invasion into vasculature, various biological factors, such as different cells, extracellular matrix, and growth factors, can be programmed into cancer models.[38]

Even though 3D bioprinting has been used to establish multiple cancer models,[39] its application in BC research is very limited. Although several reports on 3D printing of a bladder have been published,[27,40] 3D printing in BC research is yet to be explored.

Other Three-dimensional Culture Systems

In addition to organoids, several other in vitro 3D cultures have also been studied and reported. Amaral and colleagues[41,42] reported a hanging drop method and floating method using ultralow attachment plates. Drug sensitivity of BC cells using these methods is comparable with that using patient-derived xenografts.

Pumpless microfluid chambers or microchambers have recently been developed as a cheaper, convenient, and highly efficient method to culture primary BC cells. Unlike most other in vitro culture methods of primary cells, which usually need special medium supplemented with growth factors and/or feeding cells, microchambers culture cells in a restricted miniscule physical space with a height of 75 μm, which prevents the dilution/diffusion of autocrine and paracrine growth factors and allows the culture of difficult-to-culture cells, such as hepatocytes and stem cells, without the need of special medium.[43] Hepatocytes can be maintained in these microchamber devices without perfusion for up to 3 weeks with minimal loss of phenotype or function. In BC, primary cancer cell microchamber culture was developed in all 6 specimens.[44] Drug sensitivity to single drugs and combinations was comparable between microchambers and patient-derived xenografts, suggesting microchambers can possibly supplement patient-derived xenografts in screening for effective drug candidates.

IN VIVO MODELS
In vivo Tumors from Cell Lines

In vivo tumors derived from cell lines are probably the most used model in cancer research. It is easy to manipulate, cheap, and fast. Almost all cell lines can be used to generate in vivo models in BC. If cell lines are of human and dog origins, they are implanted in immunocompromised animals, such as nude mice, SCID (severe combined immune deficient) mice, or nonobese diabetic (NOD) mice (NOD.Cg-Prkdc^{sci-} ^{dlL2rgtm1Wjl}/Sz [null; NSG]). If cell lines are of mouse and rat origins, they can be implanted in immunocompetent syngeneic mice or rats, which have been widely used for research in immunotherapy as well as other research.

Cells are usually implanted subcutaneously because they are easily accessible for measurement and manipulation. However, BC is unique in that more than 70% of cases at diagnosis are at the NMIBC stages and are treated locally, including intravesical instillation. Hence, subcutaneous models may not be applicable for research in NMIBC. Furthermore, the microenvironment of BC at the bladder may be different from that at the subcutaneous space. Hence, orthotopic cancer models are needed for BC research.

There are several approaches to establish orthotopic BC models. The most intuitive approach is to instill BCs cells through the urethra directly into the bladder cavity. Because of the tight junction of urothelial cells, cancer cells rarely attach to and develop orthotopic cancer. To increase cancer cell attachment to the urothelial layer and engraftment, the bladder is usually treated with another agent, such as trypsin, poly-L-lysine, HCl, or even electrocautery.[45,46] Because of the structure of the urethra and bladder in mice and rats, female animals are preferred for easier access. Another approach is to expose the bladder through a lower abdominal incision and directly inject BC cells into the bladder with a needle.[47,48] To minimize surgical trauma, a minimally invasive ultrasonography-guided intramural inoculation was used to establish orthotopic models with high success.[49]

Because BC is a wide spectrum of cancer, ranging from low-grade noninvasive cancer to high-grade, locally advanced and metastatic cancer, orthotopic BC models provide unique opportunities to study and monitor cancer progression. Huebner and colleagues[50] established a BC in situ model by using fluorescein-labeled highly invasive BC cell line UM-UC-3, and tracked the migration and invasion of BC cells in real time with bioluminescence imaging, MRI, PET and other technologies. Lorenzatti and colleagues[48] labeled human BC cells with a variety of fluorescein markers to observe the invasion of BC in orthotopic models. Erman and colleagues[51] used nanoparticles, immunofluorescein, and electron micrograph labeling technologies to observe the early-stage BC, and clearly observed the interaction and adhesion between BC cells and normal urinary epithelial cells.

Carcinogen-induced Model

BC develops from urothelial cells that have direct contact with carcinogens in urine. Hence, chemicals, either carcinogenic directly or indirectly through in vivo metabolism, have been widely used to induce BC. After the initial report of carcinogen-induced BC in rats,[52] BC has been induced with carcinogens in several other species (reviewed by Cohen[53]). N-butyl-N-(4-hydroxybutyl) nitrosamine (BBN) is one of the first and most commonly used carcinogens. Several other carcinogens have been identified and used, including amines(such as N-nitrosamine),[54,55] anthracenes (such as 20-methylcholanthrene),[56] and formamide FANFT(N-[4-(5-nitro-2-furyl)-2-thiozolyl]formamide).[57] Most of the carcinogens have aromatic amine components. They are genotoxic and therefore induce DNA damage in bladder urothelial cells.[58,59]

BBN is clinically relevant because it can be detected in tobacco smoke, the environment, and infectious metabolites,[60] and BC is induced through chronic feeding/exposure of BBN, similar to chronic exposure of carcinogens in human patients. Pathologically, BBN exposure induces progressively pathologic changes from hyperplasia, dysplasia, cancer in situ, invasive cancer, as well as metastasis, similar to the BC progression in human patients.[60]

Genomically, carcinogen-induced BC has similar genetic alterations to those found in human BC. *TP53*, *KMT2D*, and *KDM6A* are the most common mutated genes in human BC.[61] Yamamoto and colleagues[62] analyzed mutational events of BBN-induced BC and found that BBN caused mutations of the *p53* gene heterogeneity at the early stage, and clonal *p53* mutations, commonly with $C \rightarrow T$ to $G \rightarrow A$ mutations, at the late stage. Fantini and colleagues[63] showed that the most common mutations were *Trp53* (80%), *Kmt2d* (70%), and *Kmt2c* (90%), which were similar to the mutation spectrum of human BC.

Gene expression profiling analysis suggests that the gene expression spectrum of BBN-induced BC is similar to that of the human basal subtype.[63,64] Pathways that are consistently affected in human BC and carcinogen-induced rodent BC include cell cycle regulation, apoptosis, angiogenesis, and MYC.[65] In human, BC can be classified into several subtypes based on the gene expression profiles.[66] Comparing genes with corresponding homologs across the species of humans and mice, most BBN-induced BCs can be clustered into the basal-like tumors of The Cancer Genome Atlas (TCGA; n = 408).[13]

In summary, carcinogens can consistently induce BC across species. Carcinogen-induced BC resembles that of human BC based on the mechanisms of carcinogenesis, pathologic features, genetical alterations, and gene expression profiles. Because these cancers develop in immunocompetent mice, they can be used to study BC immunotherapy in addition to other aspects of cancer research.

Genetically engineered mouse models

In genetically engineered mouse models (GEMMs), mice that carry cloned oncogenes or knocked out tumor suppressor genes allow the investigation of the effects of individual genes or gene combinations on oncogenesis. Mice with germline knock-in or knock-out can be used to study how alterations of specific genes affect cancer development of the whole body, and this study may not be feasible if perturbation of the genes causes premature death or embryonic lethality. In order to study the effects of genes on specific organs/tissues, a tissue-specific promoter is used to drive the expression of the target gene. In BC GEMM, the most used promoter that drives the bladder-specific expression of a target gene is the mouse Uroplakin II (*UpkII*) promoter. Uroplakins are membrane integral proteins expressed in urothelial cells. Multiple oncogenes under the control of the *UpkII* promoter has been widely studied in BC oncogenesis, such as *SV40 T*, *RAS*, cyclin D1 (*CCND1*), fibroblast growth factor receptor (*FGFR*), and epidermal growth factor receptor (*EGFR*). For example, expression of SV40 T antigen under the control of the *UpkII* promoter leads to the development of cancer in situ with low copy numbers and invasive to metastatic transitional carcinoma with high copy numbers.[67] Expression of *H-Ras* leads to urothelial hyperplasia to low-grade papillary noninvasive BC.[68] Nevertheless, double transgenic mice carrying both *SV40 T* and *H-Ras* develop high-grade invasive urothelial carcinoma within 1 month and succumb to this disease around 7 weeks of age.[69]

To further increase the flexibility of gene manipulation, such as temporal and spatial control of gene expression and introduction of mutation, the *Cre-LoxP* system is widely used in generating GEMM. Cre is a recombinase that acts on palindromic sequences called LoxP sites that have been genetically engineered at specific sites in the mouse genome. Hence, when the expression of Cre is under the control of a tissue-specific promoter or an inducible promoter, the Cre-LoxP system can control gene expression or introduce mutation in target tissues/cells or when an inducer molecule is introduced. More recently, instead of controlling Cre expression with a tissue-specific promoter, adenovirus expressing Cre recombinase is delivered directly into the bladder cavity to temporally and spatially control gene expression.[70]

GEMM has been making a tremendous contribution in BC research, especially in studying how perturbation of specific genes and gene combinations affects the oncogenesis of BC. The major drawback of GEMM is that it does not recapitulate highly complicated oncogenic processes. Cancers developed in GEMM lack the heterogenicity seen in clinical BC. Because of the unique location and exposure of urothelium to carcinogens and their metabolites in urine, BC oncogenesis is a highly complicated process with integrated genetic and epigenetic alterations that cannot be replicated in GEMM. In fact, BC has the third highest mutation rate among all cancer types after skin melanoma and lung cancers.[71]

PATIENT-DERIVED XENOGRAFT MODELS

The patient-derived xenograft (PDX) technique originated in the 1980s. Through continuous improvement, the success rate of transplantation gradually increases and the establishment time has also shortened.[72] Compared with other models, PDXs can better retain the characteristic of BC cells and its microenvironment in vivo, and have been widely used in the BC mechanism study, drug screening, and so forth.[73,74]

The establishment and characterization of BC PDXs have been published (**Fig. 2**).[74] Briefly, fresh clinical BC tissues from patients are collected and minced into fragments of 3 to 5 mm^3, then transplanted subcutaneously into 4-week-old to 5-week-old NOD.Cg-$Prkdc^{scid}$ $Il2rg^{tm1Wjl}$/SzJ (NSG) mice. Cancer tissues can also be digested

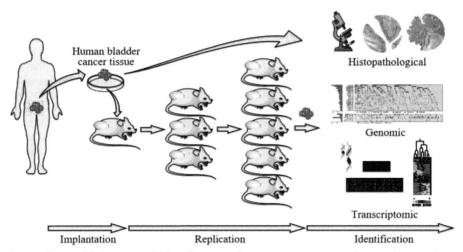

Fig. 2. The establishment and identification of PDX. BC tissues are collected from patients with BC, and implanted into immunodeficient mice to generate Passage 0 (P0) PDXs. After characterization and validation, P01 PDXs are reimplanted and expanded for cryopreservation and for research use.

into cell suspension and implanted into the bladder wall to establish orthotopic models. Mice are then monitored for tumor growth. For the first PDX establishment (P0), it usually takes 2 to 6 months. It takes a much shorter time for subsequent implantation. The engraftment rate for P0 PDXs is around 40%. To improve the engraftment rate, Jager and colleagues[75] implanted human BC tissue under the renal capsule of immunocompromised mice. All 7 tumor tissues developed PDXs, and 6 out of 7 could be successfully expanded in more mice. After PDXs are established, immunohistochemical, molecular, and genomic characterizations should be performed. The authors found that both subcutaneous and orthotopic PDXs retained the morphologic fidelity of their parental patient cancers, and that PDXs retained 92% to 97% of genetic alterations of parental patient cancers.[74] Occasionally, instead of PDXs, lymphoid tissue may grow out and need to be ruled out before using PDXs for further research. Use of the anti-CD20 antibody rituximab has decreased the development of lymphoid implant.

In addition to direct development from patient cancer tissues, PDXs and other patient-derived models of cancer can be interconvertible. For example, PDXs can be developed from CRC, microchamber cultures, hanging drop cultures, and organoids, and PDXs and their corresponding models had comparable response to the same drugs.[21,41,42,44] Lee and colleagues[31] also showed that drug response in organoids was recapitulated with their corresponding in vivo organoid-derived orthotopic BC PDXs. Furthermore, PDXs and their derived CRC cultures shared similar genetic alterations,[21] suggesting some of the in vitro patient-derived cultures can possibly complement PDXs in BC research.

Because PDXs morphologically and genomically recapitulate patient cancers, there are many potential applications in translational research in BC. First, PDXs can potentially be used to screen and select effective chemotherapy. In BC, the GC (gemcitabine and cisplatin/carboplatin) regimen is one of the 2 first-line chemotherapy regimens. It is assumed that these 2 drugs contribute to anticancer activity. However, when their activity is analyzed individually in PDXs, in 6 out of 8 PDXs, 1 drug contributes most of the anticancer activity, whereas the other has very little activity, and the remaining 2 PDXs are resistant to both drugs.[74] To study the mechanisms of chemoresistance, Wei and colleagues[76] found that cisplatin resistance is associated with alterations in genes including *MLH1*, *BRCA2*, and *CASP8* in BC PDXs derived from patients with BC who are resistant to chemotherapy. Moreover, these samples highly expressed *SLC7A11*, *TLE4*, and *IL1A*. Martin and colleagues[77] established that the levels of methionine adenosyltransferase 1a (*MAT1A*) gradually increased during GC treatment and overexpression of *MAT1A* increased tolerance to gemcitabine. Instead of studying individual genes, novel biomarkers of chemotherapy-induced DNA adduct levels for chemosensitivity have been translated from preclinical studies in PDXs into clinical trials.[78–84] For example, platinum drugs (cisplatin, carboplatin, and oxaliplatin) kill cancer cells mainly through induction of platinum-induced DNA damage/adducts, whereas gemcitabine kills cancer cells through incorporation into DNA and termination of DNA replication. Hence measurement of platinum/gemcitabine-DNA adduct levels can potentially predict chemoresistance. PDX studies showed that platinum/gemcitabine-DNA adduct levels indeed correlate with drug sensitivity to platinum/gemcitabine chemotherapy which is further supported by clinical trials.

PDXs can also be used to screen for effective molecularly targeted therapy. Based on the BC TCGA database, more than 70% of BCs harbor actionable genetic alterations.[7] However, in many cancers, targeted therapies matching the underlying genetic alterations have low response rates.[85,86] The major reason is that many of the genetic alterations are not molecular drivers and current computational biology cannot distinguish drivers from passenger mutations. Similar findings can be observed in BC. PDXs can potentially be used to screen for effective therapies.[74] Cirone and colleagues[87] used the phosphoinositide 3-kinase (PI3K) inhibitor PF-04691502 and MEK inhibitor PD-0325901 to inhibit the growth of BC PDXs, and the efficiency was similar to that of cisplatin at the maximum clinical dose, providing an experimental basis for preclinical targeted drug testing. FGFR3 and EGFR are commonly altered in BC.[61] Mahe and colleagues[88] treated BC PDXs with FGFR3 and PI3K inhibitors, and these inhibitors significantly prevented the growth and progression of the BC cells highly expressing FGFR3. Similarly, our previous research results showed that the EGFR/HER2 dual inhibitor lapatinib was also effective in preventing the growth of BC PDXs. The combination of a PI3K/AKT inhibitor and mitogen-activated protein kinase (MAPK)/ERK inhibitor was still effective on BC PDXs even if they developed secondary resistance to an EGFR/HER2 inhibitor.[74] Furthermore, serial biopsies with deep sequencing can be used to decipher resistance mechanisms. For example, downregulation of lymphocyte-specific protein 1 (LSP1) was associated with resistance to the PI3K small molecule blocker pictilisib.[89]

Another potential use of PDXs is for drug development. Traditionally, drug development uses cell lines and their derived tumor implants. It has been shown that even a few passages of in vitro culture leads to irreversible genetic alterations.[16] Hence, only 11% of drugs entering phase I clinical trials are eventually approved by the Food and Drug Administration, and it was less than 10% for oncology drugs.[90] The unique advantage of PDXs is that they are directly derived from clinical patient specimens and retain the morphology and genomic fidelity of their parental patient cancers.[74] Hence PDXs are being increasingly studied for drug development. Although extensive data on how PDXs affect drug development are still missing, several PDX coclinical trials showed promising results (reviewed elsewhere[91,92]). For example, Stebbing and colleagues[93] showed a strong correlation between PDX model responses and clinical outcomes (81%, 13 out of 16). In BC, PDXs have been used in several studies of drug development, which has reached the pre-IND/IND (investigational new drug) stage.[47,94–99]

Even though the PDX platform holds tremendous promise in translational research and drug development, there are several shortcomings. Compared with some of the in vitro models, PDXs are costly, it is difficult to manipulate cancer cells in vivo, they take a long time to develop (4–6 months), and have altered tumor microenvironment. Some of the supporting cells and stroma are retained during the establishment of PDXs but are replaced with mouse ones during subsequent passaging. Another important factor, especially in the immunotherapy era, is lack of human immune system.

HUMANIZED MODELS

Lack of competent immune system in the host animals makes the PDX platform unsuitable for study of immunotherapy, a cornerstone therapy for cancer in the modern era. Several approaches have been taken to overcome this drawback. One approach is to combine PDX studies with immunocompetent mouse models. For example, based on the TCGA database, approximately 80% of BCs have alterations along the cyclin-dependent kinase (CDK) 4/6 pathway that can possibly be targeted for the treatment of BC.[100] After accomplishment of the PDX studies, a CDK4/6 inhibitor was tested in an immunocompetent syngeneic mouse model with a mouse BC cell line and showed the synergistic antitumor activity with immunotherapy targeting the PD-1/PD-L1 pathway. Another approach is to generate transgenic mice expressing human

Table 1
Preclinical systems to develop bladder cancer therapeutics

	Source	Advantage	Deficiency
In vitro 2D models	Cell lines from human, mouse, rat, and dog	• Easy to culture • Economical • Readily available • Easy to manipulate • Mouse and rat cell lines can be implanted into immunocompetent host to study immunotherapy • The most widely used model in BC research	• Different genetic and epigenetic compositions from those of human cancers because of long-term in vitro culture • Relatively pure cancer cell population • Lack of supporting cells and TME • Human cancer lines can only be implanted into immunocompromised mice and are not suitable to study immunotherapy
	CRC culture	• Retention of genetic alterations of the parental cancer cells • Capability to differentiate into the tissue that CRC is originally developed from • High concordance of drug sensitivity with parental cancers • High success rate in establishing CRC culture	• Coculture with feeding cells • Need to irradiate feed cells • Lack of 3D structure and tumor microenvironment • Lack of immune system
In vitro 3D models	Organoids	• 3D structure with supporting cells and TME • Similar genetic alterations to the parental cancer cells • High concordance of drug sensitivity with parental cancers • Cheaper and easier than in vivo models	• Lack of in vivo factors, such as blood circulation • Lack of dynamic immune system • Special medium with growth factor support
	3D printing	• 3D structure with supporting cells and TME • Precise control of cancer cells, stromal cells, and stroma • Rapid production of large numbers of tumor 3D printings	• Need for special 3D printer • Lack of in vivo factors • Difference of 3D structure in 3D printing compared with native cancers • Lack of dynamic immune system as in vivo
In vivo models	Carcinogen-induced model	• Similar carcinogenesis process to human BC • Similar genetic alterations • Native cancer microenvironment • Competent immune system	• Time consuming and expensive • Difficult to do large-scale tests • Random events • Unique cancer in each mouse
	GEMM	• Relatively uniform cancers/mice • Generation of large identical mice	• Time consuming and expensive • Lack of heterogenicity of cancer

(*continued on next page*)

Table 1
(continued)

Source	Advantage	Deficiency
PDX	• Native cancer microenvironment • Competent immune system • Closest replication of human cancers • Morphologic and genetic fidelity of human cancers • High concordance of drug sensitivity with human cancers • 3D structure and TME	• Different carcinogenic mechanisms from human cancers • Expensive, time consuming • Lack of immune system • Difficulty to manipulate • Replacement with mouse stroma during establishment and passaging
Humanized models	• Combination of human immune system with human cancer implants • Capability to study immunotherapy and other therapies	• Complicated, expensive, and time consuming • Possibly partially defective immune system with lack of fully functional thymus • Difficulty to obtain HLA-matched immune system and PDXs • xGVHD

immune-oncology target molecules, such as human PD-1, PD-L1, CTLA4 (cytotoxic T-lymphocyte-associated protein 4), TIGIT (T cell immunoreceptor with Ig and ITIM domains), and so forth. Even though triple-humanized and even tetrahumanized immune-checkpoint transgenic mice have been generated and these mice respond to immunotherapeutic interventions against human targets, these mice and their syngeneic tumors have a mouse origin and the findings in these mice may not apply to human patients.

To better recapitulate human cancer immune response, truly humanized mice have been studied in which both the immune cells and cancer cells are derived from humans. The first generation of humanized mice is established via direct transfusion of human peripheral blood mononuclear cells into immunodeficient mice.[101,102] This humanized mouse model recapitulates the anticancer immune response when the antihuman PD-1 antibody nivolumab is administered. However, robust human xenograft-versus-host disease (xGVHD) develops within a few weeks that prevents long-term studies. To address this issue, humanized mice using human CD34+ hematopoietic progenitor and stem cells (HPSCs) were developed.[103] In this project, HPSCs are infused into 3-week-old female NSG mice 4 hours after 140 cGy of total body radiation.[104,105] B lymphocytes usually develop around 9 weeks after HPSC infusion followed by T cells 3 weeks later. The unique advantage of humanized mice from HPSCs is that xGVHD is usually mild, and the authors have kept those mice for more than 1 year.

After human T and B lymphocytes have developed in humanized mice, PDXs can then be implanted for immune-oncology research. It has been shown that the anti–human PD1 antibody pembrolizumab elicited antitumor response in the humanized NSG mice carrying human BC PDXs and induced CD8 T-cell infiltration into PDXs.[105] Different responses are observed in the same batch of humanized mice that were developed from the same CD34 HPSCs and PDXs, similar to the heterogenous response observed among metastatic cancers in the same patients.

Some of the major drawbacks of humanized mice is that they are expensive and take a long time to develop, almost 20 weeks from the time of HPSC infusion to the time of study. Furthermore, it is difficult to have human leukocyte antigen (HLA)–matched HPSCs and PDXs unless both of them are obtained from the same patients. However, it seems from the published study that HLA match is not needed.[105] Another major concern is whether immune cells in humanized mice are as fully functional as the immune cells in human patients. One major reason is that NSG mice may not have a fully functional thymus, which is needed for proper T-cell development.

SUMMARY

There are many in vitro and in vivo BC models. Each has its own unique features. This article summarizes the pros and cons of each model (**Table 1**). For example, traditional BC cell lines and their derived in vivo models are economical and easy to operate and manipulate, and remain the most commonly used models in BC research, but they may differ dramatically from human cancers in clinic; carcinogen-induced models and GEMM have competent immune systems for research in immunotherapy, but the findings at the mouse background may not be applicable to that in human patients; patient-derived organoids and PDXs recapitulate patient cancers better than other models, but lack of immune system means that they have limited applications for research in immunotherapy; humanized mice carrying PDXs have both human cancer and immune system, but it is not clear how much the immune system in those mice differ from that in human beings. In summary, there is no single model that fits all the research needs. Researchers need to take into account their research needs to select the appropriate models.

DISCLOSURE

There is no conflict of interest for this publication.

Work was supported in part by U54 grant (grant no. U54CA233306; Multi-PI: Pan), R01 grant (grant no. 1R01CA176803; PI: Pan), and Merit Review (award #I01 BX003840, PI: Pan) from the US Department of Veterans Affairs Biomedical Laboratory Research and Development Program. The contents do not represent the views of the US Department of Veterans Affairs or the US government.

REFERENCES

1. Bray F, Ferlay J, Soerjomataram I, et al. Global cancer statistics 2018: GLOBO-CAN estimates of incidence and mortality worldwide for 36 cancers in 185 countries. CA Cancer J Clin 2018;68(6):394–424.
2. Cumberbatch MGK, Jubber I, Black PC, et al. Epidemiology of Bladder Cancer: A Systematic Review and Contemporary Update of Risk Factors in 2018. Eur Urol 2018;74(6):784–95.
3. Chavan S, Bray F, Lortet-Tieulent J, et al. International variations in bladder cancer incidence and mortality. Eur Urol 2014;66(1):59–73.
4. Steinmaus C, Ferreccio C, Acevedo J, et al. Increased lung and bladder cancer incidence in adults after in utero and early-life arsenic exposure. Cancer Epidemiol Biomarkers Prev 2014;23(8):1529–38.
5. Chamie K, Litwin MS, Bassett JC, et al. Recurrence of high-risk bladder cancer: a population-based analysis. Cancer 2013;119(17):3219–27.
6. James ND, Hussain SA, Hall E, et al. Radiotherapy with or without chemotherapy in muscle-invasive bladder cancer. N Engl J Med 2012;366(16):1477–88.

7. Robertson AG, Kim J, Al-Ahmadie H, et al. Comprehensive molecular characterization of muscle-invasive bladder cancer. Cell. 2017;171(3):540–56.e5.
8. Bellmunt J, de Wit R, Vaughn DJ, et al. Pembrolizumab as second-line therapy for advanced urothelial carcinoma. N Engl J Med 2017;376(11):1015–26.
9. DeGraff DJ, Robinson VL, Shah JB, et al. Current preclinical models for the advancement of translational bladder cancer research. Mol Cancer Ther 2013;12(2):121–30.
10. Forbes SA, Tang G, Bindal N, et al. COSMIC (the Catalogue of Somatic Mutations in Cancer): a resource to investigate acquired mutations in human cancer. Nucleic Acids Res 2010;38(Database issue):D652–7.
11. Barretina J, Caponigro G, Stransky N, et al. The Cancer Cell Line Encyclopedia enables predictive modelling of anticancer drug sensitivity. Nature 2012; 483(7391):603–7.
12. Garnett MJ, Edelman EJ, Heidorn SJ, et al. Systematic identification of genomic markers of drug sensitivity in cancer cells. Nature 2012;483(7391):570–5.
13. Saito R, Smith CC, Utsumi T, et al. Molecular subtype-specific immunocompetent models of high-grade urothelial carcinoma reveal differential neoantigen expression and response to immunotherapy. Cancer Res 2018;78(14):3954–68.
14. Dhawan D, Ramos-Vara JA, Stewart JC, et al. Canine invasive transitional cell carcinoma cell lines: in vitro tools to complement a relevant animal model of invasive urinary bladder cancer. Urol Oncol 2009;27(3):284–92.
15. Cohen SM, Yang JP, Jacobs JB, et al. Transplantation and cell culture of rat urinary bladder carcinoma. Invest Urol 1981;19(3):136–41.
16. Daniel VC, Marchionni L, Hierman JS, et al. A primary xenograft model of small-cell lung cancer reveals irreversible changes in gene expression imposed by culture in vitro. Cancer Res 2009;69(8):3364–73.
17. Johnson JI, Decker S, Zaharevitz D, et al. Relationships between drug activity in NCI preclinical in vitro and in vivo models and early clinical trials. Br J Cancer 2001;84(10):1424–31.
18. Liu X, Krawczyk E, Suprynowicz FA, et al. Conditional reprogramming and long-term expansion of normal and tumor cells from human biospecimens. Nat Protoc 2017;12(2):439–51.
19. Palechor-Ceron N, Krawczyk E, Dakic A, et al. Conditional reprogramming for patient-derived cancer models and next-generation living biobanks. Cells 2019;8(11):1327.
20. Jiang S, Wang J, Yang C, et al. Continuous culture of urine-derived bladder cancer cells for precision medicine. Protein Cell 2019;10(12):902–7.
21. Mondal AM, Ma AH, Li G, et al. Fidelity of a PDX-CR model for bladder cancer. Biochem Biophys Res Commun 2019;517(1):49–56.
22. Said N. Establishing and characterization of human and murine bladder cancer organoids. Transl Androl Urol 2019;8(Suppl 3):S310–3.
23. Okuyama H, Yoshida T, Endo H, et al. Involvement of heregulin/HER3 in the primary culture of human urothelial cancer. J Urol 2013;190(1):302–10.
24. Yoshida T, Singh AK, Bishai WR, et al. Organoid culture of bladder cancer cells. Investig Clin Urol 2018;59(3):149–51.
25. Yoshida T, Okuyama H, Nakayama M, et al. High-dose chemotherapeutics of intravesical chemotherapy rapidly induce mitochondrial dysfunction in bladder cancer-derived spheroids. Cancer Sci 2015;106(1):69–77.
26. Mullenders J, de Jongh E, Brousali A, et al. Mouse and human urothelial cancer organoids: A tool for bladder cancer research. Proc Natl Acad Sci U S A 2019; 116(10):4567–74.

27. Kim MJ, Chi BH, Yoo JJ, et al. Structure establishment of three-dimensional (3D) cell culture printing model for bladder cancer. PLoS One 2019;14(10):e0223689.
28. Mantovani A, Sica A. Macrophages, innate immunity and cancer: balance, tolerance, and diversity. Curr Opin Immunol 2010;22(2):231–7.
29. Perdiguero EG, Geissmann F. The development and maintenance of resident macrophages. Nat Immunol 2016;17(1):2–8.
30. Miyake M, Hori S, Morizawa Y, et al. CXCL1-mediated interaction of cancer cells with tumor-associated macrophages and cancer-associated fibroblasts promotes tumor progression in human bladder cancer. Neoplasia 2016;18(10): 636–46.
31. Lee SH, Hu W, Matulay JT, et al. Tumor evolution and drug response in patient-derived organoid models of bladder cancer. Cell 2018;173(2):515–528 e517.
32. Ringuette Goulet C, Bernard G, Chabaud S, et al. Tissue-engineered human 3D model of bladder cancer for invasion study and drug discovery. Biomaterials 2017;145:233–41.
33. Soman P, Kelber JA, Lee JW, et al. Cancer cell migration within 3D layer-by-layer microfabricated photocrosslinked PEG scaffolds with tunable stiffness. Biomaterials 2012;33(29):7064–70.
34. Gupta MK, Meng F, Johnson BN, et al. 3D Printed Programmable Release Capsules. Nano Lett 2015;15(8):5321–9.
35. Datta P, Ayan B, Ozbolat IT. Bioprinting for vascular and vascularized tissue biofabrication. Acta Biomater 2017;51:1–20.
36. Norotte C, Marga FS, Niklason LE, et al. Scaffold-free vascular tissue engineering using bioprinting. Biomaterials 2009;30(30):5910–7.
37. Jakab K, Norotte C, Marga F, et al. Tissue engineering by self-assembly and bioprinting of living cells. Biofabrication 2010;2(2):022001.
38. Meng F, Meyer CM, Joung D, et al. 3D Bioprinted In Vitro Metastatic Models via Reconstruction of Tumor Microenvironments. Adv Mater 2019;31(10):e1806899.
39. Datta P, Dey M, Ataie Z, et al. 3D bioprinting for reconstituting the cancer microenvironment. NPJ Precis Oncol 2020;4:18.
40. Yoon WH, Lee HR, Kim S, et al. Use of inkjet-printed single cells to quantify intratumoral heterogeneity. Biofabrication 2020;12(3):035030.
41. Amaral RLF, Miranda M, Marcato PD, et al. Comparative analysis of 3D bladder tumor spheroids obtained by forced floating and hanging drop methods for drug screening. Front Physiol 2017;8:605.
42. Amaral R, Zimmermann M, Ma AH, et al. A simple three-dimensional in vitro culture mimicking the in vivo-like cell behavior of bladder patient-derived xenograft models. Cancers (Basel) 2020;12(5).
43. Guild J, Haque A, Gheibi P, et al. Embryonic stem cells cultured in microfluidic chambers take control of their fate by producing endogenous signals including lif. Stem Cells 2016;34(6):1501–12.
44. Gheibi P, Zeng S, Son KJ, et al. Microchamber cultures of bladder cancer: a platform for characterizing drug responsiveness and resistance in PDX and primary cancer cells. Sci Rep 2017;7(1):12277.
45. Chan ES, Patel AR, Smith AK, et al. Optimizing orthotopic bladder tumor implantation in a syngeneic mouse model. J Urol 2009;182(6):2926–31.
46. Lee JS, Bae MH, Choi SH, et al. Tumor establishment features of orthotopic murine bladder cancer models. Korean J Urol 2012;53(6):396–400.
47. Lin TY, Zhang H, Luo J, et al. Multifunctional targeting micelle nanocarriers with both imaging and therapeutic potential for bladder cancer. Int J Nanomedicine 2012;7:2793–804.

48. Lorenzatti Hiles G, Cates AL, El-Sawy L, et al. A surgical orthotopic approach for studying the invasive progression of human bladder cancer. Nat Protoc 2019; 14(3):738–55.

49. Jager W, Moskalev I, Janssen C, et al. Ultrasound-guided intramural inoculation of orthotopic bladder cancer xenografts: a novel high-precision approach. PLoS One 2013;8(3):e59536.

50. Huebner D, Rieger C, Bergmann R, et al. An orthotopic xenograft model for high-risk non-muscle invasive bladder cancer in mice: influence of mouse strain, tumor cell count, dwell time and bladder pretreatment. BMC Cancer 2017; 17(1):790.

51. Erman A, Kapun G, Novak S, et al. How cancer cells attach to urinary bladder epithelium in vivo: study of the early stages of tumorigenesis in an orthotopic mouse bladder tumor model. Histochem Cell Biol 2019;151(3):263–73.

52. Druckrey H, Preussmann R, Ivankovic S, et al. [Selective Induction of Bladder Cancer in Rats by Dibutyl- and N-Butyl-N-Butanol(4)-Nitrosamine]. Z Krebsforsch 1964;66:280–90.

53. Cohen SM. Urinary bladder carcinogenesis. Toxicol Pathol 1998;26(1):121–7.

54. Okada M, Suzuki E, Hashimoto Y. Carcinogenicity of N-nitrosamines related to N-butyl-N-(4-hydroxybutyl)nitrosamine and N,N,-dibutylnitrosamine in ACI/N rats. Gan 1976;67(6):825–34.

55. Althoff J, Kruger FW. Carcinogenicity of 4-hydroxybutyl-butylnitrosamine in Syrian hamsters. Cancer Lett 1975;1(1):15–9.

56. Campobasso O, Pecora M, Palestro G, et al. [Induction of bladder tumours in the mouse by direct implantation of 20-methylcholanthrene. (author's transl)]]. Tumori 1975;61(1):17–28.

57. Daskal Y, Soloway MS, DeFuria MD, et al. Morphological effects of mitomycin C administered intravesically to normal mice and mice with N-[4-(5-nitro-2-furyl)-2-thiazolyl]-formamide-induce bladder neoplasms. Cancer Res 1980;40(2):261–7.

58. Cohen SM, Ohnishi T, Clark NM, et al. Investigations of rodent urinary bladder carcinogens: collection, processing, and evaluation of urine and bladders. Toxicol Pathol 2007;35(3):337–47.

59. Oliveira PA, Vasconcelos-Nobrega C, Gil da Costa RM, et al. The N-butyl-N-4-hydroxybutyl nitrosamine mouse urinary bladder cancer model. Methods Mol Biol 2018;1655:155–67.

60. Vasconcelos-Nobrega C, Colaco A, Lopes C, et al. Review: BBN as an urothelial carcinogen. In Vivo 2012;26(4):727–39.

61. Hurst C, Rosenberg J, Knowles M. SnapShot: bladder cancer. Cancer Cell 2018;34(2):350–350.e3.

62. Yamamoto K, Nakata D, Tada M, et al. A functional and quantitative mutational analysis of p53 mutations in yeast indicates strand biases and different roles of mutations in DMBA- and BBN-induced tumors in rats. Int J Cancer 2000; 85(6):898.

63. Fantini D, Glaser AP, Rimar KJ, et al. A Carcinogen-induced mouse model recapitulates the molecular alterations of human muscle invasive bladder cancer. Oncogene 2018;37(14):1911–25.

64. Williams PD, Lee JK, Theodorescu D. Molecular credentialing of rodent bladder carcinogenesis models. Neoplasia 2008;10(8):838–46.

65. Lu Y, Liu P, Wen W, et al. Cross-species comparison of orthologous gene expression in human bladder cancer and carcinogen-induced rodent models. Am J Transl Res 2010;3(1):8–27.

66. Choi W, Porten S, Kim S, et al. Identification of distinct basal and luminal subtypes of muscle-invasive bladder cancer with different sensitivities to frontline chemotherapy. Cancer Cell 2014;25(2):152–65.

67. Zhang ZT, Pak J, Shapiro E, et al. Urothelium-specific expression of an oncogene in transgenic mice induced the formation of carcinoma in situ and invasive transitional cell carcinoma. Cancer Res 1999;59(14):3512–7.

68. Zhang ZT, Pak J, Huang HY, et al. Role of Ha-ras activation in superficial papillary pathway of urothelial tumor formation. Oncogene 2001;20(16):1973–80.

69. Garcia-Espana A, Salazar E, Sun TT, et al. Differential expression of cell cycle regulators in phenotypic variants of transgenically induced bladder tumors: implications for tumor behavior. Cancer Res 2005;65(4):1150–7.

70. Seager C, Puzio-Kuter AM, Cordon-Cardo C, et al. Mouse models of human bladder cancer as a tool for drug discovery. Curr Protoc Pharmacol 2010. https://doi.org/10.1002/0471141755.ph1414s49. Chapter 14:Unit14 14.

71. Lawrence MS, Stojanov P, Polak P, et al. Mutational heterogeneity in cancer and the search for new cancer-associated genes. Nature 2013;499(7457):214–8.

72. Inoue T, Terada N, Kobayashi T, et al. Patient-derived xenografts as in vivo models for research in urological malignancies. Nat Rev Urol 2017;14(5):267–83.

73. John BA, Said N. Insights from animal models of bladder cancer: recent advances, challenges, and opportunities. Oncotarget 2017;8(34):57766–81.

74. Pan CX, Zhang H, Tepper CG, et al. Development and Characterization of Bladder Cancer Patient-Derived Xenografts for Molecularly Guided Targeted Therapy. PLoS One 2015;10(8):e0134346.

75. Jager W, Xue H, Hayashi T, et al. Patient-derived bladder cancer xenografts in the preclinical development of novel targeted therapies. Oncotarget 2015;6(25):21522–32.

76. Wei L, Chintala S, Ciamporcero E, et al. Genomic profiling is predictive of response to cisplatin treatment but not to PI3K inhibition in bladder cancer patient-derived xenografts. Oncotarget 2016;7(47):76374–89.

77. Martin KA, Hum NR, Sebastian A, et al. Methionine adenosyltransferase 1a (MAT1A) enhances cell survival during chemotherapy treatment and is associated with drug resistance in bladder cancer PDX mice. Int J Mol Sci 2019;20(20):4983.

78. Henderson PT, Li T, He M, et al. A microdosing approach for characterizing formation and repair of carboplatin-DNA monoadducts and chemoresistance. Int J Cancer 2011;129(6):1425–34.

79. Cimino GD, Pan CX, Henderson PT. Personalized medicine for targeted and platinum-based chemotherapy of lung and bladder cancer. Bioanalysis 2013;5(3):369–91.

80. Scharadin TM, Zhang H, Zimmermann M, et al. Diagnostic microdosing approach to study gemcitabine resistance. Chem Res Toxicol 2016;29(11):1843–8.

81. Zimmermann M, Wang SS, Zhang H, et al. Microdose-induced drug-DNA adducts as biomarkers of chemotherapy resistance in humans and mice. Mol Cancer Ther 2017;16(2):376–87.

82. Scharadin TM, Malfatti MA, Haack K, et al. Toward predicting acute myeloid leukemia patient response to 7 + 3 induction chemotherapy via diagnostic microdosing. Chem Res Toxicol 2018;31(10):1042–51.

83. Wang S, Scharadin TM, Zimmermann M, et al. Correlation of platinum cytotoxicity to drug-DNA adduct levels in a breast cancer cell line panel. Chem Res Toxicol 2018;31(12):1293–304.

84. Zimmermann M, Li T, Semrad TJ, et al. Oxaliplatin-DNA adducts as predictive biomarkers of FOLFOX response in colorectal cancer: a potential treatment optimization strategy. Mol Cancer Ther 2020;19(4):1070–9.

85. Tsimberidou AM, Wen S, Hong DS, et al. Personalized medicine for patients with advanced cancer in the phase I program at MD anderson: validation and landmark analyses. Clin Cancer Res 2014;20(18):4827–36.

86. Andre F, Bachelot T, Commo F, et al. Comparative genomic hybridisation array and DNA sequencing to direct treatment of metastatic breast cancer: a multicentre, prospective, trial (SAFIR01/UNICANCER). Lancet Oncol 2014;15(3):267–74.

87. Cirone P, Andresen CJ, Eswaraka JR, et al. Patient-derived xenografts reveal limits to PI3K/mTOR- and MEK-mediated inhibition of bladder cancer. Cancer Chemother Pharmacol 2014;73(3):525–38.

88. Mahe M, Dufour F, Neyret-Kahn H, et al. An FGFR3/MYC positive feedback loop provides new opportunities for targeted therapies in bladder cancers. EMBO Mol Med 2018;10(4).

89. Zeng SX, Zhu Y, Ma AH, et al. The Phosphatidylinositol 3-Kinase Pathway as a Potential Therapeutic Target in Bladder Cancer. Clin Cancer Res 2017;23(21):6580–91.

90. Takebe T, Imai R, Ono S. The current status of drug discovery and development as originated in United States Academia: The Influence of Industrial and Academic Collaboration on Drug Discovery and Development. Clin Transl Sci 2018;11(6):597–606.

91. Koga Y, Ochiai A. Systematic review of patient-derived xenograft models for preclinical studies of anti-cancer drugs in solid tumors. Cells 2019;8(5):418.

92. Gao H, Korn JM, Ferretti S, et al. High-throughput screening using patient-derived tumor xenografts to predict clinical trial drug response. Nat Med 2015;21(11):1318–25.

93. Stebbing J, Paz K, Schwartz GK, et al. Patient-derived xenografts for individualized care in advanced sarcoma. Cancer 2014;120(13):2006–15.

94. Zhang H, Aina OH, Lam KS, et al. Identification of a bladder cancer-specific ligand using a combinatorial chemistry approach. Urol Oncol 2012;30(5):635–45.

95. Lin TY, Zhang H, Wang S, et al. Targeting canine bladder transitional cell carcinoma with a human bladder cancer-specific ligand. Mol Cancer 2011;10(1):9.

96. Lin TY, Li YP, Zhang H, et al. Tumor-targeting multifunctional micelles for imaging and chemotherapy of advanced bladder cancer. Nanomedicine (Lond) 2013;8(8):1239–51.

97. Lin TY, Li Y, Liu Q, et al. Novel theranostic nanoporphyrins for photodynamic diagnosis and trimodal therapy for bladder cancer. Biomaterials 2016;104:339–51.

98. Li Y, Lin TY, Luo Y, et al. A smart and versatile theranostic nanomedicine platform based on nanoporphyrin. Nat Commun 2014;5:4712.

99. Pan A, Zhang H, Li Y, et al. Disulfide-crosslinked nanomicelles confer cancer-specific drug delivery and improve efficacy of paclitaxel in bladder cancer. Nanotechnology 2016;27(42):425103.

100. Long Q, Ma AH, Zhang H, et al. Combination of cyclin-dependent kinase and immune checkpoint inhibitors for the treatment of bladder cancer. Cancer Immunol Immunother 2020;69(11):2305–17.
101. Fisher TS, Kamperschroer C, Oliphant T, et al. Targeting of 4-1BB by monoclonal antibody PF-05082566 enhances T-cell function and promotes anti-tumor activity. Cancer Immunol Immunother 2012;61(10):1721–33.
102. Sanmamed MF, Rodriguez I, Schalper KA, et al. Nivolumab and urelumab enhance antitumor activity of human T Lymphocytes Engrafted in Rag2-/-IL2R-gammanull Immunodeficient Mice. Cancer Res 2015;75(17):3466–78.
103. Yang SM, Wen DG, Hou JQ, et al. [Establishment and application of an orthotopic murine bladder cancer model]. Ai Zheng 2007;26(4):341–5.
104. Shultz LD, Lyons BL, Burzenski LM, et al. Human lymphoid and myeloid cell development in NOD/LtSz-scid IL2R gamma null mice engrafted with mobilized human hemopoietic stem cells. J Immunol 2005;174(10):6477–89.
105. Wang M, Yao LC, Cheng M, et al. Humanized mice in studying efficacy and mechanisms of PD-1-targeted cancer immunotherapy. FASEB J 2018;32(3):1537–49.

Developing Precision Medicine for Bladder Cancer

Brendan J. Guercio, MD[a],*, Gopa Iyer, MD[b,c], Jonathan E. Rosenberg, MD[c,d,e]

KEYWORDS

- Precision medicine • Bladder cancer • Urothelial carcinoma • Targeted therapy
- Biomarkers • Immunotherapy • Chemotherapy

KEY POINTS

- Biomarkers such as alteration of *FGFR3* and expression of programmed death ligand 1 have led to advances in precision medicine for bladder cancer.
- Additional candidate biomarkers to personalize bladder cancer care are under investigation, but significant obstacles must be overcome before they can be implemented in clinical practice.
- Promising innovations likely to advance precision medicine in bladder cancer include multi-omic approaches, innovative trials designs, cell-free DNA, and machine learning algorithms.

INTRODUCTION

Bladder cancer is a major cause of cancer-related morbidity and mortality and is characterized by significant molecular and histologic heterogeneity.[1] Despite exhibiting a high rate of potentially actionable genomic alterations[1] (**Fig. 1**), outside of FGFR3 inhibition, efforts to tailor therapy based on such biomarkers have had limited success. The failure of many initially promising biomarkers to impact the clinical care of patients with bladder cancer thus far highlights the importance of thorough biomarker validation before implementation in clinical practice. In this review, we summarize precision medicine efforts to date for patients with bladder cancer and review ongoing work in this area (**Table 1**). We also review obstacles to the advancement of precision medicine and potential solutions.

[a] Department of Medicine, Memorial Sloan Kettering Cancer Center, 1275 York Avenue, Box #8, New York, NY 10065, USA; [b] Department of Medicine, Memorial Sloan Kettering Cancer Center, 300 East 66th Street, New York, NY 10065, USA; [c] Weill Cornell Medical College, New York, NY, USA; [d] Department of Medicine, Memorial Sloan Kettering Cancer Center, New York, NY, USA; [e] MSK Sidney Kimmel Center for Prostate and Urologic Cancers, 353 E 68th Street, New York, NY 10065, USA
* Corresponding author.
E-mail address: guerciob@mskcc.org

Hematol Oncol Clin N Am 35 (2021) 633–653
https://doi.org/10.1016/j.hoc.2021.02.008
0889-8588/21/© 2021 Elsevier Inc. All rights reserved.

hemonc.theclinics.com

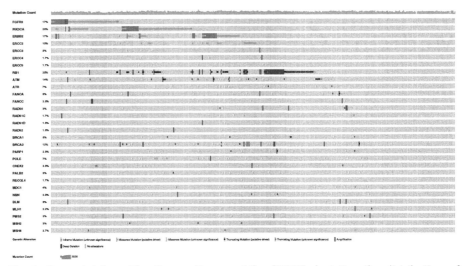

Fig. 1. Oncoprint from The Cancer Genome Atlas (TCGA) depicting the distribution of potentially predictive genomic biomarkers in muscle-invasive bladder cancer (MIBC).[1,106,107] Each column depicts the genomic profile of an individual patient. The y-axis labels include the percentage of MIBCs in the TCGA with alterations in each gene. TCGA patients without alterations in 1 or more of the selected genes are not shown.

DISCUSSION
Early Efforts: Personalizing Treatment Based on p53 Status

Prior studies showed dysregulation of the tumor suppressor p53 to be a marker of poor prognosis in bladder cancer[2] and that p53 inactivation may predict benefit from DNA-damaging chemotherapy.[3,4] In the first trial in bladder cancer to assign treatment based on molecular alterations,[5] patients with p53-mutant tumors were randomized to adjuvant methotrexate, vinblastine, doxorubicin, and cisplatin (MVAC) versus observation, whereas p53 wild-type patients were observed. Accrual was stopped after a futility analysis demonstrated no difference in recurrence by p53 status. However, the study suffered from notable limitations, including a low event rate, frequent patient refusal to receive adjuvant chemotherapy, and a high number of patients who did not receive their assigned therapy. The trial also relied on defining p53 expression by immunohistochemistry (IHC). Although wild-type p53 is not detectable by IHC owing to rapid degradation, mutant p53 is stabilized and detectable in the nucleus.[6] However, this method fails to detect p53 mutations that prevent expression of p53 and cannot differentiate between tumors with heterozygous versus homozygous loss of p53 function. These limitations can now be circumvented with genetic sequencing of *TP53*.[5]

Personalizing Therapy Based on FGFR Alterations and Expression

Deregulated fibroblast growth factor (FGF) signaling, often through gain-of-function alterations of FGF receptor (*FGFR*) 3, contributes to tumorigenesis in multiple cancers, including 32% of urothelial carcinomas (UC).[7] *FGFR* alterations occur in up to 37% of patients with upper tract UC[8] and are especially common in UC of the luminal I subtype.[9] FGFR signaling is crucial to tissue homeostasis and angiogenesis.[9] Upon binding of extracellular FGF ligands, the FGFR family of transmembrane receptor tyrosine

Table 1
Summary of notable biomarkers investigated in bladder cancer and associated study findings

Biomarker	Studies	Key Findings
p53	Stadler et al,[5] 2011	p53 status did not predict recurrence after adjuvant MVAC
FGFR3 alterations	Loriot et al,[14] 2019 Milowsky et al,[10] 2014 Pal et al,[11] 2018	Erdafitinib became the only targeted therapy approved for *FGFR* altered UC Dovitinib failed to demonstrate significant activity in unselected patients with mUC Infigratinib demonstrated modest activity in *FGFR3* altered UC
FGFR3 mRNA overexpression	Schuler et al,[16] 2019 Rosenberg et al,[17] 2020	Rogaratinib is active in UC with *FGFR3* mRNA overexpression
HER2	Hussain et al,[26] 2007 Powles et al,[29] 2017 Wulfing et al,[105] 2009 Choudhury et al,[30] 2016	Trastuzumab plus chemotherapy in HER2+ UC was active but toxic Lapatinib failed as maintenance therapy in HER2+ mUC Afatinib showed promising activity in a subset of mUC patients with altered *HER2/ERBB3*
EGFR	Petrylak et al,[23] 2010 Philips et al,[24] 2009 Pruthi et al,[25] 2010	Gefitinib was not active in unselected patients with UC Neoadjuvant erlotinib showed promise in a small cohort of unselected patients with MIBC
PIK3CA	Munster et al,[39] 2012 Seront et al,[40] 2016 McPherson et al,[41] 2020	Pan-isoform PI3K inhibitors show minimal or modest activity in advanced mUC with PI3K pathway alterations. Dosing was limited by significant toxicity
Molecular subtypes/gene expression profiling	Choi et al,[42] 2014 McConkey et al,[51] 2016 Seiler et al,[43] 2017 Rosenberg et al,[52] 2016 Sharma et al,[53] 2017 Kim et al,[54] 2019 Flaig et al,[59] 2019	Basal subtype tumors benefit most from neoadjuvant chemotherapy Activated wild-type p53 gene expression signature may confer resistance to neoadjuvant chemotherapy Luminal I subtype responds to immunotherapy less often than luminal subtype II Neuronal subtype may respond well to immunotherapy The COXEN score may predict for pathologic downstaging after neoadjuvant chemotherapy

(continued on next page)

Table 1
(continued)

Biomarker	Studies	Key Findings
DDR gene alterations	Van Allen et al,[65] 2014 Plimack et al,[69] 2015 Miron et al.[71] 2020 Teo et al,[70] 2017 Iyer et al,[72] 2018 Teo et al,[75] 2018	Sensitivity to platinum-based therapy is associated with alterations of DDR genes such as *ERCC2, ATM, FANCC,* and *RB1* DDR gene alterations are associated with benefit from immunotherapy
PD-L1	Powles et al,[80] 2018 Galsky et al,[81] 2020	Low PD-L1 expression in mUC predicts inferior survival on PD-1/PD-L1 inhibitors compared with platinum-based chemotherapy in the first-line
Tumor mutational burden	Balar et al,[55] 2017 Galsky et al,[83] 2017	High TMB is associated with high response rate and longer survival on immunotherapy in mUC
MSI	Iyer et al,[87] 2017	MSI is associated with excellent response to immunotherapy in mUC

Abbreviations: adjuvant MVAC, methotrexate, vinblastine, doxorubicin, and cisplatin; DDR, DNA damage response and repair; EGFR, epidermal growth factor receptor; FGFR, fibroblast growth factor receptor; MSI, microsatellite instability; mUC, metastatic or advanced urothelial carcinoma; PD-1, programmed cell death 1; PI3K, phosphoinositide 3-kinase; TMB, tumor mutational burden; UC, urothelial carcinoma.

kinases, consisting of FGFR1-4, trigger intracellular signaling via multiple pathways including RAS/MAPK/ERK, PI3K/AKT, PLCγ, and STAT.[9]

Early efforts to target FGFR3 using small molecule inhibitors included a phase II trial of dovitinib, a multitargeted tyrosine kinase inhibitor, in patients with advanced and metastatic UC (mUC) with and without FGFR3 mutations detected using a mass spectrometry assay.[10] Dovitinib failed to show significant activity, regardless of mutation status.[10] Moreover, only 12 *FGFR3*-mutant patients were enrolled, owing in part to some false-positive results requiring reclassification as wild type and because the rate of *FGFR3* mutations is 15% to 20% in invasive disease.[10] This study highlights the crucial importance of a reliable assay to detect the biomarker of relevance, as well as the need for drugs that effectively inhibit the target of interest.

Other FGFR inhibitors are also being investigated in the context of *FGFR* alterations. In a population of 67 patients with mUC and *FGFR3* alterations who were platinum refractory, intolerant, or ineligible, the FGFR1-4 inhibitor infigratinib demonstrated modest activity, with a response rate of 25.4%, a median progression-free survival of 3.75 months, and an overall survival of 7.75 months.[11] A randomized trial of adjuvant infigratinib versus placebo for invasive UC with specific *FGFR3* alterations is now ongoing (PROOF 302; NCT04197986). The FGFR1-3 inhibitor, pemigatinib, has been approved in cholangiocarcinoma with *FGFR2* fusions[12] and has shown clinical activity in UC with an objective response rate (ORR) of 25%.[13] Ongoing or planned studies of pemigatinib for *FGFR*-altered UC include FIGHT-205, a trial of pemigatinib with or without pembrolizumab for mUC (NCT04003610), and PEGASUS, a study of adjuvant pemigatinib for high-risk UC (NCT04294277).

The phase II BLC2001 trial tested the pan-FGFR tyrosine kinase inhibitor erdafitinib in metastatic *FGFR2/3* altered UC and demonstrated a confirmed ORR of 40%.[14] Median progression-free and overall survival rates were 5.5 and 13.8 months, respectively.[14] These results led to approval by the US Food and Drug Administration (FDA) of erdafitinib as the first targeted therapy for mUC with a specific genetic alteration.[15] A confirmatory phase III study (THOR) is currently open and randomizes patients with mUC and prespecified *FGFR* alterations to erdafitinib versus vinflunine, docetaxel, or pembrolizumab after receipt of 1 to 2 prior lines of therapy (NCT03390504).

FGFR inhibitors are also being explored in patients with FGFR messenger RNA (mRNA) overexpression. A phase I dose escalation and dose expansion study explored the pan-FGFR inhibitor rogaratinib for patients with advanced cancers, including 52 with UC, characterized by *FGFR1-3* mRNA overexpression and activating mutations, and demonstrated that rogaratinib had a favorable safety profile and promising antitumor activity.[16] In the cohort of patients with UC, 24% (n = 11) had an objective response, including 1 complete response; 49% had stable disease and 14% had progressive disease. All but one of the patients with UC who experienced an objective response were positive for *FGFR3* mRNA expression. Of the 11 responders, 6 had no alterations of the *FGFR* gene. In the FORT-2 trial of first-line rogaratinib plus atezolizumab for cisplatin-ineligible patients with mUC and *FGFR1/3* mRNA overexpression, the ORR in 23 evaluable patients was 39%, with a complete response rate of 13%.[17] Notably, most patients in FORT-2 were *FGFR* wild type, and 96% had little to no expression of programmed cell death ligand 1 (PD-L1).

The mechanisms of FGFR inhibitor resistance remain incompletely understood. Preclinical studies have suggested the existence of both on-target mechanisms, such as mutations of the tyrosine kinase domain and the adenosine triphosphate binding cleft, and off-target mechanisms, including the upregulation of parallel signaling pathways (RAS/PI3K).[18] Cell-free DNA (cfDNA) sequencing in patients treated with infigratinib identified adenosine triphosphate binding cleft mutations, or so-called gatekeeper mutations, in 4 patients whose disease ultimately progressed.[11] A further characterization of resistance mechanisms is necessary to optimize patient selection for FGFR-targeted therapies and to design the means of overcoming FGFR inhibitor resistance.

A primary limitation of current FGFR tyrosine kinase inhibitors is the spectrum of toxicity produced by the simultaneous inhibition of multiple FGFRs, resulting in hand–foot syndrome, nail toxicities, hyperphosphatemia, gastrointestinal side effects, and central serous retinopathy.[12,14,16,19] FGFR isoform-specific inhibitors, for example, inhibitors specific to FGFR3, may substantially decrease the toxicity burden, allowing for increased dosing levels to enhance target inhibition. Also, anti-FGFR3 antibody therapy may represent a less toxic means of signaling inhibition. Vofatamab is a fully human monoclonal antibody to FGFR3 that blocks both wild-type and mutant receptors.[20] Preliminary results from the FIERCE-21 study indicated that vofatamab with or without docetaxel in mUC with *FGFR3* mutations or fusions was well-tolerated, with only 1 patient discontinuing treatment owing to an adverse event.[20] However, only 7 of 55 patients had an objective response, suggesting insufficient efficacy.[20]

HER2-Targeted Therapy in Urothelial Carcinomas

The ErbB family of receptor tyrosine kinases consists of epidermal growth factor receptor (EGFR), HER2, ErbB3, and ErbB4.[21] Amplifications and somatic alterations of the ErbB family occur in a significant percentage of UC, including *EGFR* amplification (11%), *ERBB2* amplification (7%), *ERBB2* mutations (12%), and *ERBB3* mutations (10%).[1,22] Trials targeting the ErbB family in UC have produced mixed results, including 2 negative trials for gefitinib in chemotherapy-resistant UC[23,24] and 1 trial of neoadjuvant erlotinib in muscle-invasive bladder cancer (MIBC) that showed pathologic downstaging in 12 of 20 patients.[25] A single arm phase II trial of trastuzumab plus chemotherapy for patients with mUC and HER2 positivity—defined as HER2 overexpression by IHC, *ERBB2* amplification, or elevated serum HER2—resulted in a response rate of 70% but also grade 1 to 3 cardiotoxicity in 22.7% of patients (7% grade 3 toxicity).[26] Notably, the trial's primary end point was the rate of cardiotoxicity, and the trial was not powered to detect differences in ORR or survival by HER2 expression or amplification subgroups. In the phase IIa basket study MyPathway, 9 patients with advanced refractory bladder cancer with *ERBB2* amplification or overexpression were treated with trastuzumab plus pertuzumab, resulting in 1 complete response that is ongoing at 15 months, 2 partial responses lasting 1 and 6 months, and 2 patients with stable disease lasting more than 4 months.[27] A separate multicenter, phase II trial randomized 61 patients with advanced or metastatic urothelial cancer overexpressing HER2 to gemcitabine plus platinum with trastuzumab versus without trastuzumab and found that the addition of trastuzumab was well-tolerated.[28] However, there was no statistically significant difference in progression-free or overall survival.[28] A phase III, double-blind, randomized trial of maintenance lapatinib versus placebo after first-line chemotherapy in patients with EGFR- or HER2-positive UC failed to show a statistically significant difference in clinical outcomes, including in the subgroup of patients with 3+ expression by IHC.[29]

Promising findings were reported by a phase II trial of afatinib for platinum-refractory UC.[30] The median progression-free survival of patients with *ERBB2* and/or *ERBB3* alterations (n = 6) treated with afatinib was 6.6 months, a 3-fold improvement over historical controls.[30,31] One patient with both *ERBB3* mutation and *ERBB2* amplification never progressed, but did discontinue therapy at 10.3 months owing to cardiac toxicity.[30] Notably, all patients without alterations of either *ERBB2* or *ERBB3* (n = 15) progressed or died within 3 months, including patients with *EGFR* amplification and EGFR protein overexpression, perhaps because the *EGFR* exon 19 and 21 alterations for which aftanitib is approved in non–small cell lung cancer were not found in these patients.[32]

Notably, a consensus on the optimal method of measuring HER2 positivity in UC is lacking owing to the poor correlation between *ERBB2* gene amplification and HER2 overexpression in this disease.[33] Moreover, studies regarding which method is of greater prognostic relevance have yielded conflicting results.[34–36] Although earlier trials of HER-targeted therapy primarily used IHC for patient selection,[23,26] the results of the aforementioned afatinib trial suggested that *ERBB2* amplification as measured by quantitative polymerase chain reaction or fluorescence in situ hybridization may be superior in UC.[30] Although 75% of patients in the afatinib study with *ERBB2* amplification reached a progression-free survival of at least 3 months, this only occurred in 25% of patients with 2+ or 3+ HER2 overexpression by IHC.[30]

Promising trials of HER2-directed therapy for mUC continue, including a phase Ib study (NCT03523572) of nivolumab plus the highly active antibody–drug conjugate trastuzumab deruxtecan, which was recently approved by the FDA for the treatment of metastatic HER2-positive breast cancer.[37,38] Trastuzumab deruxtecan has shown efficacy in HER2-positive breast cancer even after treatment with the earlier HER2-directed antibody–drug conjugate, ado-trastuzumab emtansine, likely owing to the higher cytotoxic payload of trastuzumab deruxtecan and its efficacy at lower levels of HER2 expression.[37]

Personalizing Therapy Based on Alterations in PIK3CA

PIK3CA is altered in approximately 20% of MIBC.[1] Early stage trials of PI3K inhibitors in bladder cancer have shown significant treatment-related toxicity, but also occasional treatment responses.[39–41] Some studies suggest that responses to PI3K inhibition in bladder cancer do not always occur in the context of PI3K pathway alterations.[39,40] Recently, a phase II trial testing the pan-isoform class I PI3K inhibitor buparlisib for mUC with PI3K pathway alterations reported modest activity in patients with somatic loss of function of *TSC1*, achieving a partial response in 1 such patient and stable disease in 3.[41] However, trial accrual was halted early after no evaluable patients achieved disease control at 8 weeks. Treatment efficacy was likely impaired by dose reductions for toxicity in 40% of trial participants. The authors concluded that future trials should use isoform-selective PI3K inhibitors in genomically selected patients to increase on-target efficacy and minimize off-target toxicity.[41]

Molecular Subtypes Based on Gene Expression Profiling

The application of gene expression profiling to UC tumors defined discrete molecular subtypes, broadly categorized as luminal and basal similar to breast cancer subtypes, which are being explored intensely for correlation with response to various therapies.[1,22,42–45] Although basal tumors display aggressive behavior and expression patterns similar to less differentiated stemlike or mesenchymal cells, luminal tumors express FOXA1 and GATA3 in similar fashion to luminal-differentiated breast cancer cells and often display superficial papillary growth patterns.[42,46–49] Additional neuronal or neuroendocrine-like subtypes of UC are characterized by a gene expression profile consistent with neuronal and neuroendocrine differentiation, often in the absence of neuroendocrine histopathologic features.[1,50]

Multiple studies have reported that basal subtype tumors derive the greatest benefit from neoadjuvant cisplatin-based chemotherapy, whereas tumors with a p53-like phenotype, characterized by an activated wild-type p53 gene expression signature, are resistant to neoadjuvant chemotherapy.[42,43,51] The sensitivity of basal subtype UC to cisplatin-based chemotherapy may be attributable to an inherently higher proliferation rate given its aggressive natural history.[51]

Studies investigating the capacity of molecular subtyping to predict response to immunotherapy have generated conflicting results. In the phase II trial IMvigor 210, the ORR to the anti–PD-L1 inhibitor atezolizumab was greatest in patients with the TCGA luminal cluster II subtype at 34%.[52] However, results from CheckMate 275 suggested that patients with basal I subtype benefited most often from the anti–programmed cell death 1 (PD-1) inhibitor nivolumab with an ORR of 30%.[53] Both trials showed responses to anti–PD-1/PD-L1 therapy across all subtypes and suggested that, compared with the luminal II subtype, tumors of the luminal I subtype respond less often to immunotherapy.[52,53] Notably, luminal I tumors are characterized by absence of tumor-infiltrating immune cells, low expression of PD-L1, and enrichment for FGFR3 mutations.[52,53]

In IMvigor 210, patients with tumors of the neuronal molecular subtype experienced impressive benefit from atezolizumab, with a partial response rate of 75% and complete response rate of 25%, compared with 14% and 9% in the overall trial population, respectively,[54,55] even though these tumors lacked features otherwise associated with immunotherapy response, such as a high mutational burden and immune inflammation.[54] The response to immunotherapy was especially noteworthy given the poor prognosis associated with the neuroendocrine-like subtype in other contexts.[56]

A recent publication described a consensus classification consisting of 6 molecular subtypes of MIBC that will hopefully serve as a basis for prospective validation in future clinical trials.[57]

The predictive capacity of a different expression-based signature was tested in SWOG S1314 (NCT02177695), a phase II trial in which 237 patients with MIBC were randomized to neoadjuvant dose dense MVAC versus gemcitabine and cisplatin. The investigators tested for associations between pathologic response and the COXEN score, a dichotomized gene expression model that accurately predicted sensitivity to cisplatin-based therapy in a prior cohort of patients with bladder cancer.[58] Preliminary results from S1314 indicated that the COXEN scores were not significant predictors of response in the individual arms, though the COXEN gemcitabine-cisplatin score did predict for pathologic downstaging in pooled arms.[59] No interaction between COXEN score and chemotherapy regimen as a predictor of treatment response was identified.[59] Additional analyses focusing on genomic predictors of response are planned from S1314 specimens.

Alterations in DNA Damage Response and Repair Genes

Although successive randomized trials have demonstrated a survival benefit with neoadjuvant cisplatin-based chemotherapy for MIBC, uptake in community practice has been low given regimen toxicity and an inability to predict which patients are most likely to benefit.[60–64] Subsequent investigations have attempted to identify biomarkers of chemotherapy response to aid in patient selection. A study of whole-exome sequencing in patients with MIBC treated with neoadjuvant cisplatin-based chemotherapy identified an association between somatic *ERCC2* mutations and cisplatin sensitivity.[65] *ERCC2*, a nucleotide excision repair gene, is mutated in 10% to 18% of bladder cancers, higher than in any other cancer type.[66] *ERCC2* helicase domain mutations seem to be especially critical markers of cisplatin sensitivity.[67] The association between alteration of *ERCC2* and platinum sensitivity was validated in a later study[68] and was followed by identification of defects in other DNA repair genes as predictors of response to cisplatin-based therapy.[69,70] In a study of patients enrolled in clinical trials of neoadjuvant cisplatin-based chemotherapy, Plimack and colleagues[69] found that alterations in any one of 3 DNA repair genes—*ATM*, *RB1*, and *FANCC*—predicted pathologic response with 87% sensitivity and 100% specificity, as well as a longer overall survival.[71] In a subsequent analysis of patients with mUC, Teo and colleagues[70] found that the presence of deleterious alterations in various DNA damage response and repair (DDR) genes was associated with longer progression-free and overall survival on platinum-based therapy (overall survival 23.7 months in DDR mutant patients vs 13 months among DDR wild-type patients). Finally, a multicenter phase II trial of neoadjuvant dose-dense gemcitabine plus cisplatin for MIBC found the presence of deleterious DDR gene alterations to have positive predictive value for pathologic downstaging of 89%.[72] At a median follow-up of 2 years, no patients with deleterious DDR gene alterations had developed disease recurrence.

Two groups are currently testing a bladder-sparing approach after neoadjuvant cisplatin-based chemotherapy for patients with DDR gene-altered MIBC. In Alliance A031701 (NCT03609216), patients with MIBC whose tumors harbor deleterious DDR alterations who experience a clinical complete response or noninvasive residual disease after neoadjuvant chemotherapy are offered bladder-sparing surveillance in place of definitive local therapy. The RETAIN trial (NCT02710734) is also investigating bladder preservation for MIBC after neoadjuvant accelerated MVAC in patients with alterations in *ATM*, *RB1*, *FANCC*, or *ERCC2* and no clinical evidence of disease after neoadjuvant chemotherapy.[73] Other patients in the trial receive bladder-directed therapy in the form of intravesical therapy, chemoradiation, or cystectomy. If proven effective, such biomarker-driven bladder-sparing approaches could substantially improve patient quality of life by avoiding the morbidity of cystectomy or chemoradiation.

DDR gene alterations may also predict clinical benefit from immune checkpoint inhibitors.[74] In a study of 60 patients with mUC treated with nivolumab or atezolizumab, the presence of deleterious alterations in DDR genes proved superior to mutational load as a predictor of treatment response, overall survival, and progression-free survival.[75] Deleterious DDR alterations were associated with a response rate of 80% versus 19% among DDR gene wild-type patients.[75] At a median follow-up of 19.6 months, the median overall and progression-free survival for patients with deleterious DDR alterations were not reached[75] versus 9.3 months and 2.9 months, respectively, in DDR gene wild-type patients.[75] The association between DDR alterations and immunotherapy response is thought to be related to an increased frequency of immune-stimulating cancer neoantigens caused by defective DNA damage repair, as supported by an association between DDR alterations and higher mutational load.[75] Alterations in DDR genes may also predict immunotherapy response in other cancer types, such as esophagogastric and non–small cell lung cancer.[76,77]

Predictors of Immune Checkpoint Response in Clinical Use: Programmed Cell Death-Ligand 1, Tumor Mutational Burden, and Microsatellite Instability

Five anti–PD-1/PD-L1 immune checkpoint inhibitors are now approved by the FDA for the treatment of mUC in the second-line setting. However, approximately 80% of patients do not respond to these agents, and the ability to predict response is limited.[78] As in many solid tumors, the most extensively studied biomarker in this context is expression of PD-L1. Although high levels of tumor and immune cell PD-L1 expression are more frequently found in immune checkpoint inhibitor responders, responses have been observed in the absence of PD-L1 expression. Therefore, PD-L1 is not used to guide treatment decisions in the second-line setting.[78] A significant barrier to defining the predictive capacity of PD-L1 is the lack of standardization in PD-L1 assessment. This includes variations in PD-L1 assays, thresholds for PD-L1 positivity, and inclusion versus exclusion of PD-L1 expression on tumor-infiltrating immune cells.[78] For example, although the expression of PD-L1 is used to decide between carboplatin-based chemotherapy versus checkpoint blockade with pembrolizumab or atezolizumab in cisplatin-ineligible patients with treatment-naïve mUC, pembrolizumab is only used if the combined positive score is 10 or higher, integrating PD-L1 expression on both tumor and tumor-infiltrating immune cells as determined by the Dako 22C3 Assay, whereas atezolizumab requires PD-L1 staining of immune cells covering 5% or more of the tumor area as determined by the Ventana SP142 Assay.[79–81]

As in other tumor types, a high tumor mutational burden (TMB) has also been explored extensively as a predictor of immunotherapy response in bladder cancer.[78,82] Elevated TMB is thought to correlate with an increased frequency of neoantigens that may prompt antitumor immune recognition and response.[78] In IMvigor 210, patients treated with atezolizumab in the highest TMB quartile experienced longer overall survival compared with the rest of the trial cohort.[55] Patients treated with nivolumab in Checkmate 275 with tumors in the highest tertile of TMB also experienced a higher ORR of 31.9% compared with patients in the middle tertile (17.4%) and lowest tertile (10.9%).[83]

Of note, the anti–PD-1 agent pembrolizumab was recently approved by the FDA for all patients with advanced solid tumors with 10 or more mutations per megabase who have progressed on prior treatment and have no satisfactory alternative therapies[84] based on results from KEYNOTE-158, which enrolled patients with high microsatellite instability (MSI)/deficient mismatch repair noncolorectal tumors.[84,85] Although this approval does not impact the management of mUC, it does apply to patients with advanced bladder cancers with high TMB and nonurothelial histology.

Similar to TMB, MSI or mismatch repair deficiency is also a marker of immunotherapy response.[86] The FDA approved pembrolizumab for all solid tumors with MSI that have already progressed on prior therapies without satisfactory alternative treatments options.[86] MSI or mismatch repair deficiency occurs in 3% to 5% of UC, predominantly upper tract UC tumors in patients with Lynch syndrome or somatic MMR deficiency.[75,87,88] A retrospective study identified 13 of 424 UC patients with MSI. Of the 5 who received immune checkpoint blockade for metastatic disease, all achieved near-complete or complete responses, and all were alive at 27 months of follow-up.[87]

Innovative Trial Designs and Associated Limitations

Validation of biomarkers within single cancer types can prove challenging, especially given that such biomarkers are typically found in the minority of tumors, robust preclinical data confirming their biologic relevance and mechanism of action are often limited, and because a standardized method to screen for these biomarkers may not be established. In response to these limitations, innovative trial designs have been developed, including basket trials, umbrella trials, and adaptive platform trials (**Fig. 2**). Collectively, these methods have been referred to as master protocols.[89] Basket trials enroll patients with cancers of various types on the basis of a shared targetable trait—for example, alteration of a specific gene—to investigate a single targeted therapy. Umbrella trials focus on a single cancer histology or lineage and match patients by theoretically targetable alterations, such as *FGFR* alteration or *HER2* amplification, to one of several rational targeted therapies. Adaptive platform trials feature multiple interventions in a single disease that may enter or exit the platform over time as directed by a decision algorithm (**Fig. 3**). Such adaptive platform trials allow investigators to revise study designs in light of newly generated data in real time.[89] The potential limitations of master protocols include the simultaneous testing of multiple hypotheses leading to decreased statistical power, longer trial timelines that may suffer owing to changes in standard of care during the study period, and the increased planning required for trial complexity.[89] Examples of master protocols

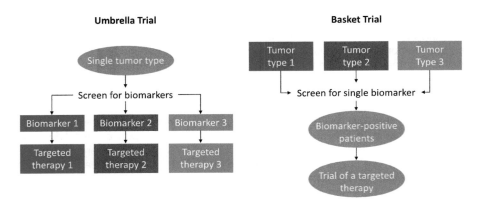

Fig. 2. Umbrella trials match patients with a single disease to one of multiple rational targeted therapies based on the presence of informative biomarkers. Basket trials enroll patients with various diseases based on a shared targetable trait to facilitate investigation of a single targeted therapy.

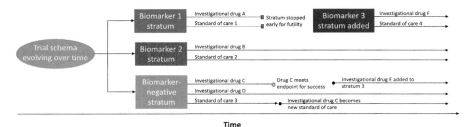

Time

Fig. 3. Example schema for an adaptive platform trial. The schema depicts evolution of a platform trial's design over time. In this example, patients are screened and matched to a trial stratum based on the presence or absence of targetable biomarkers. Each stratum features 1 or more investigational therapies personalized to patient biomarker status compared with a standard of care. As evidence from the trial accrues, each stratum or arm within a stratum can be individually stopped early for success or futility, while the remaining strata and arms may be left open for continued enrollment. New strata (eg, biomarker 3 stratum) and treatment arms (eg, investigational drug E) can be added as the trial proceeds. If a stratum closes early, patients enrolled in that stratum can be enrolled in another (eg, transition from biomarker 1 stratum to the biomarker-negative stratum). The overall trial does not necessarily feature a fixed stop date.

include NCI-MATCH (NCT02465060) and MPACT (NCT01827384), ongoing National Cancer Institute–funded, histology–agnostic, multicenter basket trials of targeted therapies for patients with advanced cancers.

The phase Ib BISCAY study is a multidrug, biomarker-directed, umbrella trial for patients with muscle-invasive UC that has progressed on prior therapy.[90] Treatments investigated in this study include the PD-L1 inhibitor durvalumab alone or in combination with various targeted agents, including the FGFR1-3 inhibitor AZD4547 for patients with *FGFR* alterations, the PARP inhibitor olaparib for patients with alterations in *BRCA1/2*, *ATM*, and homologous recombination repair gene alterations, the mammalian target of rapamycin inhibitor vistusertib, the Wee1 inhibitor AZD1775, and the antisense oligonucleotide STAT3 inhibitor AZD9150.[90] Patients without targetable biomarkers received durvalumab monotherapy.[90] Preliminary results from BISCAY showed that the combinations of durvalumab with targeted therapies were reasonably tolerated and that treatment responses occurred across all study arms, with ORRs ranging from 20.0% to 35.7%.[90] However, ORRs in all arms reported to date have failed to meet the prespecified efficacy end point of 50%. The trial is ongoing and will have additional arms to report in the future.

The BISCAY trial's failure to meet its prespecified end points despite the matching of multiple targeted therapies to rationally selected biomarkers highlights an important obstacle to precision oncology: differences in drug efficacy often depend on tumor lineage. For example, whereas the PARP inhibitor olaparib is an effective standard agent in the management of prostate and epithelial ovarian cancers with homologous recombination repair deficiency,[91,92] the BISCAY trial reported an ORR to olaparib plus durvalumab of 35.7% despite a PD-L1 positivity rate in this cohort of 50%.[90] Disappointing findings for PARP inhibition in bladder cancer were also reported in preliminary results of the ATLAS trial, in which rucaparib monotherapy failed to demonstrate significant activity in unselected patients with previously treated mUC.[93] Notably, 20.6% of the 66 patients were ultimately determined to have homologous recombination deficiency. Although additional trials of PARP inhibition in bladder cancers with somatic DDR alterations are ongoing (NCT03448718, NCT03375307), the currently available findings suggest that PARP inhibition may not succeed in bladder cancer even in genomically selected patients.

A possible explanation for the failure of PARP inhibitors and other targeted agents in bladder cancer may lie in the results of a study by Jonsson and colleagues.[94] The study characterized BRCA-mediated phenotypes across a variety of cancer lineages and found that BRCA1/2 mutations only conferred sensitivity to PARP inhibition in cancer types with increased heritable risk in BRCA1/2 carriers.[94] The authors concluded that BRCA1/2 alterations in non–BRCA-associated cancers are often passenger mutations that play little role in tumor pathogenesis, and therefore do not predict response to BRCA-targeted therapies.[94] If these findings prove generalizable to biomarkers beyond BRCA1/2, then targeted agents may only succeed in specific tumor types where their respective targets are foundational drivers of oncogenesis. Basket trials are therefore needed to interrogate genomic alterations in the context of multiple tumor lineages simultaneously. For example, although HER2 mutations are prevalent in UC, a basket trial of the HER kinase inhibitor neratinib failed to achieve a partial response in any of 16 patients with ERBB2 mutant UC.[95]

Overcoming Tumor Heterogeneity

Intertumor and intratumor genomic heterogeneity poses a major barrier to precision medicine in bladder cancer.[96] Biopsy specimens from a single tumor site may miss informative alterations present in synchronous metastases or even subclonal alterations within the biopsied tumor.[96] Such heterogeneity can lead to the proliferation of resistant subclones, limiting the usefulness of the targeted therapies. The application of cfDNA sequencing may complement mutation data extracted from the primary tumor and encompass subclonal alterations missed by single site sampling.[97] By sampling tumor DNA from blood and urine, cfDNA sequencing provides a noninvasive means to detect somatic alterations potentially shed by any tumor site in the body.[97] Such liquid biopsies also offer a means to noninvasively assess the genomic evolution of tumors over time, which under selective pressures inevitably generates mechanisms of resistance to precision cancer therapies.[97] In mUC, cfDNA has already proven useful in studies of FGFR inhibition, wherein plasma cfDNA sequencing detected FGFR3 alterations in 79% of patients with FGFR3 altered tumors.[98] Plasma cfDNA from patients on infigratinib also identified the emergence of putative resistance mutations and tracked changes in plasma mutant FGFR3 allele fractions that correlated with changes in tumor volume.[11]

Multi-Omic Platforms and Computational Methods

Efforts to define biomarkers of treatment response in bladder cancer are ongoing. A key example is the multi-omic investigation underway within the completed trial CALGB 90601.[99] This phase III trial of gemcitabine and cisplatin plus either bevacizumab or placebo for mUC failed to demonstrate a significant improvement in overall survival with the addition of bevacizumab. However, the large, well-annotated trial cohort of 506 patients provides an opportunity to investigate biomarkers of response to cisplatin-based and anti-VEGF therapy. A multi-institutional endeavor is underway to define the predictive capacity of DDR alterations, angiogenesis signatures and expression subtypes, germline single nucleotide polymorphisms, circulating angiokines, and other alterations associated with treatment sensitivity. Ultimately, this collaboration aims to develop composite biomarkers of response for investigation in future studies. Although many biomarkers investigated in bladder cancer are enriched in responders, such as DDR alterations in the case of cisplatin-based therapy or PD-L1 in immunotherapy, the positive and negative predictive value of most individual biomarkers is limited. Composite biomarkers may allow prediction of response with precision sufficient for clinical decision making. Historically, many bladder cancer biomarker studies have been limited in size. The use of larger cohorts such as CALGB 90601 are critical to characterize definitive composite biomarkers of response, which may require the integration of larger datasets across multi-omic platforms.

Multi-omic analyses are essential to the development of successful precision medicine approaches in bladder cancer, allowing for the integration of aberrations at the genetic, trascriptomic, epigenetic, and proteomic levels that may all influence sensitivity to therapy. For example, resistance to the antibody–drug conjugate enfortumab-vedotin may be mediated in some cases by loss of surface expression of nectin-4, enfortumab-vedotin's cell surface target.[100] Therefore, characterization of expression and localization of proteins such as nectin-4 through transcriptomics and proteomics may be necessary to fully understand response and resistance to oncologic therapies. The multi-omic platforms used by TCGA, PanCancer Atlas, and others offer role models for future endeavors.[1,101]

Such complex multi-omic analyses will only be feasible with increasingly sophisticated computation methods.[102] Machine learning has already shown promise in precision oncology as an investigatory means of improving central nervous system tumor classification, a historically challenging task fraught with interobserver variability.[103] Such advanced computational methods will allow rapid analysis of vast datasets, as demonstrated by a PanSoftware analysis of 9423 tumor exomes from the PanCancer Atlas that identified 59 novel likely oncodriver genes.[104]

SUMMARY

Ongoing efforts to implement precision medicine in bladder cancer have yielded pivotal improvements in the care of patients with mUC through targeting FGFR2/3 alterations with the pan-FGFR inhibitor, erdafitinb. Investigation of PD-L1 expression has also led to improvements in patient selection for first-line immunotherapy for mUC. A variety of other promising biomarkers to further advance precision medicine in bladder cancer remain investigational. Such biomarkers offer the potential for personalization of care in both the neoadjuvant and metastatic settings and include molecular subtypes of UC, DDR gene alterations, and alterations of PIK3CA and genes encoding the ErbB family of receptor tyrosine kinases. Barriers to the advancement of precision medicine in bladder cancer remain, but innovative trial designs, cfDNA sequencing, multi-omic platforms, and increasingly sophisticated computational methods offer promising solutions for future studies.

CLINICS CARE POINTS

- Alterations of FGFR2/3 are the only genetic feature of metastatic urothelial cancer currently used to select patients for targeted therapy. Erdafitinib is the only targeted therapy specifically approved for FGFR-altered urothelial cancer.

- The selection of patients with metastatic urothelial carcinoma to receive first-line immunotherapy is informed by expression of PD-L1. Such patients must also be cisplatin ineligible, but may be carboplatin eligible if PD-L1 expression is sufficiently high.

- Patients with metastatic urothelial carcinoma who are ineligible for any platinum-based chemotherapy may receive immunotherapy in the first-line regardless of PD-L1 expression.

- High TMB and MSI may be used to select patients for treatment with immunotherapy in cases of advanced bladder cancer with some nonurothelial histologies in which patients have already progressed on all other satisfactory alternatives. Such cases are rare.

- Promising biomarkers may eventually lead to greater personalization of care for patients with bladder cancer, but remain investigational. These include but are not limited to molecular subtypes of urothelial carcinoma, alterations of DDR genes, FGFR amplifications, alterations/amplifications of genes encoding ErbB receptor tyrosine kinases, and alterations of PIK3CA.

DISCLOSURE

All authors receive institutional support from Memorial Sloan Kettering's NIH/NCI Cancer Center Support Grant P30 CA008748. Dr B.J. Guercio is supported by NIH/NCI award No. T32-CA009207). Drs G. Iyer and J.E. Rosenberg are supported by MSK's NCI SPORE in Bladder Cancer (award No. P50 CA221745–01) and a DOD Congressionally Directed Medical Research Program Translational Team Science Award. Dr J.E. Rosenberg is also supported by the NCI Biomarker, Imaging and Quality of Life Studies Funding Program (BIQSFP). Dr B.J. Guercio reports honoraria from Medscape and institutional research funding from Bristol-Myers Squibb, Genentech, Eli Lilly, Pfizer, and Sanofi, outside the submitted work. Dr G. Iyer reports grants and personal fees from Mirati Therapeutics, grants from Novartis, grants from DeBioPharm, grants and personal fees from Janssen, outside the submitted work.

Dr J.E. Rosenberg reports honoraria, consulting/advisory role, and expenses from Bristol-Myers Squibb, institutional research funding, honoraria, and consulting/advisory role from AstraZeneca, honoraria from Chugai Pharma, consulting/advisory role for Lilly, consulting/advisory role for Merck, consulting/advisory role and institutional research funding from Astellas, consulting/advisory role, expenses, and institutional research funding from Genentech/Roche, consulting/advisory role for Pfizer, consulting/advisory role and institutional research funding from Seattle Genetics, consulting/advisory role and institutional research funding from Bayer, consulting/advisory role for BioClin Therapeutics, consulting/advisory role and institutional research funding from QED Therapeutics, consulting/advisory role for Pharmacyclics, consulting/advisory role for GlaxoSmithKline, consulting/advisory role for Janssen Oncology, consulting/advisory role for Boehringer Ingelheim, consulting/advisory role for Mirati Therapeutics, outside the submitted work. In addition, Dr J.E. Rosenberg has a patent Predictor of platinum sensitivity owned by Memorial Sloan Kettering Cancer Center.

REFERENCES

1. Robertson AG, Kim J, Al-Ahmadie H, et al. Comprehensive molecular characterization of muscle-invasive bladder cancer. Cell 2017;171(3):540–56.e5.
2. Goebell PJ, Groshen SG, Schmitz-Drager BJ, et al. p53 immunohistochemistry in bladder cancer–a new approach to an old question. Urol Oncol 2010;28(4):377–88.
3. Ferreira CG, Tolis C, Giaccone G. p53 and chemosensitivity. Ann Oncol 1999; 10(9):1011–21.
4. Cote RJ, Esrig D, Groshen S, et al. p53 and treatment of bladder cancer. Nature 1997;385(6612):123–5.
5. Stadler WM, Lerner SP, Groshen S, et al. Phase III study of molecularly targeted adjuvant therapy in locally advanced urothelial cancer of the bladder based on p53 status. J Clin Oncol 2011;29(25):3443–9.
6. Esrig D, Spruck CH 3rd, Nichols PW, et al. p53 nuclear protein accumulation correlates with mutations in the p53 gene, tumor grade, and stage in bladder cancer. Am J Pathol 1993;143(5):1389–97.

7. Helsten T, Elkin S, Arthur E, et al. The FGFR landscape in cancer: analysis of 4,853 tumors by next-generation sequencing. Clin Cancer Res 2016;22(1): 259–67.

8. Li Q, Bagrodia A, Cha EK, et al. Prognostic genetic signatures in upper tract urothelial carcinoma. Curr Urol Rep 2016;17(2):12.

9. Haugsten EM, Wiedlocha A, Olsnes S, et al. Roles of fibroblast growth factor receptors in carcinogenesis. Mol Cancer Res 2010;8(11):1439–52.

10. Milowsky MI, Dittrich C, Duran I, et al. Phase 2 trial of dovitinib in patients with progressive FGFR3-mutated or FGFR3 wild-type advanced urothelial carcinoma. Eur J Cancer 2014;50(18):3145–52.

11. Pal SK, Rosenberg JE, Hoffman-Censits JH, et al. Efficacy of BGJ398, a fibroblast growth factor receptor 1-3 inhibitor, in patients with previously treated advanced urothelial carcinoma with FGFR3 Alterations. Cancer Discov 2018; 8(7):812–21.

12. Abou-Alfa GK, Sahai V, Hollebecque A, et al. Pemigatinib for previously treated, locally advanced or metastatic cholangiocarcinoma: a multicentre, open-label, phase 2 study. Lancet Oncol 2020;21(5):671–84.

13. Necchi A, Pouessel D, Leibowitz-Amit R, et al. Interim results of FIGHT-201, a phase 2, open-label, multicenter study of INCB054828 in patients (pts) with metastatic or surgically unresectable urothelial carcinoma (UC) harboring fibroblast growth factor (FGF)/FGF receptor (FGFR) genetic alterations (GA). Ann Oncol 2018;29(suppl_8):viii303–31.

14. Loriot Y, Necchi A, Park SH, et al. Erdafitinib in Locally Advanced or Metastatic Urothelial Carcinoma. N Engl J Med 2019;381(4):338–48.

15. U.S. Food & Drug Administration. FDA grants accelerated approval to erdafitinib for metastatic urothelial carcinoma. 2019. Available at: https://www.fda.gov/ drugs/resources-information-approved-drugs/fda-grants-accelerated-approval-erdafitinib-metastatic-urothelial-carcinoma - :~:text=On%20April%2012%2C% 202019%2C%20the,progressed%20during%20or%20following%20platinum% 2D. Accessed August 2, 2020.

16. Schuler M, Cho BC, Sayehli CM, et al. Rogaratinib in patients with advanced cancers selected by FGFR mRNA expression: a phase 1 dose-escalation and dose-expansion study. Lancet Oncol 2019;20(10):1454–66.

17. Rosenberg JE, Gajate P, Morales-Barrera R, et al. Safety and preliminary efficacy of rogaratinib in combination with atezolizumab in a phase Ib/II study (FORT-2) of first-line treatment in cisplatin-ineligible patients (pts) with locally advanced or metastatic urothelial cancer (UC) and FGFR mRNA overexpression. J Clin Oncol 2020;38(15_suppl):5014.

18. Babina IS, Turner NC. Advances and challenges in targeting FGFR signalling in cancer. Nat Rev Cancer 2017;17(5):318–32.

19. Joerger M, Cassier P, Penel N, et al. Rogaratinib treatment of patients with advanced urothelial carcinomas prescreened for tumor FGFR mRNA expression. J Clin Oncol 2018;36(6_suppl):494.

20. Necchi A, Castellano DE, Mellado B, et al. Fierce-21: phase II study of vofatmab (B-701), a selective inhibitor of FGFR3, as salvage therapy in metastatic urothelial carcinoma (mUC). J Clin Oncol 2019;37(7_suppl):409.

21. Mooso BA, Vinall RL, Mudryj M, et al. The role of EGFR family inhibitors in muscle invasive bladder cancer: a review of clinical data and molecular evidence. J Urol 2015;193(1):19–29.

22. Cancer Genome Atlas Research N. Comprehensive molecular characterization of urothelial bladder carcinoma. Nature 2014;507(7492):315–22.

23. Petrylak DP, Tangen CM, Van Veldhuizen PJ Jr, et al. Results of the Southwest Oncology Group phase II evaluation (study S0031) of ZD1839 for advanced transitional cell carcinoma of the urothelium. BJU Int 2010;105(3):317–21.

24. Philips GK, Halabi S, Sanford BL, et al. A phase II trial of cisplatin (C), gemcitabine (G) and gefitinib for advanced urothelial tract carcinoma: results of Cancer and Leukemia Group B (CALGB) 90102. Ann Oncol 2009;20(6):1074–9.

25. Pruthi RS, Nielsen M, Heathcote S, et al. A phase II trial of neoadjuvant erlotinib in patients with muscle-invasive bladder cancer undergoing radical cystectomy: clinical and pathological results. BJU Int 2010;106(3):349–54.

26. Hussain MH, MacVicar GR, Petrylak DP, et al. Trastuzumab, paclitaxel, carboplatin, and gemcitabine in advanced human epidermal growth factor receptor-2/neu-positive urothelial carcinoma: results of a multicenter phase II National Cancer Institute trial. J Clin Oncol 2007;25(16):2218–24.

27. Hainsworth JD, Meric-Bernstam F, Swanton C, et al. Targeted therapy for advanced solid tumors on the basis of molecular profiles: results from MyPathway, an open-label, phase IIa multiple basket study. J Clin Oncol 2018;36(6):536–42.

28. Oudard S, Culine S, Vano Y, et al. Multicentre randomised phase II trial of gemcitabine+platinum, with or without trastuzumab, in advanced or metastatic urothelial carcinoma overexpressing Her2. Eur J Cancer 2015;51(1):45–54.

29. Powles T, Huddart RA, Elliott T, et al. Phase III, double-blind, randomized trial that compared maintenance lapatinib versus placebo after first-line chemotherapy in patients with human epidermal growth factor receptor 1/2-positive metastatic bladder cancer. J Clin Oncol 2017;35(1):48–55.

30. Choudhury NJ, Campanile A, Antic T, et al. Afatinib activity in platinum-refractory metastatic urothelial carcinoma in patients with ERBB alterations. J Clin Oncol 2016;34(18):2165–71.

31. Sonpavde G, Pond GR, Fougeray R, et al. Time from prior chemotherapy enhances prognostic risk grouping in the second-line setting of advanced urothelial carcinoma: a retrospective analysis of pooled, prospective phase 2 trials. Eur Urol 2013;63(4):717–23.

32. Chaux A, Cohen JS, Schultz L, et al. High epidermal growth factor receptor immunohistochemical expression in urothelial carcinoma of the bladder is not associated with EGFR mutations in exons 19 and 21: a study using formalin-fixed, paraffin-embedded archival tissues. Hum Pathol 2012;43(10):1590–5.

33. Kruger S, Weitsch G, Buttner H, et al. Overexpression of c-erbB-2 oncoprotein in muscle-invasive bladder carcinoma: relationship with gene amplification, clinicopathological parameters and prognostic outcome. Int J Oncol 2002;21(5):981–7.

34. Fleischmann A, Rotzer D, Seiler R, et al. Her2 amplification is significantly more frequent in lymph node metastases from urothelial bladder cancer than in the primary tumours. Eur Urol 2011;60(2):350–7.

35. Bellmunt J, Werner L, Bamias A, et al. HER2 as a target in invasive urothelial carcinoma. Cancer Med 2015;4(6):844–52.

36. Jimenez RE, Hussain M, Bianco FJ Jr, et al. Her-2/neu overexpression in muscle-invasive urothelial carcinoma of the bladder: prognostic significance and comparative analysis in primary and metastatic tumors. Clin Cancer Res 2001;7(8):2440–7.

37. Modi S, Saura C, Yamashita T, et al. Trastuzumab Deruxtecan in Previously Treated HER2-Positive Breast Cancer. N Engl J Med 2020;382(7):610–21.

38. U.S. Food & Drug Administration. FDA approves fam-trastuzumab deruxtecan-nxki for unresectable or metastatic HER2-positive breast cancer. 2019. Available at: https://www.fda.gov/drugs/resources-information-approved-drugs/fda-approves-fam-trastuzumab-deruxtecan-nxki-unresectable-or-metastatic-her2-positive-breast-cancer. Accessed August 17, 2020.

39. Munster P, van der Noll R, Voest E, et al. PI3K kinase inhibitor GSK2126458 (GSK458): clinical activity in select patient (PT) populations defined by predictive markers (STUDY P3K112826). Ann Oncol 2012;23(suppl_9):IX153–4.

40. Seront E, Rottey S, Filleul B, et al. Phase II study of dual phosphoinositol-3-kinase (PI3K) and mammalian target of rapamycin (mTOR) inhibitor BEZ235 in patients with locally advanced or metastatic transitional cell carcinoma. BJU Int 2016;118(3):408–15.

41. McPherson V, Reardon B, Bhayankara A, et al. A phase 2 trial of buparlisib in patients with platinum-resistant metastatic urothelial carcinoma. Cancer 2020; 126(20):4532–44.

42. Choi W, Porten S, Kim S, et al. Identification of distinct basal and luminal subtypes of muscle-invasive bladder cancer with different sensitivities to frontline chemotherapy. Cancer Cell 2014;25(2):152–65.

43. Seiler R, Ashab HAD, Erho N, et al. Impact of Molecular Subtypes in Muscle-invasive Bladder Cancer on Predicting Response and Survival after Neoadjuvant Chemotherapy. Eur Urol 2017;72(4):544–54.

44. Damrauer JS, Hoadley KA, Chism DD, et al. Intrinsic subtypes of high-grade bladder cancer reflect the hallmarks of breast cancer biology. Proc Natl Acad Sci U S A 2014;111(8):3110–5.

45. Sjodahl G, Lauss M, Lovgren K, et al. A molecular taxonomy for urothelial carcinoma. Clin Cancer Res 2012;18(12):3377–86.

46. Papafotiou G, Paraskevopoulou V, Vasilaki E, et al. KRT14 marks a subpopulation of bladder basal cells with pivotal role in regeneration and tumorigenesis. Nat Commun 2016;7:11914.

47. Dadhania V, Zhang M, Zhang L, et al. Meta-Analysis of the Luminal and Basal Subtypes of Bladder Cancer and the Identification of Signature Immunohistochemical Markers for Clinical Use. EBioMedicine 2016;12:105–17.

48. Volkmer JP, Sahoo D, Chin RK, et al. Three differentiation states risk-stratify bladder cancer into distinct subtypes. Proc Natl Acad Sci U S A 2012;109(6): 2078–83.

49. Warrick JI, Walter V, Yamashita H, et al. FOXA1, GATA3 and PPAR cooperate to drive luminal subtype in bladder cancer: a molecular analysis of established human cell lines. Sci Rep 2016;6:38531.

50. Sjodahl G, Eriksson P, Liedberg F, et al. Molecular classification of urothelial carcinoma: global mRNA classification versus tumour-cell phenotype classification. J Pathol 2017;242(1):113–25.

51. McConkey DJ, Choi W, Shen Y, et al. A prognostic gene expression signature in the molecular classification of chemotherapy-naive urothelial cancer is predictive of clinical outcomes from neoadjuvant chemotherapy: a phase 2 trial of dose-dense methotrexate, vinblastine, doxorubicin, and cisplatin with bevacizumab in urothelial cancer. Eur Urol 2016;69(5):855–62.

52. Rosenberg JE, Hoffman-Censits J, Powles T, et al. Atezolizumab in patients with locally advanced and metastatic urothelial carcinoma who have progressed following treatment with platinum-based chemotherapy: a single-arm, multi-centre, phase 2 trial. Lancet 2016;387(10031):1909–20.

53. Sharma P, Retz M, Siefker-Radtke A, et al. Nivolumab in metastatic urothelial carcinoma after platinum therapy (CheckMate 275): a multicentre, single-arm, phase 2 trial. Lancet Oncol 2017;18(3):312–22.

54. Kim J, Kwiatkowski D, McConkey DJ, et al. The Cancer Genome Atlas Expression Subtypes Stratify Response to Checkpoint Inhibition in Advanced Urothelial Cancer and Identify a Subset of Patients with High Survival Probability. Eur Urol 2019;75(6):961–4.

55. Balar AV, Galsky MD, Rosenberg JE, et al. Atezolizumab as first-line treatment in cisplatin-ineligible patients with locally advanced and metastatic urothelial carcinoma: a single-arm, multicentre, phase 2 trial. Lancet 2017;389(10064):67–76.

56. Batista da Costa J, Gibb EA, Bivalacqua TJ, et al. Molecular characterization of neuroendocrine-like bladder cancer. Clin Cancer Res 2019;25(13):3908–20.

57. Kamoun A, de Reynies A, Allory Y, et al. A consensus molecular classification of muscle-invasive bladder cancer. Eur Urol 2020;77(4):420–33.

58. Kothari S, Gustafson D, Killian K, et al. COXEN prediction of antineoplastic drug sensitivity in bladder cancer patients. J Clin Oncol 2016;34(2_suppl):365.

59. Flaig TW, Tangen CM, Daneshmand S, et al. SWOG S1314: a randomized phase II study of co-expression extrapolation (COXEN) with neoadjuvant chemotherapy for localized, muscle-invasive bladder cancer. J Clin Oncol 2019; 37(15_suppl):4506.

60. Sternberg CN, Skoneczna I, Kerst JM, et al. Immediate versus deferred chemotherapy after radical cystectomy in patients with pT3-pT4 or N+ M0 urothelial carcinoma of the bladder (EORTC 30994): an intergroup, open-label, randomised phase 3 trial. Lancet Oncol 2015;16(1):76–86.

61. Advanced Bladder Cancer Meta-analysis C. Neoadjuvant chemotherapy in invasive bladder cancer: a systematic review and meta-analysis. Lancet 2003; 361(9373):1927–34.

62. Winquist E, Kirchner TS, Segal R, et al, Genitourinary Cancer Disease Site Group CCOPiE-bCPGI. Neoadjuvant chemotherapy for transitional cell carcinoma of the bladder: a systematic review and meta-analysis. J Urol 2004; 171(2 Pt 1):561–9.

63. Advanced Bladder Cancer Meta-analysis Collaboration. Neoadjuvant chemotherapy in invasive bladder cancer: update of a systematic review and meta-analysis of individual patient data advanced bladder cancer (ABC) meta-analysis collaboration. Eur Urol 2005;48(2):202–5 [discussion: 205–6].

64. Raj GV, Karavadia S, Schlomer B, et al. Contemporary use of perioperative cisplatin-based chemotherapy in patients with muscle-invasive bladder cancer. Cancer 2011;117(2):276–82.

65. Van Allen EM, Mouw KW, Kim P, et al. Somatic ERCC2 mutations correlate with cisplatin sensitivity in muscle-invasive urothelial carcinoma. Cancer Discov 2014;4(10):1140–53.

66. Abbosh PH, Plimack ER. Molecular and Clinical Insights into the Role and Significance of Mutated DNA Repair Genes in Bladder Cancer. Bladder Cancer 2018;4(1):9–18.

67. Li Q, Damish AW, Frazier Z, et al. ERCC2 Helicase Domain Mutations Confer Nucleotide Excision Repair Deficiency and Drive Cisplatin Sensitivity in Muscle-Invasive Bladder Cancer. Clin Cancer Res 2019;25(3):977–88.

68. Liu D, Plimack ER, Hoffman-Censits J, et al. Clinical validation of chemotherapy response biomarker ERCC2 in muscle-invasive urothelial bladder carcinoma. JAMA Oncol 2016;2(8):1094–6.

69. Plimack ER, Dunbrack RL, Brennan TA, et al. Defects in DNA repair genes predict response to neoadjuvant cisplatin-based chemotherapy in muscle-invasive bladder cancer. Eur Urol 2015;68(6):959–67.

70. Teo MY, Bambury RM, Zabor EC, et al. DNA damage response and repair gene alterations are associated with improved survival in patients with platinum-treated advanced urothelial carcinoma. Clin Cancer Res 2017;23(14):3610–8.

71. Miron B, Hoffman-Censits JH, Anari F, et al. Defects in DNA repair genes confer improved long-term survival after cisplatin-based neoadjuvant chemotherapy for muscle-invasive bladder cancer. Eur Urol Oncol 2020;3(4):544–7.

72. Iyer G, Balar AV, Milowsky MI, et al. Multicenter prospective phase II trial of neoadjuvant dose-dense gemcitabine plus cisplatin in patients with muscle-invasive bladder cancer. J Clin Oncol 2018;36(19):1949–56.

73. Geynisman DM, Abbosh P, Zibelman MR, et al. A phase II trial of risk-adapted treatment for muscle invasive bladder cancer after neoadjuvant accelerated MVAC. J Clin Oncol 2018;36(6_suppl):TPS537.

74. Mouw KW, Goldberg MS, Konstantinopoulos PA, et al. DNA Damage and Repair Biomarkers of Immunotherapy Response. Cancer Discov 2017;7(7):675–93.

75. Teo MY, Seier K, Ostrovnaya I, et al. Alterations in DNA Damage Response and Repair Genes as Potential Marker of Clinical Benefit From PD-1/PD-L1 Blockade in Advanced Urothelial Cancers. J Clin Oncol 2018;36(17):1685–94.

76. Hsiehchen D, Hsieh A, Samstein RM, et al. DNA repair gene mutations as predictors of immune checkpoint inhibitor response beyond tumor mutation burden. Cell Rep Med 2020;1(3):100034.

77. Zhang J, Shih DJH, Lin SY. Role of DNA repair defects in predicting immunotherapy response. Biomark Res 2020;8:23.

78. Zhu J, Armstrong AJ, Friedlander TW, et al. Biomarkers of immunotherapy in urothelial and renal cell carcinoma: PD-L1, tumor mutational burden, and beyond. J Immunother Cancer 2018;6(1):4.

79. U.S. Food and Drug Administration. FDA alerts health care professionals and oncology clinical investigators about an efficacy issue identified in clinical trials for some patients taking Keytruda (pembrolizumab) or Tecentriq (atezolizumab) as monotherapy to treat urothelial cancer with low expression of PD-L1. 2018. Available at: https://www.fda.gov/drugs/drug-safety-and-availability/fda-alerts-health-care-professionals-and-oncology-clinical-investigators-about-efficacy-issue. January 18, 2020.

80. Powles T, Loriot Y, Gschwend JE, et al. KEYNOTE-361: phase 3 trial of pembrolizumab ± chemotherapy versus chemotherapy alone in advanced urothelial cancer. Eur Urol supplements 2018;17(2):e1147–8.

81. Galsky MD, Arija JAA, Bamias A, et al. Atezolizumab with or without chemotherapy in metastatic urothelial cancer (IMvigor130): a multicentre, randomised, placebo-controlled phase 3 trial. Lancet 2020;395(10236):1547–57.

82. Samstein RM, Lee CH, Shoushtari AN, et al. Tumor mutational load predicts survival after immunotherapy across multiple cancer types. Nat Genet 2019;51(2):202–6.

83. Galsky MD, Saci A, Szabo PM, et al. Impact of tumor mutation burden on nivolumab efficacy in second-line urothelial carcinoma patients: exploratory analysis of the phase II checkmate 275 study. Ann Oncol 2017;28(suppl_5):296–7.

84. U.S. Food and Drug Administration. FDA approves pembrolizumab for adults and children with TMB-H solid tumors. Available at: https://www.fda.gov/drugs/drug-approvals-and-databases/fda-approves-pembrolizumab-adults-and-children-tmb-h-solid-tumors. Accessed July 24, 2020.

85. Marabelle A, Fakih MG, Lopez J, et al. Association of tumor mutational burden with outcomes in patients with select advanced solid tumors treated with pembrolizumab in KEYNOTE-158. Ann Oncol 2019;30(suppl_5):v475–532.

86. U.S. Food and Drug Administration. FDA approves first cancer treatment for any solid tumor with a specific genetic feature. 2017. Available at: https://www.fda.gov/news-events/press-announcements/fda-approves-first-cancer-treatment-any-solid-tumor-specific-genetic-feature. Accessed August 1, 2020.

87. Iyer G, Audenet F, Middha S, et al. Mismatch repair (MMR) detection in urothelial carcinoma (UC) and correlation with immune checkpoint blockade (ICB) response. J Clin Oncol 2017;35(15_suppl):4511.

88. Pradere B, Lotan Y, Roupret M. Lynch syndrome in upper tract urothelial carcinoma: significance, screening, and surveillance. Curr Opin Urol 2017;27(1): 48–55.

89. Woodcock J, LaVange LM. Master protocols to study multiple therapies, multiple diseases, or both. N Engl J Med 2017;377(1):62–70.

90. Powles TB, Balar A, Gravis G, et al. An adaptive, biomarker directed platform study in metastatic urothelial cancer (BISCAY) with durvalumab in combination with targeted therapies. Ann Oncol 2019;30(suppl_5):v356–402.

91. Tew WP, Lacchetti C, Ellis A, et al. PARP inhibitors in the management of ovarian cancer: ASCO Guideline. J Clin Oncol 2020;38(30):3468–93.

92. U.S. Food and Drug Administration. FDA approves olaparib for HRR gene-mutated metastatic castration-resistant prostate cancer. 2020. Available at: https://www.fda.gov/drugs/drug-approvals-and-databases/fda-approves-olaparib-hrr-gene-mutated-metastatic-castration-resistant-prostate-cancer. Accessed August 16, 2020.

93. Grivas P, Loriot Y, Feyerabend S, et al. Rucaparib for recurrent, locally advanced, or metastatic urothelial carcinoma (mUC): results from ATLAS, a phase II open-label trial. J Clin Oncol 2020;38(6_suppl):440.

94. Jonsson P, Bandlamudi C, Cheng ML, et al. Tumour lineage shapes BRCA-mediated phenotypes. Nature 2019;571(7766):576–9.

95. Hyman DM, Piha-Paul SA, Won H, et al. HER kinase inhibition in patients with HER2- and HER3-mutant cancers. Nature 2018;554(7691):189–94.

96. Meeks JJ, Al-Ahmadie H, Faltas BM, et al. Genomic heterogeneity in bladder cancer: challenges and possible solutions to improve outcomes. Nat Rev Urol 2020;17(5):259–70.

97. Corcoran RB, Chabner BA. Application of cell-free DNA analysis to cancer treatment. N Engl J Med 2018;379(18):1754–65.

98. Pal SK, Bajorin D, Dizman N, et al. Infigratinib in upper tract urothelial carcinoma versus urothelial carcinoma of the bladder and its association with comprehensive genomic profiling and/or cell-free DNA results. Cancer 2020;126(11): 2597–606.

99. Rosenberg JE, Ballman KV, Halabi S, et al. CALGB 90601 (Alliance): randomized, double-blind, placebo-controlled phase III trial comparing gemcitabine and cisplatin with bevacizumab or placebo in patients with metastatic urothelial carcinoma. J Clin Oncol 2019;37(15_suppl):4503.

100. Rosenberg JE, O'Donnell PH, Balar AV, et al. Pivotal trial of enfortumab vedotin in urothelial carcinoma after platinum and anti-programmed death 1/programmed death ligand 1 therapy. J Clin Oncol 2019;37(29):2592–600.

101. Cancer Genome Atlas Research N, Weinstein JN, Collisson EA, et al. The Cancer Genome Atlas Pan-Cancer analysis project. Nat Genet 2013;45(10): 1113–20.

102. Azuaje F. Artificial intelligence for precision oncology: beyond patient stratification. NPJ Precis Oncol 2019;3:6.
103. Capper D, Jones DTW, Sill M, et al. DNA methylation-based classification of central nervous system tumours. Nature 2018;555(7697):469–74.
104. Bailey MH, Tokheim C, Porta-Pardo E, et al. Comprehensive Characterization of Cancer Driver Genes and Mutations. Cell 2018;173(2):371–85.e3.
105. Wulfing C, Machiels JP, Richel DJ, et al. A single-arm, multicenter, open-label phase 2 study of lapatinib as the second-line treatment of patients with locally advanced or metastatic transitional cell carcinoma. Cancer 2009;115(13): 2881–90.
106. Cerami E, Gao J, Dogrusoz U, et al. The cBio cancer genomics portal: an open platform for exploring multidimensional cancer genomics data. Cancer Discov 2012;2(5):401–4.
107. Gao J, Aksoy BA, Dogrusoz U, et al. Integrative analysis of complex cancer genomics and clinical profiles using the cBioPortal. Sci Signal 2013;6(269):pl1.

Future Directions in Bladder Cancer Treatment and Research—The Patient Advocates' Perspective

Rick Bangs, MBA[a,b],*, Diane Zipursky Quale, JD[b,1]

KEY WORDS

- Bladder • Cancer • Patient • Treatment • Research • Priorities • Gaps • Trials

KEY POINTS

- Despite significant advancements in the past 10 years in the understanding of the biology of bladder cancer and the development and approval of many new therapies, bladder cancer in 2021 remains a deadly disease with low public awareness, inequitable and inadequate funding, and a limited number of effective treatment options.
- Research advances should be focused on improving the quality of life for bladder cancer patients from the time of initial diagnosis through the end of life, with an emphasis on improving the ability to stratify patients into the appropriate risk categories for recurrence and invasion and developing effective treatments to eliminate the need for bladder removal.
- From the patient advocacy perspective, future research opportunities should be prioritized into these areas: prevention of disease, improved diagnostics, increased understanding of variant histologies and subgroups and targeting treatments, more effective therapies across disease states, advances in survivorship care to improve quality of life, and improved access to clinical trials.
- Continued emphasis on multidisciplinary collaboration and team science will ensure limited financial resources are used most efficiently and effectively.

INTRODUCTION
The Bladder Cancer Clinical and Research Fields Have Advanced

The primary goal of medical research is to provide meaningful improvement in the duration and quality of life for the underlying patient population. Basic, translational, and clinical research should sequentially drive new guidelines for the standard of care, and those standards should inform and support the resulting pattern of practice. Gaps within or between these stages reflect opportunities for continuous improvement and exploration.

---

[a] SWOG, Pittsford, NY, USA; [b] Bladder Cancer Advocacy Network, Bethesda, MD, USA
[1] Present address: 4520 East-West Highway, Suite 610, Bethesda, MD 20814.
* Corresponding author. 10 Widewaters Lane, Pittsford, NY 14534.
E-mail address: chezrick@comcast.net

Hematol Oncol Clin N Am 35 (2021) 655–664
https://doi.org/10.1016/j.hoc.2021.01.006
0889-8588/21/© 2021 Elsevier Inc. All rights reserved.
hemonc.theclinics.com

Until the beginning of the twenty-first century, bladder cancer largely was ignored. Despite its prevalence—the fourth most diagnosed cancer among men[1]—bladder cancer received no public attention and was among the lowest funded cancers by the National Cancer Institute. Substantial gaps in basic, translational, clinical, and cancer care delivery research existed—as well as the integration among them. There were no new treatments and no promising medical advances. Overall, the science was immature; the funding was at best anemic. From a career perspective, the field for years was perceived as stagnant, boring, and unrewarding. Three leading bladder cancer researchers once aptly described bladder cancer survivors in the first-line setting as having been "stranded on a shallow plateau for nearly a generation."[2]

The creation of the Bladder Cancer Advocacy Network (BCAN) in 2005 by John and Diane Quale provided a needed platform on which the bladder cancer clinical and research community would mobilize. Prior to this, no national advocacy group for bladder cancer existed—the voice of its survivor community was silent.

BCAN's annual Bladder Cancer Think Tank meetings started in 2006 with 50 attendees. By 2019, close to 300 members of the clinical and research communities spanning the range of stakeholders in bladder cancer research were in attendance. These meetings focus on collaboration to advance the field and improve outcomes for bladder cancer patients. To date, BCAN has provided more than $5 million in funding to young investigators as well as senior researchers to advance the science of bladder cancer.[3]

In addition, in 2014, 2 new research organizations dedicated to bladder cancer were opened: the Johns Hopkins Greenberg Bladder Cancer Institute[4] and the Leo and Anne Albert Institute for Bladder Cancer Care and Research at University of Kansas.[5] The work of these institutions further highlights the transformation of bladder cancer research from its humble baseline 20 years ago.

Equally important, since 2016, approvals for new bladder cancer drugs (atezolizumab, avelumab, durvalumab, enfortumab vedotin-ejfv, erdafitinib, mitomycin gel, nivolumab, and pembrolizumab) provide substantive evidence that today this is a highly desirable and exciting portfolio with great potential and reward.

Critical Gaps in Bladder Cancer Research and Treatment Remain Today

Despite these significant advancements in bladder cancer research and treatment options, bladder cancer in 2021 remains a deadly disease with limited public awareness, inadequate funding, and a dearth of broadly and uniformly effective treatment options. It is estimated that in 2021 alone, more than 83,000 people will be diagnosed in the United States with bladder cancer, with 17,000 deaths.[6]

From a patient advocate perspective, bladder cancer remains a complicated disease, with a multitude of challenges:

- Rather than being a single disease, bladder cancer appears to be many diseases. Not only is there a significant distinction between non–muscle-invasive bladder cancer and muscle-invasive disease but also there are multiple histologies and subgroups, many of which are uncommon, making research into the biology and treatment of those subgroups more difficult.
- With its high recurrence rate, requiring lifetime surveillance, bladder cancer is the most expensive cancer to treat per patient lifetime (even before immunotherapy), resulting in significant financial toxicity that is acknowledged but neither well understood nor sufficiently studied.[7–9]
- Although the bladder offers a readily accessible platform for biopsy via the urethra, this procedure can be extremely uncomfortable and invasive, especially if it is required to be performed multiple times each year.

- For most patients with non–muscle-invasive bladder cancer, treatment with bacillus Calmette-Guérin (BCG) is standard of care.[10] The mechanisms of action of BCG, one of the oldest therapies for bladder cancer and one of the earliest uses of immunotherapy in the cancer setting, remain mysterious and understudied. Moreover, there is a long-standing shortage of BCG in the United States and other countries, which is not expected to be alleviated any time soon.
- One-quarter of bladder cancer patients already are stage 2 or higher when diagnosed,[11] which in this context is described as muscle-invasive bladder cancer. The current standard of care for muscle-invasive bladder cancer is removal of the bladder and reconstruction of a new urinary diversion, a major life-transforming surgery with great risk of complications and significant impact on quality of life.[12]
- Bladder preservation therapies have been available for years, but the United States has been slow to adopt them.
- The prognosis for patients with advanced disease remains grim.[13]

These challenges collectively drive a compelling case for change and offer significant opportunity for clinicians and researchers to have an impact on the field while greatly improving the lives of patients and their families. This article articulates critical gaps needing closure across the landscape of treatment and research and some critical success factors for making that closure possible.

Recommended Research Priorities

Despite the improved research footprint and presence confirmed by the previous context, the opportunities for research remain significant. From an advocacy perspective, research priorities fall into the following categories (not listed in order of priority):

- Prevention of disease
- Improved diagnostics
- Increased understanding of variant histologies and subgroups and targeting treatments
- Safer and more effective therapies across disease states with increased focus on bladder-preserving therapies
- Advances in survivorship care to improve quality of life
- Improved access to clinical trials
- Continued partnerships and collaborations

These priorities reflect the current state of the science and the delivery of standard of care and pattern of practice to the bladder cancer community in 2021. They should not be cast in concrete but evolve with changes in the ways research and bladder cancer care are conducted and findings from new research and the bladder cancer ecosystem.

DISCUSSION
Prevention of Bladder Cancer is the Obvious Starting Point

Focus on more effective smoking cessation programs
To significantly reduce the burden of bladder cancer, preventing it from happening must be addressed first. With its strong linkage to smoking, tactics to reduce the incidence of smoking are logical but remain challenging. Progress has been made, but the beast still has not been tamed. To the extent that the initiation of smoking cannot be prevented, public health efforts should focus on smoking cessation and reduction. Although ideally this happens well before bladder cancer has occurred, a patient

who stops smoking after a bladder cancer diagnosis has an improved prognosis and reduced mortality. The need for research into developing and implementing effective smoking cessation programs for bladder cancer patients continues. These programs then need to be made readily available to primary care physicians, urologists, and oncologists, both in community and in academic practices.

Improved understanding of environmental causes of bladder cancer is essential

Although firsthand smoking and secondhand smoking are at the root of many bladder cancers, there are other known environmental causes. Occupational exposures to carcinogens known to trigger bladder cancer are common for hairdressers, firefighters, and workers in the rubber and chemical industries. Mechanisms to protect individuals from risk factors and screen exposed individuals are not widespread but could enable earlier detection. Research to leverage such tools efficiently and effectively and to build higher levels of awareness within the general population needs to continue, in particular those integrating electronic health records.

Improving Diagnostics Will Improve Outcomes and Quality of Life

Need improved screening techniques

Too many bladder cancer survivors are diagnosed extremely late in the course of the disease and have poorer outcomes as a result. Research into risk-based screening techniques that are cost effective and accurate must continue.

In addition, primary care physicians, gynecologists, and urologists need to be better trained in identifying and assessing the well-known symptoms of bladder cancer, without regard to the typical bladder cancer patient profile. Although most bladder cancer patients are men over the age of 70, the incidence of bladder cancer in women and in younger men is significant. Too often, women who present with blood in their urine initially are treated for a urinary tract infection, only to find later that the bleeding was caused by a bladder tumor. Many men—of all ages—have been misdiagnosed with prostatitis, then later found to have bladder cancer. Early diagnosis of bladder cancer, with appropriate referral to a urologic oncologist, is essential to improving patient outcomes.

Need improved biomarkers to stratify patients effectively

Given the complex heterogeneity of bladder cancer, identifying effective biomarkers and corresponding tests to allow for the appropriate risk stratification among bladder cancer patients is greatly needed. Although it is understood that bladder cancer has a high recurrence rate, patients deserve a better understanding of whether a recurrence likely is life-threatening, requiring more diligent surveillance and perhaps more active treatment. Diagnostic tests are needed that consistently and accurately drive the right therapeutic recommendation for every patient. Finding actionable biomarkers is fundamental to making the shift to precision medicine in bladder cancer.

Cystoscopy is one of the essential tools for bladder cancer diagnosis, allowing urologists to evaluate the bladder itself. Although there have been great improvements to this procedure recently, it is an invasive procedure, which for most patients brings varying levels of anxiety and discomfort. Improved biomarkers for bladder cancer may reduce the need for repeated cystoscopies over a patient's lifetime.

In addition, improved biomarkers will help identify those patients who are likely to benefit from more aggressive treatment. At diagnosis, many patients are presented with one or more treatment options and the associated risks and benefits to consider. Risk and reward today, however, sometimes are unclear. For example, a patient with a high-grade T2 urothelial tumor typically is offered neoadjuvant chemotherapy prior to radical cystectomy, which has been adopted as the standard of care based on clinical trials.[12] A better approach at this crossroads would be knowing in advance if a patient is likely to benefit from chemotherapy at all, with additional clarity around the specific agent(s) that will work best for this patient.

Improvement in pathology reporting is essential to patient comprehension of diagnosis

In addition, improvements in pathology reporting are greatly needed to improve patients' understanding of their diagnoses. A project to address that deficiency by creating graphics and plain language explanations of stage and grade explored the potential for patient-centric pathology reporting.[14] Data showed improved ability by patients to describe stage and identify cancer grade. Research in this area needs to continue so that more patient-centric reporting is created and deployed universally. That outcome likely will trigger similar and very necessary work in other cancers.

Increased Understanding of Variant Histologies and Subgroups

Need to broaden focus beyond urothelial cancer

Although a better understanding of bladder cancer has been gained in the past decade, most of the research has by necessity focused on the more mainstream urothelial cancer histology without variants or subtypes. Knowledge of the incidence of variants and subtypes is limited, and consensus does not always exist. An inability to consistently identify the correct pathology across histologies, variants, and subtypes has extremely negative implications for patient outcomes.

To address this, more uniformity in pathology reporting must be developed. Pathology analyses should be consistent across institutions, and incidence rates need more precision. The lack of consensus on this fundamental knowledge must be triaged, and from there the work to understand the biology and treatments will have the solid foundation necessary to proceed.

Although improved outcomes have been seen for many patients with plain vanilla urothelial carcinoma, expanding beyond that footprint and extending the lives of those patients who have one of the many variants of bladder cancer are needed. Identifying more effective treatments for squamous, micropapillary, adenocarcinoma, and small cell bladder cancer is needed. In addition, better options for upper tract disease, which does not always behave nor respond like bladder cancer, are needed.

Need improved understanding of disease impact on women and minorities

Although bladder cancer is more common in men than in women, women have a poorer prognosis.[15] It cannot simply be assumed this is because women often are delayed in diagnosis. A better understanding of the underlying biology of the disease and whether it has a different impact based on gender is needed.

It also is known that African Americans have poorer outcomes than whites,[16] but again, there is not an adequate understanding of why. A better understanding is needed of whether race has an impact on the underlying biology. Access to care issues for underserved communities of people of color also needs to be addressed.

Safer and More Effective Therapeutic Options for all Disease Stages Are Needed

Need alternatives to bacillus Calmette-Guérin

Bladder cancer was among the first cancers to benefit from an immunotherapy treatment, well before the current influx of immunotherapy treatments for cancer. BCG, an attenuated form of tuberculosis, has been approved for intravesical treatment since 1990 for non–muscle-invasive bladder cancer.[17] It generally is effective and tolerated. In addition, it is relatively inexpensive for a cancer treatment.

In the past decade, however, the global supply of available strains has struggled to keep up with demand. Three major shortages between 2012 and 2021 have had a severe impact on the bladder cancer community, with unquantifiable but significant harm and distress. The forecast for recovery from these shortages is uncertain.

Furthermore, the mechanism of action and the optimal dosing are, to this day, not fully understood. Research into alternative strains and alternative drugs must accelerate; research into alternative (lower) dosing, which potentially could extend supply at a time when alternatives are not available, is needed. Knowledge about the mechanism of action of BCG must increase.

Need increased focus on bladder preservation

For those patients for whom BCG is not effective, or those who are diagnosed with muscle invasive bladder cancer, the standard of care in the United States has been radical cystectomy—removal of the bladder and prostate for male patients and, in the majority of cases of female patients, removal of the bladder along with a complete hysterectomy. This not only is a complicated, lengthy operation from a surgical standpoint with significant risks and side effects but also is a life-transforming surgery. The patient loses his or her native, biological bladder and must adjust to a new normal of living with a urinary diversion. Although the success rate for this surgery is high—and patients make the necessary adjustments—patients always prefer to keep their biological bladders. Every effort should be made to find more effective treatments that enable patients to keep their own bladders and their sexual function while safely eradicating their cancer. These treatments will likely be guided by clinical, molecular, and radiographic information.

In the United States, the use of multimodality therapy—bladder preservation through the combined use of chemotherapy and radiation—has increased (albeit slowly) over the past decade, reflecting better data, patient demand, strong advocacy, and research prioritization from the National Cancer Institute.[18] More attention needs to be paid to this multimodality treatment tract so that it becomes standard of care. Continued refinement of the patient population that will benefit as much or more from bladder preservation versus radical cystectomy or systemic therapies will be necessary. In addition, the treatments and treatment regimens in the bladder preservation space must advance. The creation and support of multidisciplinary practices in cancer centers as well as at community practices will ensure that more patients are given the option of bladder preservation.

Need effective combination therapies for advanced disease

For patients with metastatic bladder cancer, non-BCG immunotherapy changed the landscape in bladder cancer. Since 2016, five immunotherapy drugs have been approved for advanced disease. This is unprecedented growth for patients who had been characterized as "stranded on a shallow plateau for nearly a generation."[2] Yet challenges remain with immunotherapy. Most patients do not respond to these therapies. Like all drugs, there are side effects that cannot always be predicted, and they may occur much later than the completion of the therapy. Research is needed that will manipulate the biology to overcome or offset the resistance of tumors in many patients, combine immunotherapy with other treatments to extend the population that benefits, and predict who will have which side effects and to have offsetting treatments ready when they are needed. The resulting therapies also must be safer.

One of the larger challenges in delivering treatments to bladder cancer patients is that platinum-based chemotherapies and radical cystectomy are not viable for many patients. With an average age of 73 years, they cannot safely tolerate chemotherapy, surgery, or both. Less toxic treatments clearly are needed along with the related research. The shift to bladder preservation as a viable option in the United

States will help address this for some patients, but research into safer, more tolerable options for patients who both do and do not benefit from chemotherapy is critical to serving a significant portion of the bladder cancer community.

Advances in Survivorship Care Needed to Improve Quality of Life

Need better understanding and treatment of side effects

Bladder cancer is a life-changing disease for many patients. Whether treatments are delivered over many years or provided with high intensity in a relatively short time frame, patients experience side effects. Side effects extend beyond urinary continence, frequency, and urgency to encompass sexual function, neuropathy, immune-related disorders, gastrointestinal problems, depression, and other adverse impacts.

Treatments to alleviate short-term side effects of cancer treatments have improved. For example, although not completely controlled in all cases, the impact of nausea on patients has been reduced in the past 20 years. That said, nausea and other side effects are debilitating for too many patients and need further advances. Immunotherapy has unleashed an entirely new dimension of side effects. Being able to predict who will have and how to prevent and manage side effects during treatment must continue to be a priority. Bladder cancer likely will be the beneficiary of work in other cancers, but some side effects are unique to bladder cancer treatments. Research on preventing, minimizing, or eliminating side effects specific to the bladder cancer context needs to be done by the bladder cancer community.

Need better understanding of the long-term impact of treatments

Beyond the immediate side effects of treatment, the long-term effects of treatments need more attention. In addition to the long-run impacts of chemotherapy and immunotherapy, a better understanding of the long-term metabolic impacts of neobladders, Indiana pouches, and ileal conduits is needed.

Additional study also is needed to mature survivorship plans. Patients who have completed treatment need clear guidance on the appropriate surveillance plan for them. Today those plans are provided inconsistently. In addition, the standards typically are silent on surveillance beyond the 5-year mark, and the potential long-term impacts of treatment on ongoing monitoring are not well understood (for example, the need for testing vitamin B_{12} levels for neobladder recipients).

Need to address caregiver needs

Caregivers remain an underserved population in cancer studies, and bladder cancer is no exception. Better tools are needed to diagnose the problems of this population as are proactive interventions to either prevent those problems from occurring in the first place or minimize their negative consequences.

Need to address financial toxicity

The potential for bladder cancer survivors to experience severe financial toxicities is significant and not well studied. As a cancer population burdened with the highest cost per patient lifetime of any cancer,[7–9] this is a shocking result that needs corrective action—research that will clarify and provide countermeasures for considerable financial toxicity.

Improved Access to Clinical Trials and Efficient Clinical Trial Designs Are Needed

Changes to the standard of care are predicated on data and evidence collected during clinical trials. Significant opportunities for prevention, diagnostics, treatments, and survivorship are discussed in this article, all of which are dependent on thoughtful and compelling clinical trial concepts and robust implementation plans. The key to successful clinical trials is successful accrual. The key to successful accrual is improved access, making it easier for patients to learn about clinical trials, enroll in trials, and participate without significant personal burden.

The first step in increasing patient accrual is making certain patients know about the availability of clinical trials for which they may be eligible. Improved collaboration between community urologic and oncology practices (where most bladder cancer patients are treated) and the major cancer centers (where most trials are originated) is essential. Clinical trials must demonstrate safety and efficacy for the studied population regardless of location and volume. Solutions must work in the community.

Triggering clinical trial accrual with electronic health record prompts has long been a vision for many clinicians and patients.[19] The complexity of inclusions and exclusions makes it exceedingly difficult and sometimes impossible to discern if trials are relevant to a patient. Efforts to connect inclusions and exclusions with clinical records must advance.

Educating and informing patients about clinical trials would be greatly advanced with continued research to identify the most efficient and effective uses of targeted social media to support accrual. This would be particularly impactful for the rarer histologies, variants, and subtypes, because no single institution is likely to have a sufficient pool of patients to conduct a trial in these subpopulations.

Finally, the use of basket, umbrella, and platform trials in bladder cancer has not yet been fully realized, and these models offer significant potential. In particular, they can address the rarer forms of bladder cancer efficiently. They also would be beneficial in developing alternatives to BCG. These trial structures currently are in use in other cancers, including rare cancer treatments, and should be leveraged in bladder cancer now.

Supporting Partnerships and Collaboration Will Accelerate Advancements

Given the breadth and depth of bladder cancer treatments, multidisciplinary teams must continue to be employed and will be a critical factor in ensuring optimal outcomes for patients. Much of the progress in bladder cancer has resulted from a strong culture of collaboration, and that will be the key to continued progress. Efforts to include community perspectives in these collaborations must increase because most bladder cancer patients receive their treatment in that setting.

Conceiving great concepts and nurturing great partners are important building blocks to better outcomes for bladder cancer patients. But the process of prioritizing, developing, and delivering those concepts often defines success or failure. In recent years, much has been written about implementation and implementation science. The establishment of a high-performance team at all stages of the research lifecycle must be a priority, leveraging the principles of team science. Team science is a "new interdisciplinary field that empirically examines the processes by which large and small scientific teams, research centers, and institutes organize, communicate, and conduct research. It is concerned with understanding and managing circumstances that facilitate or hinder the effectiveness of collaborative research, including translational research. This includes understanding how teams connect and collaborate to achieve scientific breakthroughs that would not be attainable by either individual or simply additive efforts."[20] Better trained and multidisciplinary research study teams will deliver better concepts faster and more efficiently.

In addition, collaboration external to bladder cancer will become increasingly important. The trend toward multicancer and pan-cancer biomarkers, therapies, and interventions is here to stay. Monitoring activities external to bladder cancer will enable continual benchmarking of bladder cancer opportunities and their prioritization within the portfolio while facilitating synergy and better return on investment from research funding.

Delivering on the roadmap and recalibrating it accurately across time also will require the continued integration of patients and advocacy. A study that fails to accrue to its target generally is a waste of time, money, and resources—none of which can be recouped after the fact. Inclusion of patients helps accelerate accrual and ensure meaningful outcomes are achieved. But it is not a natural act for many. The current level of integration in bladder cancer is comparatively robust but will continue to expand. Methodologies and training for this engagement are starting to appear within and external to bladder cancer. Inclusion of patients in establishment of scientific priorities, during the initial development of concepts, and across the clinical trial lifecycle is becoming the norm within the BCAN sphere of influence. Patient inclusion must increase within and certainly beyond the BCAN sphere.

SUMMARY

Bladder cancer research has experienced phenomenal growth in the past 10 years, growth that previously would not have been anticipated. With that growth has come a richer understanding of the biology of bladder cancer and clarity about the gaps and opportunities that have been insufficiently explored.

This article highlights opportunities from the patient advocate perspective and provides a roadmap to delivering significant change across the bladder cancer landscape. That roadmap builds on the substantial work thus far to establish a more solid scientific and collaborative foundation. Going forward, the roadmap will require recalibration to accommodate new findings and evidence. The authors are as excited to implement the roadmap as to make recalibrations and look forward to moving all bladder cancer survivors off their respective shallow plateaus.

DISCLOSURE

The authors have nothing to disclose.

REFERENCES

1. Available at: https://www.cancer.org/cancer/bladder-cancer/about/key-statistics.html Accessed August 9, 2020

2. Shah J, Mcconkey D, Dinney C. New strategies in muscle-invasive bladder cancer: on the road to personalized medicine. Clin Cancer Res 2011;2608–12. https://doi.org/10.1158/1078-0432.CCR-10-2770.

3. Available at: https://bcan.org/the-bladder-cancer-advocacy-network-announces-awardees-of-its-2020-new-discoveries-young-investigator-awards/#more-809603 Accessed August 15, 2020

4. Available at: https://www.hopkinsmedicine.org/greenberg-bladder-cancer-institute/about/ Accessed August 15, 2020

5. Available at: https://www.charitynavigator.org/ein/471075307. Accessed August 15, 2020 and https://www.ctopendata.com/1145280-the-leo-and-anne-albert-institute-for-bladder-cancer-care-and-research-inc Accessed August 15, 2020.

6. Available at: https://www.cancer.org/cancer/bladder-cancer/about/key-statistics.html#: ~ :text=The%20American%20Cancer%20Society's%20estimates,men%20and%204%2C930%20in%20women. Accessed February 22, 2021.

7. Botteman MF, Pashos CL, Redaelli A, et al. The health economics of bladder cancer: a comprehensive review of the published literature. Pharmacoeconomics 2003;21(18):1315–30.

8. Mossanen M, Gore JL. The burden of bladder cancer care: direct and indirect costs. Curr Opin Urol 2014;24(5):487–91.

9. Sloan FA, Yashkin A, Akushevich I, et al. The cost to medicare of bladder cancer care. Eur Urol Oncol 2020. https://doi.org/10.1016/j.euo.2019.01.015.

10. Chang SS, Boorjian SA, Chou R, et al. Diagnosis and treatment of non-muscle invasive bladder cancer: AUA/SUO guideline. J Urol 2016;196:1021. Statements 17 and 18.

11. Konety BR, Joyce GF, Wise M. Bladder and upper tract urothelial cancer. J Urol 2007;177(5):1636–45.

12. Chang SS, Bochner BH, Chou R, et al. Treatment of non-metastatic muscle-invasive bladder cancer: AUA/ASCO/ASTRO/SUO guideline. J Urol 2017;198:552. Statements 8, 10 and 11 and Statements 6 and 8.

13. Available at: https://www.cancer.org/cancer/bladder-cancer/detection-diagnosis-staging/survival-rates.html Accessed August 20, 2020.

14. Mossanen M, Macleod LC, Chu A, et al. Comparative effectiveness of a patient centered pathology report for bladder cancer care. J Urol 2016;196(5):1383–9.

15. Marks P, Soave A, Shariat SF, et al. Female with bladder cancer: what and why is there a difference? Transl Androl Urol 2016;5(5):668–82.

16. Wang Y, Chang Q, Li Y. Racial differences in urinary bladder cancer in the United States. Sci Rep 2018;8(1):12521.

17. Lerner SP, Bajorin DF, Dinney CP, et al. Summary and Recommendations from the National Cancer Institute's Clinical Trials Planning Meeting on Novel Therapeutics for Non-Muscle Invasive Bladder Cancer. Bladder Cancer 2016;2(2):165–202.

18. Keegan KA, Resnick MJ, Clark PE. Multimodal therapies for muscle-invasive urothelial carcinoma of the bladder. Curr Opin Oncol 2012;24(3):278–83.

19. Embi PJ, Jain A, Clark J, et al. Development of an electronic health record-based Clinical Trial Alert system to enhance recruitment at the point of care. AMIA Annu Symp Proc 2005;2005:231–5.

20. Available at: https://sites.nationalacademies.org/dbasse/bbcss/currentprojects/dbasse_080231. National Academies of Sciences, Engineering, and Medicine website Accessed July 8, 2020.